ALZHEIMER'S, STROKE, AND 29 OTHER NEUROLOGICAL DISORDERS SOURCEBOOK

ALZHEIMER'S, STROKE, AND 29 OTHER NEUROLOGICAL DISORDERS SOURCEBOOK

Basic Information for the Layperson on 31 Diseases or Disorders Affecting the Brain and Nervous System, First Describing the Illness, Then Listing Symptoms, Diagnostic Methods, and Treatment Options, and Including Statistics on Incidence and Causes

Health Reference Series
Volume Two

Edited By
Frank E. Bair

Omnigraphics, Inc. • Penobscot Building • Detroit, MI 48226

1993

BIBLIOGRAPHIC NOTE:

This volume compiles 34 individual booklets, papers, and bulletins issued by the National Institutes of Health between 1979 and 1989. These documents are identifiable as NIH publications: 79-75; 81-156; 81-159; 81-160; 81-2240; 81-2250; 82-87; 82-157; 82-307; 82-504; 82-717; 82-2406; 83-139; 83-2126; 83-2163; 83-2222; 83-2252; 83-2625; 84-158; 84-916; 84-2251; 84-2478; 84-2628; 85-1846; 85-2716; 86-76; 86-309; 86-2760; 86-2655; 87-2790; 88-2757; and 89-391.

Frank E. Bair
Editor

∞
This book is printed on acid-free paper meeting the ANSI Z39.48 Standard. The infinity symbol that appears above indicates that the paper in this book meets that standard.

ISBN 1-55888-748-2

Printed in the United States of America

CONTENTS

PREFACE

One of the most important advances in modern medical treatment involves patient knowledge. Only fifty years ago patients were largely ignorant of all but the most fundamental concepts of disease. Most knew next to nothing about treatment options until a doctor provided a terse explanation — one that patients were typically unprepared to understand. This dilemma, while understandable given the rapid expansion of medical technology, often caused the patient to delay seeking treatment and sharply retarded the treatment's effectiveness. Today, things are changing.

Now more patients enhance their recovery chances by becoming able participants in the healing process. By learning more about their body's processes and functions, and enough about the fundamental disease to understand a diagnosis, they can more actively affect the outcome of their treatment.

Alzheimer's, Stroke, and 29 Other Neurological Disorders Sourcebook is offered to support the ongoing growth in patient awareness. It is provided to help the patient who has received a diagnosis of a neurological disorder, as well as the family member or nonprofessional caregiver who must learn to care and to cope with the disease.

The brain and the neurological system

Of all areas of medicine, neurology must be the hardest for the layperson to understand. The organs it deals with are, like other body organs, formed of living tissue. But the neurological system is vastly different in function from most other structures of the body. It does not provide a "process" or produce a "product" as most other organs do, but rather originates and transmits vital signals around the body. These signals — complex enough to tax a large telephone system — comprise an information flow that involves both electrical and chemical transfers. Deciphering the complexities of this system and the disorders that afflict it is the purpose of this publication.

The *Alzheimer's Sourcebook* is a collection of information provided by the National Institute of Neurological and Communicative Disorders and Stroke (NINCDS). It is based on a public information program that was instituted a few years ago by the U.S.

Public Health Service. A dedicated staff of writers, having access to the most authoritative neurologists and neurology literature, have meticulously gathered, studiously evaluated, and clearly articulated the data contained here. Much of the information has appeared in a wide-ranging, single subject publication series, but this is its first appearance in book form, compiled and indexed with the nonprofessional user in mind.

How to use this book

The Sourcebook provides 31 chapters devoted to a wide range of neurological diseases. For each disorder, the volume offers the following information: a description of the disease, symptoms, diagnostic methods, treatment options, statistics on incidence and causes, and a list of organizations for patients and families. Together, this material offers an informed first step on the path to understanding and decision-making.

Omni's Health Reference Series

Alzheimer's, Stroke, and 29 Other Neurological Disorders Sourcebook is the second volume in the Health Reference Series published by Omnigraphics. The first volume covered cancer; later volumes in the series will include such subjects as diabetes and other metabolic disorders, diseases of the immune system (including AIDS), and disorders of the heart, vascular, and lymphatic system.

The editor welcomes the comments of readers to improve the scope and usefulness of the series.

Frank E. Bair

INTRODUCTION

This volume represents the efforts of the NINCDS — National Institute of Neurological and Communicative Disorders and Stroke — to help the layperson, whether patient, family member, or other caregiver, to understand his or her illness. The editor has assembled the expertly researched and well-written pamphlets produced by the NINCDS into a compendium of information on neurological disorders, from the most common to the most unusual. In a clear, readable style, the text provides a discussion of each disease, including etiology (if known), signs and symptoms, diagnosis, course, and treatment available. The reader learns about the latest developments in each area and is offered sources for further information.

This book is a must for caretakers involved in the management of neurologically affected people and is also a good, quick reference for medical professionals.

Edwin L. Berger, M.D.

PART ONE

COMMON DISEASES AND DISORDERS OF THE NEUROLOGICAL SYSTEM

Chapter 1

Alzheimer's Disease

Alzheimer's Disease

A generation ago, health care workers were quick — too quick — to label their elderly patients "senile." Almost anyone over age 65 who experienced marked confusion, disorientation, and memory loss was said to have "hardening of the arteries of the brain," a condition of age thought to be inevitable, progressive, and incurable.

Today we have come full circle, and health professionals — among them physicians, nurses, psychotherapists, and social workers — as well as the lay public have learned that "senility" is not inevitable. Health practitioners now know that the visible symptoms of dementia can be caused by a myriad of underlying physical disorders that affect brain functioning in the aged. This means when an elderly patient exhibits memory loss and confusion (the symptoms too often referred to as "senility"), it is usual for the physician to perform tests to rule out the causes that might be treatable — anemia, vitamin deficiency, endocrine disorder, even constipation or a bad cold. And particular attention will be paid to the two most likely causes — **depression** and **drug intoxication.**

Despite the new alertness to the possibility that the patient is suffering from one of the "reversible dementias," however, the fact is that most carefully screened cases of dementia in the aged cannot be reversed. Even after the practitioner has meticulously eliminated all possible underlying causes for the elderly patient's confusion and disorientation, unhappily, it will still remain that in four out of five cases, the diagnosis of irreversible dementia will be the one left standing. And the vast majority of those cases, perhaps as many as two-thirds, will be due to a neurological disorder known as **Alzheimer's disease.**

An estimated 1.3 million to 1.8 million Americans over the age of 65 suffer from Alzheimer's disease. Another 80,000 or so, in their forties and fifties, also are victims of Alzheimer's. Today there is neither a cure nor a treatment that can stop the progression or reverse the course of the intellectual decline. A definite diagnosis of Alzheimer's disease today carries with it a near certainty of eventual mental emptiness.

In terms of the emotional cost to the victim's family and caretakers, and the financial cost of institutional care for patients in the final stages of illness, the burden of Alzheimer's disease is overwhelming. The overall incidence of Alzheimer's disease for persons over 65 is five to seven percent, and the incidence rises steadily for each subsequent decade until it reaches about 20 percent for those in their eighties. In the next 40 years, this is the group that is expected to undergo rapid growth; the proportion of Americans over 65 will rise from 11 percent to 20 percent, and their numbers will more than double, from 26 million to more than 58 million. The result: the overall number of persons likely to suffer from Alzheimer's disease will substantially increase.

Although the progression of the disease is highly idiosyncratic — it may be 5 years before it reaches the final stages, or 10 years, or only 10 months, and there's no telling which faculties will be lost first and which maintained — the eventual result is complete disorientation and memory loss and, ultimately, death. The consequences of Alzheimer's disease generally reduce a person's normally remaining life expectancy by about one-half. Death comes probably not from the brain deterioration itself, but from physical infirmities that can accompany the profound intellectual loss of Alzheimer's disease — infirmities such as pneumonia and pulmonary embolism. In this indirect manner, Alzheimer's disease is thought to be associated with an estimated 100,000 to 120,000 deaths a year in the United States.

The behavioral hallmark of Alzheimer's disease seems to be memory loss, especially for recent events. But this is not the familiar "benign forgetfulness" of old age. When an individual with Alzheimer's disease, even in the early stages, forgets a person or event, the loss is complete; the patient cannot even recall the context of the thing that's been forgotten. Eventually, the memory loss becomes so profound that the patient cannot remember the previous sentence in a conversation, cannot follow the story line of a television show, cannot identify familiar persons or objects, and, in the last stages, cannot even remember the names of family members.

Other behavioral changes are caused by the illness as well. In its early stages, Alzheimer's disease can lead to an inability to concentrate, anxiety, irritability, agitation, withdrawal, or petulance. Later, the Alzheimer's patient may lose the ability to calculate, may exhibit lack of judgment, may become disoriented as to time and place, may be unable to understand jokes or cartoons.

Some persons with Alzheimer's disease tend to wander about and lose their way; some become prone to temper tantrums or obsessional behavior, like washing and rewashing the dishes; some are depressed or delusional, perhaps accusing their spouses of being impostors, or conversing with imaginary companions; some forget how to dress themselves or set the table, or forget words, or forget how to make change. Although the timing and sequence of lost function varies from patient to patient, those in the final stages of Alzheimer's disease tend to exhibit the same traits — apathy, disorientation, and lack of concern about others' opinions. Occasionally, though not always, Alzheimer's patients become incontinent in the final months of life.

A word about terminology

For most of this century, clinicians divided dementia into two types: presenile and senile. *Senile dementia*, often mistakenly called "hardening of the arteries of the brain," was thought to be inevitable if one lived long enough and, as the common label implies, was presumed to be a cerebrovascular disorder. The term *presenile dementia* was reserved for forgetfulness, personality deterioration, and loss of intellectual functioning with an onset before the age of 65. Presenile dementia also became known as Alzheimer's disease, named after Alois Alzheimer, the German physician who first described it in a 51-year-old patient in 1906. It was thought to differ from senile dementia in that it was a neurological disorder in which pathological brain cell changes could be found on autopsy.

As research into the brain changes characteristic of dementia progressed, it became clear that the two major lesions found in "classic" Alzheimer's disease — that is, neurofibrillary tangles and neuritic plaques — were found also in older patients with "senile dementia." In amount and distribution, the lesions of these two conditions were virtually identical. In fact, only a minority of "senile dementia" cases — some 20 percent — were found to be related to the vascular changes of age. The term *multi-infarct dementia* gradually replaced the inappropriate "hardening of the arteries of the brain" to describe this less common disorder.

It became clear, too, that of those elderly, demented patients without a vascular disorder, the vast majority — at least 60 to 65 percent — were suffering from a neurological form of the disease that looked very much like a late onset of Alzheimer's disease. This disorder then came to be called senile dementia of the Alzheimer's type, or SDAT.

The term SDAT, while more precise than "senility" or "organic brain syndrome" and more correct than "hardening of the arteries of the brain," is still needlessly cumbersome. It still distinguishes between the early-onset and late-onset forms of Alzheimer's disease — but this is a distinction that many experts now believe to be arbitrary and perhaps even meaningless. Since many leaders in the field have come to agree that the etiology, pathology, and prognosis of Alzheimer's disease is the same no matter what age its victim is, this text shall use the term *Alzheimer's disease* to mean the illness as it affects patients both older and younger than age 65.

The pathology of Alzheimer's disease

On autopsy, Alzheimer's-disease brains reveal a characteristic set of changes. Two of these changes are considered the hallmarks of the condition: neurofibrillary tangles and neuritic plaques.

Analysis of these lesions is one key step toward developing hypotheses as to what might have caused them — and how they might somehow be eliminated.

Neurofibrillary tangles are neurofibers found within brain cells which have, for some unknown reason, adopted the unusual configuration of paired helices. They may be either pieces of *normal* fibers in a novel combination, or pieces of *abnormal* fibers composed of an unfamiliar protein. Investigators are now working to determine which explanation is right.

Neurofibrillary tangles are found to some extent not only in Alzheimer's disease but in the brains of persons with postencephalitic Parkinson's disease, adults with Down syndrome, and ex-prizefighters suffering from dementia pugilistica, the "punch-drunk syndrome" observed in some boxers after too many blows to the head. Epidemiologists are stumped by the variety of diseases that have been associated with neurofibrillary tangles, since they all have different etiologies: postencephalitic Parkinson's has a viral origin, Down syndrome is genetic, and dementia pugilistica is related to trauma. Which explanation is right for Alzheimer's disease?

Neuritic plaques, when analyzed microscopically, have also raised more questions about Alzheimer's disease than they have answered. At the core of each plaque is a substance called amyloid, an abnormal protein not usually found in the brain. Amyloid formation has been linked to the presence of "free radicals," a highly reactive class of molecule fragments that combine readily with other pieces of molecules. Free radicals are thought by some scientists to be the primary culprits in aging, causing chemical reactions that lead to damage to, and plugging up of, vessels and cells throughout the body.

The neuritic plaque's amyloid core is surrounded by other brain cell pieces, most of them degenerating or abnormal in some way, such as dying mitochondria, unmyelinated presynaptic terminals, and paired helical filaments identical to those that compose the neurofibrillary tangle. Although the composition of plaques has been fairly well described, the question remains: How and why have these fragments clustered together?

The brain lesions of Alzheimer's disease seem directly related to the loss of mental functioning experienced by its victims. Recent research has associated these lesions, especially neuritic plaques, with the gradual loss of cells in the basal nucleus, the region of the forebrain that projects into the cerebral cortex and is thought to activate some of the brain's higher cognitive functions, especially memory. One theory is that as the basal nucleus cells degenerate, their axons swell and gradually evolve into plaques.

Perplexingly, many of the lesions of Alzheimer's disease, especially neurofibrillary tangles and neuritic plaques, are found to some degree in all individuals if they live long enough. With a few tangles and plaques, it seems, an aged individual can maintain normal intellectual functioning; but once the lesions reach a critical threshold, they interfere with memory and cognition, and the more lesions there are, the more severe the deficit.

Epidemiologists in Great Britain, after examining the clinical records and autopsied brains of 104 aged patients, concluded in a classic 1968 study that the more plaques and tangles an individual has, the greater his or her cognitive loss. This finding has since held up in study after study. In Switzerland, for instance, another research team found that the more extensive the concentration of plaques and tangles in the hippocampus and the neocortex, the greater the memory loss. Of a sample of nearly 650 elderly Swiss patients, 100 percent of those with very high concentrations of lesions suffered from amnesia, compared to 30 percent of those with no noticeable brain lesions.

Because there seems to be this direct connection, scientists believe that if they could stop the lesions from developing, or do away with them once they have formed, they could prevent or cure Alzheimer's disease. They are therefore directing their attention to some of the most promising theories as to how plaques and tangles might form.

What causes Alzheimer's disease?

No one knows yet what causes Alzheimer's disease, but several promising hypotheses are being investigated. Among them are that Alzheimer's disease may be caused by:

- a deficit in the brain's cholinergic system of neurotransmitters
- selective brain cell death provoked by viral or infectious agents

- selective brain cell death provoked by environmental toxins, and
- a genetic defect (or at least a genetic predisposition)

The *cholinergic hypothesis* is perhaps the most promising. In the mid-1970s, several groups of scientists independently reported a severe deficit in the brains of Alzheimer's disease patients in the enzyme used to manufacture an important neurotransmitter, acetylcholine, that is known to play a role in memory formation. Levels of this enzyme, called choline acetyltransferase, decrease somewhat during normal aging, but decrease far more dramatically — by as much as 90 percent — in Alzheimer's disease. This finding was further supported by autopsy findings that in the brains of Alzheimer's disease patients, the brain cells involved in the cholinergic system — cells found in the cerebral cortex, hippocampus, and basal forebrain in particular — have died in numbers far greater than would be expected by age alone.

The *viral hypothesis* is supported by experimental evidence that the introduction of diseased brain extracts into healthy neuronal tissue cultures can lead to the formation of neurofibrillary tangles. This brain-to-brain transmission of disease has been observed in other neurological disorders known to be caused by a virus: kuru and Creutzfeldt-Jakob disease, for example. Another clue that links Alzheimer's disease to an infectious agent is the fact that one form of the transmissible agent of scrapie (a progressive brain degeneration in animals) appears to have an amyloid structure resembling the core of the Alzheimer's plaque.

The *aluminum intoxication* hypothesis began with the observation that the injection of aluminum salts into animals, either systemically or directly into the brain, led to the proliferation of brain changes similar to the lesions of Alzheimer's disease. Subsequently, the brains of affected individuals were found to contain aluminum levels up to 30 times those of normal, age-matched people of a control group. Aluminum has also been implicated in the mental changes of dialysis dementia — a frequent side effect of long-term renal dialysis therapy — so the theory that aluminum is somehow related to senile dementia is intriguing.

Genetic theories about the etiology of Alzheimer's disease are equally intriguing, but difficult to confirm. Evidence is growing that Alzheimer's often clusters in families; some estimates are that 40 to 60 percent of the cases seen in the United States are familial in origin. The familial clustering is strongest in families where the

Alzheimer's patient developed the illness at a relatively young age. "Familial," however, is not the same as genetic. Family members have both the same genetic heritage and common exposure to the same infectious agents and environmental toxins.

Epidemiologists note that while the general population over age 65 runs a two or three percent chance of developing Alzheimer's disease, the likelihood increases to about seven or eight percent if a parent or sibling is already afflicted. Several bits of evidence support a possible genetic component to the disease. For one, plaques and tangles have been known to form in the brains of middle-aged patients suffering from trisomy 21, or Down syndrome, which is a known chromosomal disorder.

Diagnosing Alzheimer's disease

Because the diagnosis of Alzheimer's disease carries with it such a dismal prognosis, the medical practitioner must display extraordinary care before pronouncing it. And because the only way it can be diagnosed with conviction is on autopsy, the physician will approach diagnosis first by ruling out all the other illnesses that might cause dementia (see page 20). Once he knows what the diagnosis is not, he is left with just one probable explanation: Alzheimer's disease.

One complication in this method of diagnosis is that it is possible to have Alzheimer's disease in combination with other, more easily diagnosed — and often more easily treated — causes of dementia. Therefore, a diagnosis of Parkinson's disease, for example, does not absolutely eliminate a concomitant diagnosis of Alzheimer's disease. Alzheimer's disease can be ruled out with confidence only after many months of observation and attempted treatment. If the dementia progresses despite vigorous treatment of the suspected reversible cause or causes, the probable remaining diagnosis is Alzheimer's disease.

The most common cause of forgetfulness, confusion, and disorientation in the aged is **drug intoxication**. The elderly are a multimedicated group (85 percent have at least one chronic illness, and usually two or three), and the physiological changes of age often make them more prone to adverse side effects and drug-drug interactions. They have a greater proportion of fat cells than when they were younger, and their liver and kidney functions have decreased somewhat — all changes that mean drugs take longer to clear out of the systems of the elderly than they would in the middle-aged. In addition, some elderly patients have trouble taking medications appropriately, either because they did not understand the doctor's instructions in the first place (more than half of Americans over 65 did not complete high school, and great numbers of them were raised speaking a language other than English), or because they forget which pills they've taken when, or because they have an inherent distrust of the value of medicine. For all these reasons, drugs can be dangerous to old people.

The first system to break down when the drug burden becomes too great is the nervous system. Many sage physicians confronted with confused elderly patients simply eliminate all drugs for a trial period. Often, that is sufficient to clear the confusion; when drugs are reintroduced, the patient frequently is able to manage on far fewer medications.

A second common cause of dementia-like symptoms in the aged is **depression**. But depression can be a chameleon, almost as difficult to diagnose as is Alzheimer's disease. Depressed individuals of any age, lacking a strong sense of self, tend to embrace the stereotype of how they "should" behave. Depressed teenagers may act rebellious and destructive; depressed oldsters tend to act forgetful and confused. But, as with other causes of reversible dementia, a diagnosis of depression does not positively rule out a coexisting diagnosis of Alzheimer's disease. It is possible to be depressed and demented at the same time.

For elderly patients with a presumptive diagnosis of depression, many physicians offer a trial of antidepressant medications, and perhaps psychotherapy. The mere fact that patients are old does not mean they do not deserve aggressive psychological therapy when necessary to add joy and health to their final years. But after the depression clears, be alert to continued decline in intellectual function, which would indicate that Alzheimer's disease or some other dementing process might still be under way.

Many of the other conditions that can cause reversible dementia in the aged are common problems that produce no mental symptoms in the young and middle-aged. The physician will therefore be particularly attuned to this fact about symptoms: in older patients a wide range of common disorders, including heart attack, appendicitis, vitamin deficiency, thyroid dysfunction and, sometimes, even a bad case of influenza or gastroenteritis can all cause confusion, memory loss, and disorientation in persons over 65. **A word of explanation is in order. For men and women whose brains have already undergone the changes associated with normal aging, mental functioning often is maintained only through a delicate balance of compensatory mechanisms. When the balance is shifted by any external stress, even**

one as apparently benign as the flu, the brain frequently is the first organ to show signs of the strain.

The health practitioner, today, is therefore trained to suspect almost anything when an elderly patient shows some indications of being demented, especially if the symptoms have appeared suddenly rather than over a period of several months.

While the odds are that the physician will *not* find a treatable cause for the symptoms — only an estimated 15 to 30 percent of cases of dementia can be reversed — the conscientious physician will search long and hard anyway. He knows that mistaking a potentially treatable disorder for irreversible Alzheimer's disease are too devastating to allow for anything but a no-holds-barred approach in his patient's workup.

The good exam will include a scrupulous physical examination along with a comprehensive round of laboratory screening tests and diagnostic procedures. The physician will be on the alert for signs of other neurological diseases — papilledema, gait ataxia, reduced vibratory sensation, abnormalities of ankle jerks, nystagmus, and focal signs. Blood and urine tests will likely be ordered, geared to ruling out all potentially treatable explanations for the dementia. Only if warranted by earlier findings is it probable that more invasive tests will be performed, including chest X-ray, brain CT scan, and, in a rapidly developing dementia, lumbar puncture.

Some simple office tests

Once the most likely physical explanations for dementia have been eliminated, the next step is to determine how severe the dementia really is. It is common for the practitioner to wait six months and make a determination again. If the degree of dementia has not worsened significantly, the patient probably does *not* have Alzheimer's disease.

The easiest way to make a quick assessment of the degree of confusion is through the Mental Status Questionnaire (MSQ). This test comprises 10 simple questions that have been shown to be good indicators of a patient's alertness, orientation for time and place, and recent and remote memory. The physician may choose any appropriate time while examining the patient to ask the questions, but it can be expected that he will be careful to ask them all. Moreover, he will write down the patient's answers, as well as any telling signs of hostility, evasiveness, or confabulation.

The MSQ questions are:

- Where are we now?
- Where is this place located?
- What is today's date?
- What month is it?
- What year is it?
- How old are you?
- When is your birthday?
- What year were you born?
- Who is the president of the United States?
- Who was the president before him?

A score of 9 to 10 correct means the patient is not confused; 6 to 8, slightly confused; 3 to 5, moderately confused; and 0 to 2, severely confused.

The MSQ may not be adequate to pick up mild degrees of dementia, however, so the physician will normally ask other questions to gauge the patient's intellectual functioning. A standard approach is for the physician, when he introduces himself, to ask the patient to repeat his name once, and tell the patient he will, later, ask him to repeat it again, "to see how good your memory is." He will do the same with a list of three items, telling the patient to try and remember them. He will ask again in five minutes what the items were. He will also ask the patient to make change, to count backward from 100 by sevens, to interpret proverbs, and to explain cartoons. Again, none of these responses will conclusively mean that the patient does or does not have Alzheimer's disease, but the performance will serve as another piece to fit into the diagnostic puzzle.

The spouse, relative, or friend who accompanies the patient to the physician's office also can help quantify the degree of impairment. It is very likely the practitioner will interview the companion before meeting with the patient — this meeting will usually occur first, because it may be difficult for the physician to interrupt his encounter with the patient once he begins it, and if such interruption were to occur it might be met with suspicion.

The practitioner, instead of chatting informally with the companion, will be more likely to structure the interview, because a loved one's reports of a patient's mental state may be vague and colored by bias and emotions. Before the patient comes in, the physician will probably ask the companion the following questions regarding the patient's ability to cope with the activities of daily life. Can the patient:

1. Remain continent of bowel and bladder?
2. Move unassisted from bed to chair?
3. Get about on foot or by wheelchair unassisted?
4. Take care of hair, teeth, and usual toilet independently?
5. Dress and undress properly and appropriately with no help?
6. Bathe without assistance?
7. Shop, cook, and do ordinary housework?
8. Travel alone by car or public transportation?

The most severely impaired patients will not be able to do *any* of these things. Those with moderate impairment will be able at least to dress, undress, and wash themselves (activities 1 through 5). The mildly to moderately impaired will also be able to bathe, shop, and cook (activities 1 through 7), and those who can travel alone (1 through 8) probably have minimal or no impairment.

Patients with Alzheimer's disease sometimes give clues to their condition not only in the way they think and remember, but in the way they walk. Again, because of the idiosyncratic nature of the disease, no observation is applicable to everyone. But in many Alzheimer's patients, the gait is slow, the posture stooped, and the arm swing almost absent. They may take mincing steps from a flexed, wide-based stance (called the *"marche a petits pas"*), and may hold their hands cupped at their sides, thumbs adducted. Often, the patient exhibits paratonia, a resistance to the practitioner's efforts to move an arm or a leg, which worsens as the patient tries to relax.

Reflexes, too, appear in Alzheimer's disease that are not present in healthy adults. One is the snout reflex, a puckering of the lips elicited by percussing the orbicularis oris (the area around the chin and mouth). Another is the palmomental reflex, a contraction of the mentalis muscle in the chin when the palm of the hand is scratched. The grasp reflex, elicited by contact with the patient's palm, may also be present, as may the tonic foot response in which the toes turn downward in response to pressure on the sole.

Many physicians use one more office test — the Face-Hand Test — to see whether the observed disorder is organic or functional. In this assessment, the physician will sit facing the patient, and ask the patient to close his or her eyes and to place hands on knees. He will stroke the patient's cheek and, at the same time, the back of one hand. then he will alternate the face-hand combinations: right cheek and left hand, left cheek and right hand, right cheek and right hand, left cheek and left hand. Each time, the patient will be asked to report which hand and cheek are being touched. If the patient is wrong, it may be inferred that the confusion is due to Alzheimer's disease or some other neurological, organic cause. (The physician may repeat the Face-Hand Test with the patient's eyes open, but 80 percent of those who perform poorly with their eyes closed do no better when their eyes are open.)

This round of office tests will usually be repeated, at the physician's request, six months after the initial visit. The purpose of this return visit is to be sure the patient is suffering from a *progressive* deterioration. If the patient does not seem to have worsened in that time, then another diagnosis, perhaps depression, would be considered.

Treatment possibilities

As yet, no drug exists that can miraculously cure Alzheimer's disease. The best that can be done pharmacologically is treatment of the excess disability of the dementia. That is, the physician may offer medications aimed at easing the more distressing concomitants of the disease: tranquilizers to relieve agitation or violence; antidepressants to relieve a reactive depression. It should be noted that clinical trials on a few of the drugs that have looked promising have so far provided only limited encouragement. While the drugs under test are occasionally able to improve mood or state of arousal, they are unable to slow the deterioration of intellectual functioning that characterizes Alzheimer's.

Still, there is value in improving an Alzheimer's patient's mood or state of arousal. Behavioral studies have shown that such changes lead to significant improvement in the patient's quality of life, primarily because they affect the attitude of the patient's relatives and caretakers.

A chemical approach to the treatment of Alzheimer's disease, while it still eludes scientists, is nonetheless theoretically feasible, since the disease does seem to have a neurochemical base. As this text has earlier noted, the brain enzyme used to manufacture acetylcholine, which is crucial in memory formation, has been observed to fall off sharply in persons with Alzheimer's disease. Some clinical investigators have tried dietary replacement of the missing enzyme by supplying the precursor, choline, or its chemical cousin, lecithin. While the theory is that ingestion of choline or lecithin will increase the level of acetylcholine in the brain (a fact observed in experimental animals and humans), it does not seem to apply in Alzheimer's disease. Nevertheless, some do-it-yourselfers are buying lecithin in health food stores around the country, and ingesting several tablespoons of the grainy stuff each day — probably doing themselves no harm but, sadly, probably doing themselves little good.

The patient and the family

Medications and over-the-counter nostrums hold out little promise for Alzheimer's disease patients, but that does not mean there is reason to despair. The physician can probably help slow the consequences of the disease by encouraging the family and caretakers to allow the patient to perform to his or her fullest potential. This includes keeping the patient employed, mobile, and in a position to interact with others for as long as possible.

"It looks like death from boredom," the noted geriatrician Sir Martin Roth once commented about the 100,000 or more deaths a year associated with Alzheimer's disease. To help relieve the boredom — brought about inevitably when an individual loses the capacity to read, to converse, even to follow the melody line in a piece of music — friends and relatives of Alzheimer's patients are strongly counseled to encourage them to do whatever they still can do for themselves and by themselves.

Because the progression of the disease varies significantly with individuals, there is no telling what an individual patient may still be able to do three or five or seven years after the diagnosis. Long after she has lost the ability to do arithmetic, one patient may still be able to read; long after he has been forced to give up working on his car, another might still be able to sing along to old tunes on the radio. The best engrained skills tend to remain the longest: many Alzheimer's patients can manage to drive or play the piano or cook despite profound memory loss. But these "skills" often require constant guidance to be of any use. A patient who can still cook, for example, cannot be turned loose in the kitchen to bake a cake. Continuous direction may be needed: "Break the eggs," "Now beat them," etc. Health care workers and family members should be alert to the preserved abilities of these patients, and are urged by physicians to help them to develop and use the skills they still have.

A great distinction can be made between a progressive loss of *neurological* function and a progressive loss of *cognitive* function. Some intellectual skills may be maintained despite a steady deterioration of the brain itself. Consider the prognosis of another progressive, incurable neurological disease — polio. Many victims of polio, while permanently unable to regain lost nerve cells, have been rehabilitated sufficiently to regain much lost function. Similarly, while patients with Alzheimer's disease may be unable to recapture the damaged parts of the brain, they may be able to be rehabilitated and supported sufficiently to enable them to function at a decent level.

This is where the patient's family comes in. It is truly a test of a physician's tact to sensitively broach the idea of additional chores for family members, who are already going through many painful adjustments of their own. Not only must these family members take care of the patient, which can be physically and emotionally exhausting, and which requires a refocusing of the family's entire way of life — they must also come to grips with the grief, anger, self-pity, and finally acceptance that come about when their loved one turns into a new individual they barely recognize.

All of the attributes that made the Alzheimer's disease patient most loved during his or her healthy years — intellect, kindness, understanding, sense of humor, compassion — might disappear in the course of the disease. But because of their unique position of love and intimacy, family members are best able to help the patient hold on for as long as possible to those abilities that remain.

This means that skillfuly or not, the physician will be a voice urging the patient's family not to ignore their loved one. It's so easy to assume that because an individual cannot express thoughts properly, he or she cannot think or feel. Thus family members must have it made known to them the importance of a stimulating environment for the patient with Alzheimer's disease. Of course, the physician will also be warning them of the fine line between stimulating and overwhelming.

The family will be reminded that Alzheimer's patients need the comfort of routine to get from day to day, but will nevertheless be urged to incorporate new sights and feelings into the routine. They will be encouraged to delegate simple chores to give their loved one a sense of usefulness and accomplishment.

The family will be coached to push the patient a little farther than is comfortable, occasionally setting tasks that are challenging without being frustrating. A positive approach to the patient and his or her problems should be taken, but this should not encourage self-delusion. That is, the family will need to remind themselves from time to time that the mental infirmity will become more obvious and more incapacitating with time, and may eventually lead to institutionalization.

To help family members work through their complicated feelings, and to provide practical advice on the day-to-day chores associated with caring for the Alzheimer's disease patient, a self-help group for families is invaluable. For a listing of local resources, the patient's family should contact one of the self-help groups that have recently emerged. Among the most visible are:

Alzheimer's Disease and Related Disorders Association
360 North Michigan Avenue,
Suite 1102
Chicago, Ill. 60601
Telephone: 800-621-0379 (toll-free)
800-572-6037 (toll-free in Illinois)

Family Survival Project for Brain-Damaged Adults
1736 Divisadero Street
San Francisco, Calif. 94115
Telephone: 415-921-5400

Other local groups may be listed in the phone book or found through the nearest medical school, hospital, or department of health.

Should the patient need to be institutionalized, the family should recognize that some guilt feelings are unavoidable at such a time, but those feelings should ease somewhat if they will do a bit of reviewing in their minds. They should remember the positive contributions both family and caregivers had made to the patient's well-being over a long period of time. Some physicians will be able to aid this process by helping family members to talk about the disabilities — such as incontinence or night wandering — that made it clear the patient needs round-the-clock custodial care.

Throughout the illness, health professionals will help the patient's family keep in mind that the Alzheimer's victim remains first a human being, no matter how many intellectual faculties and cognitive skills may disappear. They can be expected to counsel an attitude of patience and — insofar as possible, as one watches a loved one deteriorate — objectivity. The family will be urged to employ "gentle correction" to keep the patient continually in touch with reality. The more involved Alzheimer's patients remain with the world around them, the more resourceful they become at finding ways to keep that world from slipping away.

Note to Health Care Professionals:
Specific diagnostic criteria for Alzheimer's disease are outlined in: McKhann, Guy M., et al., "Clinical Diagnosis of Alzheimer's Disease: Report of the NINCDS-ADRDA Work Group Under the Auspices of the U.S. Department of Health and Human Service's Task Force on Alzheimer's Disease," (*Neurology* 34(7), July 1984).

Reversible Causes of Mental Impairment

	Dementia	Delirium	Either or Both
Therapeutic drug intoxication			Yes
Depression	Yes		
Metabolic			
a. Azotemia or renal failure (dehydration, diuretics, obstruction, hypokalemia)			Yes
b. Hyponatremia (diuretics, excess antidiuretic hormone, salt washing, intravenous fluids)			Yes
c. Hypernatremia (dehydration, intravenous saline)		Yes	
d. Volume depletion(diuretics, bleeding, inadequate fluids)			Yes
e. Acid-base disturbance		Yes	
f. Hypoglycemia (insulin, oral hypoglycemics, starvation)			Yes
g. Hyperglycemia (diabetic ketoacidosis, or hyperosmolar coma)		Yes	
h. Hepatic failure			Yes
i. Hypothyroidism			Yes
j. Hyperthyroidism (especially apathetic)			Yes
k. Hypercalcemia			Yes
l. Cushing's syndrome	Yes		
m. Hypopituitarism			Yes
Infection, fever, or both			
a. Viral			Yes
b. Bacterial			
Pneumonia		Yes	

	Dementia	Delirium	Either or Both
Pyelonephritis		Yes	
Cholecystitis		Yes	
Diverticulitis		Yes	
Tuberculosis			Yes
Endocarditis			Yes
Cardiovascular			
a. Acute myocardial infarct		Yes	
b. Congestive heart failure			Yes
c. Arrhythmia			Yes
d. Vascular occlusion			Yes
e. pulmonary embolus		Yes	
Brain disorders			
a. Vascular insufficiency			
Transient ischemia		Yes	
Stroke			Yes
b. Trauma			
Subdural hematoma			Yes
Concussion/contusion		Yes	
Intracerebral hemorrhage		Yes	
Epidural hematoma		Yes	
c. Infection			
Acute meningitis (pyogenic, viral)		Yes	
Chronic meningitis (tuberculous, fungal)			Yes
Neurosyphilis			Yes
Subdural empyema			Yes
Brain abscess			Yes
d. Tumors			
Metastatic to brain			Yes

	Dementia	Delirium	Either or Both
Primary in brain			Yes
e. Normal pressure hydrocephalus	Yes		
Pain			
a. Fecal impaction			Yes
b. Urinary retention		Yes	
c. Fracture		Yes	
d. Surgical abdomen		Yes	
Sensory deprivation states such as blindness or deafness			Yes
Hospitalization			
a. Anesthesia or surgery			Yes
b. Environmental change and isolation			Yes
Alcohol toxic reactions			
a. Lifelong alcoholism	Yes		
b. Alcoholism new in old age			Yes
c. Decreased tolerance with age producing increasing intoxication			Yes

Chapter 2

Amyotrophic Lateral Sclerosis

Amyotrophic Lateral Sclerosis

David Niven, the late actor whose film roles entertained millions, was well known for his rich accent and his ability to glide effortlessly across a movie set. Tragically, however, the last months of this debonair performer's life were marred by the effects of a disease that caused him to lose both his ability to speak and his celebrated mobility.

That disease is amyotrophic lateral sclerosis (ALS), a progressive, usually fatal disorder that attacks the body's nerves and muscles. It is sometimes called "Lou Gehrig's disease" after the famed New York Yankee slugger whose death in 1941 was caused by the disorder.

ALS is a motor neuron disease. It affects the nerve cells that control muscles we can move voluntarily. For some undiscovered reason, nerve cells in the brain and spinal cord, known as *motor neurons*, gradually degenerate, causing the muscles under their control to weaken and waste away. ALS victims eventually become disabled, have difficulty speaking and swallowing, and may succumb to infections, particularly pneumonia.

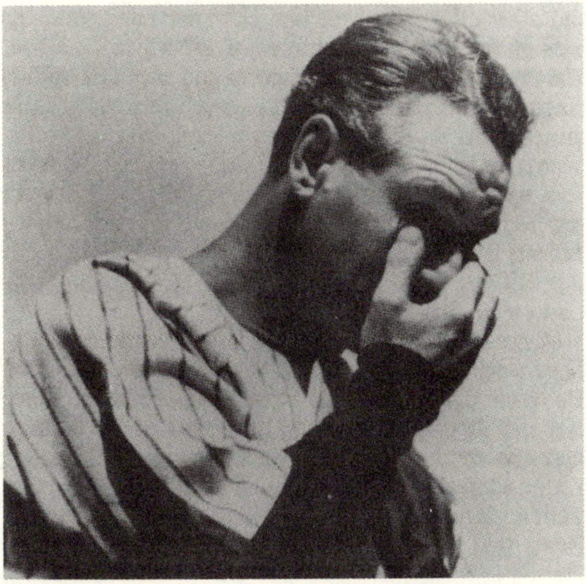

New York Yankee Lou Gehrig, who suffered from ALS, delivered his farewell speech to baseball in 1939. Gehrig told the 60,000 fans packed into Yankee Stadium, "I might have been given a bad break . . . but I've got an awful lot to live for."

While the disease paralyzes the "voluntary" muscles, patients remain alert and are able to think clearly, so that they can find ways to communicate without speech. The five senses are virtually unaffected, and most ALS patients maintain control over their bowel and bladder. For some patients, using these remaining abilities can be the springboard to coping with the disease.

The hope of all ALS patients is medical research. Within the federal government, the National Institute of Neurological and Communicative Disorders and Stroke (NINCDS) is the focal point for research on ALS and other disorders of the brain and nervous system. As part of the National Institutes of Health in Bethesda, Maryland, the NINCDS supports and conducts studies ranging from basic nerve cell research seeking possible causes of ALS, to tests of experimental drugs and other treatments in ALS patients. Thanks to research, scientists now have a better understanding of ALS and can use new technologies to discover improved ways of helping patients compensate for its effects.

Lost connections

Motor neurons are among the largest of all nerve cells. They reach from the brain to the spinal cord and from the spinal cord to muscles throughout the body. When they die, as they do in ALS, the ability of the brain to start and control muscle movement dies with them.

Consider what happens when a healthy person undertakes an action as simple as picking up a glass of water. First, the brain sends out electrical and dial "messages" to nerves destined to instruct the hand muscles. Motor neurons pick up these messages and provide a passageway for them to travel along to the hand. After the motor neuron has transported the signals to the end of the passageway, it releases the signals to the hand muscles. The muscles then recognize and respond to the command to grip the glass.

In the ALS patient, this sequence of events is eventually disrupted. Because the individual motor neuron is dead, it cannot produce and transport the vital signals to the muscle. So electrical and chemical messages originating in the brain never reach the muscles to activate them. Muscles then weaken from lack of stimulation and use.

The passageways that carry the brain's messages are comprised of delicate nerve processes as fine as wisps of thread. There are two main types of nerve processes: *dendrites* and *axons*.

Dendrites are message "receivers": short fibers that branch out from the center of the nerve cell, picking up signals being passed along from the brain or other nerve fibers.

The axon, a long fiber also extending from the center of the cell, is the message "sender." It transmits the messages received by the dendrites to muscles or other nerve cells. Each nerve cell in the body has perhaps hundreds of dendrites, but only one axon.

Messages are carried to the body's muscles through two types of motor nerve cells. "Upper" motor neurons start in the brain itself and send their nerve fibers downward within the spinal cord to "lower" motor neurons, which reside in the front of the spinal cord. Lower motor neurons send their fibers outward to arm and leg muscles.

Motor neuron axons are surrounded by a fatty covering called *myelin* which, like the protective coating of a telephone wire, insulates the nerve fibers and helps conduct messages. As motor neurons deteriorate in ALS, so does their myelin covering. Later, firm scar tissue may form in the areas where neurons degenerate.

The name *amyotrophic lateral sclerosis* accurately describes the disease state. *Amyo-trophic* comes from the Greek language and literally means "without muscle nourishment" — the "starved" appearance of muscles weakened from disuse. *Lateral* identifies the location of the affected nerve fibers which course through each side of the spinal cord. *Sclerosis,* also from a Greek word, means "hardening" — an apt description of the scar tissue that may follow neuron degeneration.

The ALS population

Scientists estimate that as many as 4,600 people in the United States develop ALS each year. With aging of the population, this incidence figure is expected to increase. Overall, as many as 17,000 Americans have the disease at any given time.

Research advances achieved in recent years have helped increase the number of years ALS patients can survive. Half of all ALS patients live 3 years or more after diagnosis. Twenty percent live 5 years or more. Up to 10 percent will survive more than 10 years.

Generally, younger ALS patients tend to live longer. Half of the patients diagnosed before age 50 live more than 7 years.

ALS is considered a disease of the middle years. The average age at the time of diagnosis is about 56 years. More men seem to get the disease than women, but a recent study reports the difference in numbers to be small. As women approach the age of menopause, they seem to be affected by ALS at the same rate as men.

ALS generally appears unpredictably and sporadically throughout the world. The geographical distribution of the disease is rather even, with only a few areas having an unusually high number of cases.

Ninety-five percent of ALS patients have no family history of the disease. The remaining 5 percent of ALS cases are considered familial. Some of these familial cases of ALS may be transmitted in a "dominant" pattern of inheritance, in which only one abnormal gene is needed from either parent for the disease to occur.

The first signs

ALS occurs in three different forms on which motor neurons are affected:

- *Bulbar ALS*. This form results from the destruction of motor neurons at the bulb-like stem of the brain. Muscles controlling speech, swallowing, and eventually breathing are rendered useless.
- *Upper motor neuron disease*. This form, also called primary lateral sclerosis, results from loss of motor neurons which extend from the brain through the spinal cord. The first signs are muscle weakness, spasticity, and exaggerated reflexes.
- *Lower motor neuron disease*. This form, also known as progressive muscular atrophy, results from the death of motor neurons originating in the spinal cord. The first signs are muscle weakness and wasting in the arms or legs, isolated muscle contractions, and a loss of reflexes.

No matter where ALS begins, the disease eventually affects almost all muscles under the patient's voluntary control.

No one form of ALS occurs more frequently than the others. In any form, the process of nerve and muscle destruction is probably well under way before most patients are aware of a problem.

Generally, the first visible signs of ALS are clumsy, weak hands or legs. Muscle twitches or spasms may occur. Patients may also begin to slur their words and have difficulty in swallowing. Some patients may overlook the first signs of ALS, thinking they are only experiencing the normal changes of aging.

The vagueness of early symptoms may also cause healthy people to assume incorrectly that they have ALS when occasional clumsiness or muscle twitches occur. Because of the dangers of self-diagnosis, people who experience any type of muscle control problems should see their family physician.

A visit to the doctor

Research advances have made it easier for physicians to tell if a patient has ALS. However, in some ALS patients — those with unusual symptoms — diagnosis is still difficult.

Since there is no clinical or laboratory test that can identify ALS, diagnosis is generally made through a careful examination of the patient's medical history and through neurological testing. Test results will vary according to which parts of the nervous system are affected and the current stage of the disease. Muscle reflexes, for example, may react more briskly than normal if upper motor neurons are most affected. Reflexes disappear when lower motor neurons are lost. Physicians may use another test of muscle activity — called an electromyogram (EMG) — to help determine if muscles are being adequately stimulated by nerves.

Once a diagnosis of ALS has been confirmed, the physician may use a variety of terms to refer to the disease. *Motor neuron disease* is a general term that refers to a group of disorders that includes ALS. Depending on their particular symptoms, patients may be told that they have ALS, spinal muscular atrophy, progressive bulbar palsy, primary lateral sclerosis, or benign focal amyotrophy. In each of these, different groups of motor neurons are damaged. Often the term ALS is used as a synonym for the general category of motor neuron disease.

What to expect

Newly diagnosed ALS patients have many specific questions for their doctors. But the first question is almost always, "What happens now?"

Because the disease progresses at different rates in different patients, it is difficult to predict how rapidly any particular person will become disabled. As muscles deteriorate, patients can still see, feel, hear, taste, and smell. Some patients are able for a time to continue their normal activities. Pain is usually not a problem.

Eventually, however, the muscles controlling speech may fail and weakened limb muscles confine ALS patients to wheelchairs or beds. Because of weakened breathing muscles, late-stage ALS patients usually face decisions about having a special breathing tube inserted in the windpipe and receiving supplementary oxygen. At this stage of ALS, infections such as pneumonia can become a threat to life. A recent NINCDS study has shown that some late-stage ALS patients may also develop complications such as hypertension and malnutrition.

The search for the culprit

Daniel Barash is a middle-aged ALS patient with a wife and two teenage sons. As an engineer and civic leader, he helped shape energy and transit policies in his hometown of Seattle. When ALS restricted his mobility, he turned to writing. Today, from his ground-floor bedroom, the former den of his two-story home, he produces letters and essays — some of them aimed at informing the public about ALS. As his condition progresses, Daniel is taking longer to bathe, dress, and eat, and he must use a walker and a wheelchair to get around. He is gradually adapting his life to the progressive constraints of the disease.

It is for Daniel and thousands of other ALS patients that the National Institute of Neurological and Communicative Disorders and Stroke conducts and supports research to find the cause of this disease.

NINCDS-supported scientists and other investigators have considered many possible culprits: bacteria, viruses, genetic factors, toxins, minerals, hormones, altered metabolism, and a defective immune system. Whatever causes the motor neuron to die has not yet been identified. But NINCDS scientists believe that clues to understanding ALS are most likely to come from research advances in basic science — through increased knowledge of the interacting parts of the nervous system.

One popular ALS theory is that motor neurons are damaged by some substance in our everyday surroundings. But if this were the whole answer, everyone living near the destructive substance would develop ALS. Since only certain people develop the fatal disease, it has been suggested that ALS may strike individuals with a particular genetic makeup or with high levels of the damaging substance.

Support for an environmental cause of ALS comes from several kinds of evidence:

The Pacific connection. ALS occurs with a higher-than-normal frequency on the island of Guam, the peninsula of Japan, and a region of West New Guinea — all areas with volcanic soil. Because these areas provide an unusually promising focus for ALS research, NINCDS scientists have been studying the environment there for clues to the cause of the disease. They have discovered lower-than-normal levels of some minerals in the soil and water, and increased levels of other minerals. A long-term NINCDS research program on Guam has also shown that the brains of Guamanians with ALS contain high levels of some of these minerals in diseased neurons.

Scientists are intrigued by other clues. They have found that the incidence of ALS in Guam has declined in the last 30 years from about 1 in 10 people to less than 1 in 100. This decline coincided with changes in the population's diet and water sources as the island modernized.

The incidence of ALS declined even further among Guamanian natives who migrated to other parts of the world, out of the range of any potentially harmful agent. Conversely, Philippines-born people who moved to Guam have been found to develop the disease more frequently than Filipinos who did not leave their country.

These patterns suggest that the environment may have some influence on the occurrence of ALS.

Blood studies. Laboratory studies also implicate the environment as a source for the cause of ALS. From ALS patients' blood, biologists have isolated substances thought to damage nerve cells when applied to cell cultures grown in the laboratory. The body may produce these substances in response to some agent in the environment. If scientists can confirm this theory and find where the substance first damages the cell, they also may discover ways to prevent or repair the damage.

An elusive virus? It is possible, say some scientists, that ALS may be caused not by a chemical substance, but by a virus present in the environment. NINCDS investigators working in New Guinea discovered that a degenerative neurological disease called kuru was caused by a virus-like organism that had entered its victims undetected many years before symptoms of the disease appeared. Scientists postulate that the same kind of slow-acting or "latent" virus might be at fault in ALS.

If an organism is involved, there is no evidence that it is contagious. It may be that people who develop ALS have weakened body defense systems that are unable to ward off the virus.

Investigators have been searching for evidence of an elusive ALS virus in diseased tissue for many years, but have not yet found a culprit. They are also attempting to identify a viral cause by transferring ALS tissue into laboratory animals to see if the animals will develop the disease.

Searching for an enemy within

Although some scientists strongly suspect that an environmental factor or virus triggers the onset of ALS, the true cause of the disease may yet lie within the body itself. One way to discover if the body is at fault in ALS is to examine the biological changes that the disease brings about.

Body chemistry. Investigators studying changes in the body fluids of ALS patients have found altered blood levels of certain substances. Norepinephrine, a hormone that causes blood vessels to constrict, is reportedly higher than normal in the blood of some ALS patients. Taurine, an amino acid, is sometimes found in high amounts in the motor cortex, the portion of the brain that controls muscle movement. Gamma-aminobutyric acid, a chemical that slows the delivery of nerve messages, is reported to be lower than normal in the spinal fluid of some patients. Scientists hope to find a common thread linking these changes to the onset of ALS.

Some investigators suspect that a lack of a chemical called a *nerve growth factor* is responsible for motor neuron death in ALS. Nerve growth factors are proteins that help keep nerve cells healthy. If, for some reason, a certain nerve growth factor is not provided, motor neurons may die. Several nerve growth factors have been isolated, and there is hope that a specific growth factor for motor neurons will be identified. If ALS is caused by the loss of such a growth factor, physicians might eventually be able to treat the disease by providing this factor to patients in much the same way that they provide insulin to diabetics.

Nerve function. Not all motor neurons are damaged in ALS. The cranial nerve that controls movement of the eye muscles almost invariably remains unharmed. Similarly, the spinal nerves that control muscles of the rectum and urinary bladder are usually preserved. If scientists can learn what causes these neurons to be spared, they may eventually be able to treat or prevent ALS.

Other intriguing events are associated with the destruction of motor nerve cells. New nerve-cell endings have been found to grow near damaged motor neurons. Other nearby neurons send out extra axon sprouts to try to compensate for those nerves lost to the disease. Some scientists think that further research on this axon-sprouting phenomenon might lead to a practical treatment for ALS.

Inside the cell. Neurobiologists are also interested in changes that occur inside the dying motor neuron. NINCDS-supported scientists are investigating why damaged motor neurons accumulate large amounts of normal nerve-cell components called neurofilaments. In healthy individuals, neurofilaments are scattered throughout the cell. In ALS patients, however, neurofilaments accumulate in the axon near the nerve cell body where they are made, causing the axon to swell. This swelling may damage the cell body.

Some scientists have suggested that motor neurons die because they lack stimulation by sex hormones. Normally, special proteins

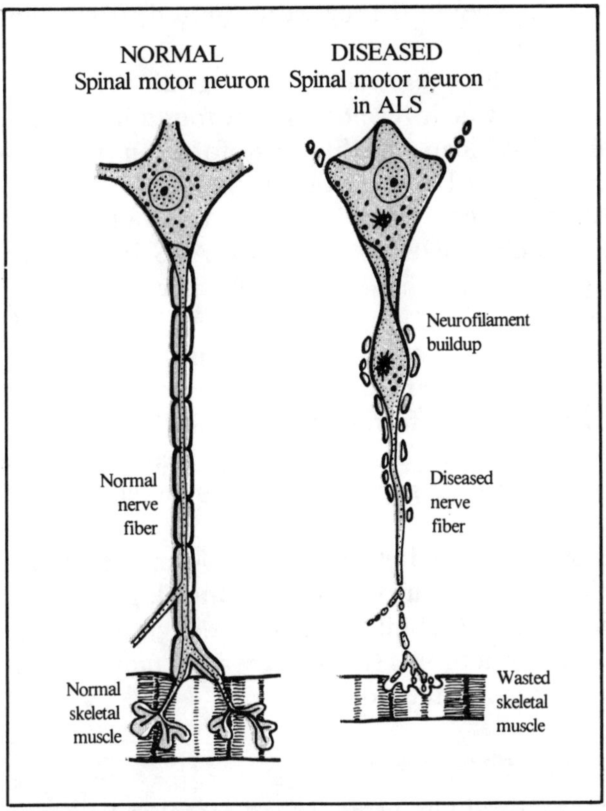

In the diseased motor neuron, neurofilaments accumulate near the nerve cell body, possibly causing damage when the axon swells.

scattered throughout the motor neuron attract sex hormones to the nerve cell. But in ALS, the nerve cell's transport system may be damaged, and these special proteins may not be distributed properly. As a result, sex hormones may not enter the neuron to provide the stimulation it needs to remain vital.

Investigators also speculate that a loss of protein might be responsible for motor neuron destruction. Research has shown that ribonucleic acid (RNA) — a compound needed for protein-making — is reduced in the motor neurons of ALS patients. In addition, the motor neuron's protein-making machinery disappears. Without protein, the nerve cell cannot survive.

A mirror image of disease

ALS is also being studied today in both chemical and animal models that mimic the human disease. These models help investigators learn far more than they could if they were limited to studying damaged neurons from patients.

Scientists have discovered several chemicals that seem to produce neuron destruction which resembles that found in ALS. A substance isolated from the African chickling pea, for example, causes a motor neuron disease like ALS. Two other chemicals are also known to damage motor neurons by causing axons to swell, disrupting neurofilaments. These chemicals do not cause ALS in most patients, but some investigators think that similar substances may be responsible for the disease.

No animal diseases have yet been identified that exactly mimic human diseases. However, there are two animal diseases which resemble ALS: these are forms of hereditary motor neuron disease in special strains of mice and in Brittany spaniels. These naturally occurring mouse and dog models may give clues to the human disease.

NINCDS-supported scientists at The Johns Hopkins University discovered that motor neuron axons in the dog model are swollen because of neurofilament buildup. The investigators theorize that the failure of the motor neuron's transport system may be responsible for the ALS-like disease in the dog.

Help from a high-tech sleuth

Major advances in brain and spinal cord research have come from an exciting new method of looking at the living brain: positron emission tomography (PET). NINCDS was an early supporter of PET scanning, which provides a safe way of observing the brain at work without opening the skull. PET images reveal changes in the brain activity of research patients as they think, see, or listen.

This research tool, when applied to the study of motor neurons, may provide useful data that could help chart the earliest changes in ALS patients.

PET scans depend on the need of brain cells to burn a sugar compound called glucose as fuel. Certain nerve cells in a diseased brain may use more or less glucose than the same cells in a normal brain. PET scans show the amount of glucose-burning activity in each part of the brain, thus pointing to areas where a problem may be occurring.

A person scanned by PET is given a harmless, short-lived radioactive compound attached to glucose. The radioactively tagged glucose emits energy as the brain uses the sugar — energy which is recorded by PET's electronic detectors. The less-active parts of the brain use less glucose and thus give off a smaller amount of radioactivity. A computer translates the pattern of released radioactivity into an image.

Using PET, NINCDS scientists have found that ALS patients have reduced activity in the part of the brain that controls movement. The investigators also noted that the area of an ALS patient's brain with the least metabolic activity was also the control center for those muscles that first showed signs of the disease.

Viewing the immediate effects of new ALS treatments is another task to which PET is well suited. Since PET shows the living brain in action, the instrument may be used to see subtle changes in motor neurons or other nerve cells as therapy is applied.

Treatment: Hope or hoax?

Over the years, the serious nature of ALS has led many patients and their families to consider a variety of experimental, and sometimes unorthodox, treatments in hopes of a cure. Until disproved, snake venom was sought by some patients as a cure for the disease. Dimethyl sulfoxide (DMSO) and various vitamin and dietary regimens are other unproven therapies hailed as beneficial to patients.

Holding more promise are several new experimental drugs now being tested by research scientists in a small number of ALS patients. The list includes thyrotropin-releasing hormone (TRH), Cronassial, and interferon.

TRH is a naturally occurring hormone produced by the brain and found in the motor neurons of the spinal cord. Because TRH was reported to be deficient in ALS patients, scientists at the National

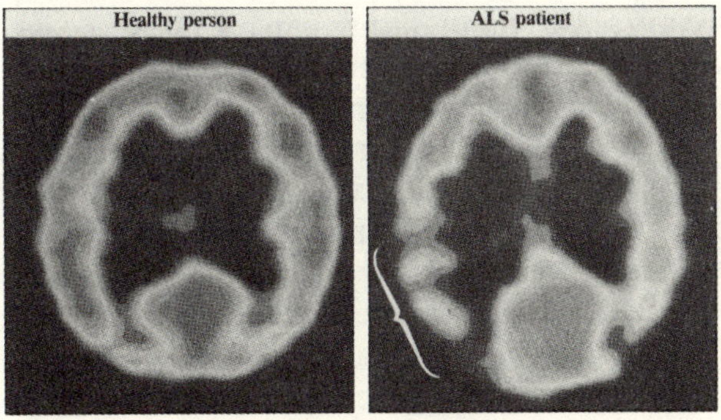

On the left, a PET scan of a healthy person's brain shows normal levels of activity. On the right, a PET scan of an ALS patient reveals decreased metabolic activity in areas (bracketed) of nerve cell damage.

Institutes of Health-supported General Clinical Research Center at the University of Southern California decided to test this hormone against the disease. When the scientists administered massive dosages of the scarce drug to selected ALS patients, muscle strength temporarily improved. Medical scientists are now testing different methods of giving the drug in attempts to lengthen its effects, and some have reported improvement in symptoms for 72 hours or more after administration. Research is continuing, to determine if TRH halts the progressive death of motor neurons or alters the expected course of the disease.

Cronassial is a drug containing natural brain compounds called gangliosides. Gangliosides, which are found in nerve cells, are thought to help repair injured neurons. Scientists are exploring the question of whether administering Cronassial will promote the regrowth of damaged motor neurons and halt the degeneration process in ALS.

Some ALS patients are suspected of having abnormalities that prevent their bodies from fighting off infections. If ALS is caused by a virus, a stronger defense system against infection might allow patients to ward off the disease. Because of this, NINCDS scientists and other investigators are now studying the effect of interferon — a compound that appears to stimulate the body's defense system and fight persistent virus infections — on selected ALS patients.

Supportive therapy

Although no miracle cure has yet been discovered for ALS, many patients and their families have had success in controlling some symptoms. Physicians today can prescribe quinine compounds to relieve muscle cramping, muscle relaxants to ease spasticity, or sedatives to control twitching. Drugs can also be effective against the excess accumulation of saliva that sometimes results when ALS patients have difficulty swallowing.

ALS patients should avoid certain other drugs such as sleeping pills, barbiturates, opiates, or excess alcohol — substances that adversely affect an already weakened nervous system.

A balanced diet can help the ALS patient maintain whatever strength has not been lost to the disease. But families should be aware that an ALS patient's swallowing problems may require a change in the way food is prepared at home. Patients may need to have their food chopped and lubricated with butter or sauces. As symptoms worsen, a nutritious, low-fiber, high-calorie diet composed of soft or liquid foods may be necessary. ALS patients who must avoid bulkier foods sometimes turn to vitamin supplements to fill out their nutritional requirements. At some point, however, tube feeding may become the most efficient way to obtain proper nourishment.

In the latter stages of the disease, patients must be on guard against the threat of choking. Weakened swallowing muscles may allow foods or fluids to become trapped in the throat. To help prevent this, some patients and their families have learned to use an aspirator, a device that suctions off excess fluid. Family members can also learn techniques for clearing the patient's throat in an emergency.

As ALS progresses, muscles that assist in breathing eventually fail. Therapy for this problem often includes an operation called a tracheostomy. In this procedure, a plastic tube is inserted in the patient's windpipe through an opening in the neck to allow easier breathing. Further breathing assistance can be provided by a respirator, a machine that artificially inflates the patient's lungs. Patients and families can be taught to perform the routine maintenance procedures that keep a respirator in good working condition.

Some problems of ALS patients are caused by inactivity and immobility. Most experts believe that mild or passive exercise can help patients keep their joints and muscles relatively healthy. Exercise can also strengthen unaffected muscles. Physicians warn, however, against exercising to fatigue. Patients should not start an exercise program without first consulting a health professional who can help balance their needs and abilities.

ALS patients should also learn ways to conserve their energy and to perform daily tasks efficiently. Oral hygiene, for example, can be improved by the use of an electric or water-jet toothbrush. A variety of mechanical aids, including braces, tools, fasteners, and wheelchairs, are available to simplify patients' lives. These devices make patients more mobile and self-sufficient.

Coping with lost abilities

Although ALS robs the body of strength and control, the loss is gradual, and the ability to think and feel is mercifully spared. Some ALS patients have used their remaining abilities to cope with the disease.

One person who has remained productive in the face of this debilitating disease is Dr. Stephen Hawking, an eminent British scientist whose life's work is studying the origins of the universe. He has struggled with ALS for more than 20 years, and continues to investigate the complex problems of astrophysics from his office at

Cambridge University. Undaunted by ALS, Dr. Hawking devotes his time to his family and his career, taking time out occasionally to fly to London and the United States for meetings.

Not all ALS patients can be expected to share Dr. Hawking's optimism. The disease places heavy burdens on patient and family alike, and serious consideration must be given to the medical, social, and financial consequences of coping with ALS in its late stages. But many patients can, if they choose, be helped to a more meaningful life despite their disabilities.

The voice of technology. Any disease that limits the ability to speak removes an important communications link to life and family. Ingenious high-technology instruments have been developed to help ALS patients overcome this handicap. Computer-connected probes, for example, can be attached to the eyebrows. By moving their eyebrow muscles in a coded pattern, ALS patients can then "speak" via the computer's voice synthesizer. Another device consists of a transparent board through which patients look, guiding the eyes of the "listener" to letters and numbers imprinted on the board's surface. In this manner, patients can spell words and communicate with the trained caretaker.

Health care at home. Physicians who specialize in treating ALS patients concentrate on keeping them as active and involved in daily life as possible. Most experts agree that ALS patients are best cared for in their own homes, where families or friends can tend to their needs.

People with ALS also need support from health professionals who can help them live longer and better. These professionals attend to health needs both related and unrelated to ALS, and they often favor the team approach to care. Physicians, nurses, dieticians, occupational therapists, physical therapists, and counselors help ALS patients adapt to the disability and continue to function.

Mental attitude. Some ALS patients have found ways to cope with the feelings of discouragement, anxiety, and discontent that can accompany a serious illness. Such methods sometimes involve reliance on religious faith or moral teachings.

Daniel Barash, the Seattle engineer, has developed his own personal "ground rules" for dealing with ALS:

1. Live by the values you have trusted.
2. Face the truths of today.
3. Believe in the possibilities of tomorrow.
4. Work on your health problems only when they actually occur.

5. Preserve the health you have — eat nutritiously, stay rested, and welcome aid from others.
6. Laugh at the world's and your own follies.
7. Fight for what you know is right and fair.
8. Serve yourself and your loved ones and the humanity of strangers.

Sounding boards. Sympathetic listening by friends and loved ones can also help patients cope. Experts say that ALS patients need to talk about their feelings of fear and anxiety, and feel relief when they do so. But they sometimes are afraid they will lose close friends if they express their deepest feelings. They speak most easily to a person who will not be threatened by their anxiety.

The problems that arise when an ALS patient is "shut out" by friends were painfully evident to one physician who himself developed the disease. As his physical disabilities became more apparent, coworkers and friends began to avoid him or, at best, to pretend that everything was normal. The physician often felt isolated and was sometimes unable to obtain the help he needed.

"What the patient and family need," he says, "is the sense that people care. No one else can assume the burden of ALS, but knowing that you are not forgotten does ease the pain."

Keeping up the fight

Both patients and doctors know the importance of hope. For patients willing to grapple with the limitations imposed by ALS, medical care can prolong and improve their lives. Respirators can assist breathing when chest muscles have weakened. Nutrition can be maintained by intravenous feeding and drugs can relieve some troublesome symptoms.

The late Senator Jacob Javits is among those ALS patients who chose to fight the disease and remain as active as possible. Senator Javits used his still considerable influence to improve the public's awareness of ALS. "I've never given up," he said about the illness, "and I'm not going to give up now. I continue to write and speak and stay in contact with my colleagues."

Senator Javits believed research to be the only hope for ALS patients. He would have been glad to participate in a research project "to do any good for others."

"I'm a risk taker," he asserted.

"My advice to others with this illness is to reconcile yourself to your condition," said Javits. "Give it a fair portion of your time and energy, but devote yourself to what you love to do. Don't be obsessed with the fact that you're sick."

Where to go for help

If you or a family member has ALS, you will need medical help and emotional support. You may want to develop a personal team of people to help you pass through this crisis in your life. You also may be rewarded by getting involved in one of the private, nonprofit agencies that provide essential aid for ALS patients and their families. These volunteer agencies offer information, support, and counseling, and may be able to provide mechanical aids. They also fund medical clinics throughout the U.S. For further information, contact:

ALS Society of America
15300 Ventura Boulevard
Suite 315
Sherman Oaks, CA 91403
(818)990-2151

National ALS Foundation, Inc.
185 Madison Avenue
New York, N.Y. 10016
(212) 679-4016

Muscular Dystrophy Association, Inc.
810 Seventh Avenue
New York, N.Y. 10019
(212) 586-0808

Human tissue banks

The study of brain tissue from persons with neurological disorders is invaluable in research, especially in conditions like ALS where the cause is obscure. NINCDS supports a national neurospecimen bank in Los Angeles and a national brain tissue bank near Boston, and the National ALS Foundation sponsors an ALS tissue bank in New York City. For information about tissue donation and collection write:

Dr. Wallace W. Tourtellotte, Director
Human Neurospecimen Bank
VA Wadsworth Hospital Center
Los Angeles, Calif. 90073

Dr. Edward D. Bird, Director
Brain Tissue Bank, Mailman Research Center
McLean Hospital
Belmont, Mass. 02178

Dr. James T. Caroscio, Director
National ALS Foundation Tissue Bank
Department of Neurology
Mount Sinai Hospital
One Gustave L. Levy Place
New York, N.Y. 10029

Additional information

For additional information about ALS research conducted at the NINCDS and through NINCDS research grant support, send your questions to:

Office of Scientific and Health Reports
National Institute of Neurological and Communicative Disorders and Stroke
National Institutes of Health
Building 31, Room 8A-16
Bethesda, Md. 20205
(301) 496-5751

Chapter 3

Aphasia

Aphasia

An elderly woman, who once delighted in reading, now struggles to make sense of the morning's headline: the newsprint is clear, but the words appear to her like random squiggles on the page. A middle-aged man speaks haltingly, groping for words that once flowed with ease and eloquence. Thousands of alert, intelligent men and women find themselves suddenly plunged into a world of jumbled communication because brain damage has left them aphasic.

Aphasia is the loss of the ability to make sense of language, including inability to understand printed words. It does not affect intelligence. Patients remain mentally alert, even though their speech may be jumbled, fragmented, or totally incoherent, and they may not be able to comprehend words spoken to them. It's like being in a foreign land, unable to speak or understand the native tongue. The problem is not one of intelligence, but of communication. To patronize an aphasic patient or otherwise treat him as though he were mentally incompetent could cause great anguish and slow his recovery.

Some Facts and Figures

It is difficult, perhaps impossible, to obtain accurate statistics on how many people in the United States have aphasia. Since aphasia is not a disease but a symptom of brain injury, it may not be reported; in fact, many times the brain injury itself is not detected. Furthermore, because aphasia is poorly understood it often goes unrecognized by physicians or is wrongly attributed to confusion or a mental disturbance. Reliable data are scarce and the true dimensions of the problem remain hidden.

Any adult who incurs brain damage might develop aphasia. Most commonly seen in adults who have suffered a stroke, aphasia can also result from a brain tumor, infection, or a head injury that damages the brain.

A very rough estimate of the number of people in the United States suffering from aphasia is 1 million. The following table breaks this estimate down by cause:

Strokes	500,000
Head wounds	200,000
Infections, exposure to toxic materials, lead poisoning, other causes	300,000
TOTAL	1,000,000

An estimated 20 percent of stroke patients develop aphasia. Since more victims now survive a stroke, the reservoir of aphasic patients is growing.

The personal, social, and economic implications of language disorders are immense. Aphasia often occurs during a person's peak years of productivity. Following the disorder's onset, previously active and vigorous men and women may be forced into early retirement. Some families must considerably alter their lifestyles to meet household expenses and the added costs of rehabilitating the patient or maintaining him in an institution. In 1969, the cost of speech and language rehabilitation for aphasics was estimated at $13.2 million a year.* This figure may have since tripled.

Besides the financial burden, many patients and families must adjust to new routines, new demands, and new family roles when an aphasic patient is cared for at home.

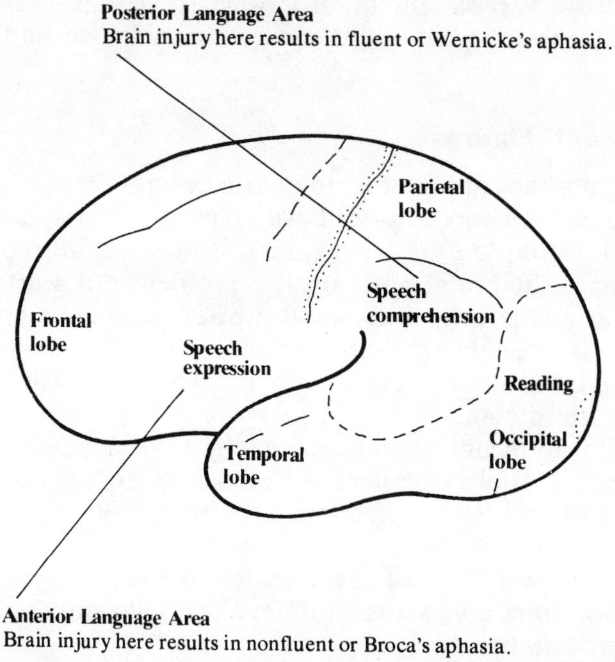

* Report of the Subcommittee on Human Communication and Its Disorders, National Advisory Neurological Diseases and Stroke Council.

What Happens in Aphasia?

The brain is master of man's ability to communicate through language. Through complex cerebral processes, people attach meaning to words, combine words to represent ideas, and understand each others' speech.

The brain is divided into two sides, or hemispheres. The hemispheres are connected and work closely together to monitor and regulate the body's functions. Certain functions are ordinarily controlled by the left hemisphere, other functions by the right hemisphere. In most people, for example, language function is governed by the left hemisphere; in a small percentage of the population, however, the right hemisphere governs this function. The exact locations of all the different language functions are not yet known, but research has revealed roughly where the major language functions are located in the left hemisphere, as diagrammed on the previous page.

Brain tissue receives oxygen from a rich network of blood vessels. When the normal flow of blood to a part of the brain is cut off, as occurs in a stroke, the cells in that region die from lack of oxygen and can no longer do their job. If the language control centers of the brain are deprived of blood, aphasia will result. Blood flow in the brain can be disrupted in several ways: See diagrams on page 49.

Language in the Aphasic Patient

Aphasia symptoms vary greatly among patients. The type and severity of language loss are related to the location and extent of brain injury. Disabilities can range from a temporary slurring of speech to total loss of communication.

Various terms are used to describe the different types of aphasia; even scientists do not fully agree on these terms or on precise methods of classification. In general, however, aphasia can be divided into four broad categories:

- *Expressive aphasia* (also called motor aphasia, nonfluent aphasia, and Broca's aphasia) involves difficulty in conveying thoughts through speech or writing. The patient knows what he wants to say but cannot find the words he needs. He has thoughts but can't recall or organize the language to express them. Patients with expressive aphasia often sound like a telegram when they speak: "Me . . . my wife . . . went . . . school, no, speech, speech, speech therapy. Oh. I don't know, I went . . . and work, work." Besides their grammatical errors, patients with expressive aphasia also have difficulty naming objects, using the telephone, spelling, counting, repeating, telling time and, in the most severe cases, even gesturing appropriately.

- *Receptive aphasia* (also called sensory aphasia, fluent aphasia, and Wernicke's aphasia) involves difficulty understanding spoken or written language. The aphasic hears the voice or sees the print but cannot make sense of the words. The ability to read, listen, concentrate, or follow instructions is usually impaired. Although these patients talk a great deal, they often don't make sense and their speech is devoid of specific meaning: "I like to do those things all the time with them, just like that." Victims of receptive aphasia often substitute sounds in their words, making the words unintelligible to others; for example, they may say "crepe recepter" for tape recorder. Also, words of similar meaning or words that are often associated may be substituted, such as "chair" for table.
- *Anomic or amnesic aphasia* occurs in the milder cases of aphasia. These patients' major difficulties are in using the correct names for particular objects, people, places or events. When such patients can't recall the precise name, they will often talk about the object or person until their listeners understand what they mean.
- *Global aphasia* results from severe and extensive damage to the language areas of the brain. Patients lose almost all language function, both in comprehension and expression. They cannot speak or understand speech, nor can they read or write.

The milder types of aphasia can cause the patient frequent annoyance and frustration, while severe aphasia can be shattering. People who are suddenly deprived of conversation with friends, or the enjoyment of reading a novel or watching a film, and who cannot even ask for a blanket when they are chilled, quickly feel isolated, helpless, and depressed.

Other Problems Associated With Aphasia

Physical Problems

Certain physical disabilities commonly result from brain damage and often accompany aphasia.

Muscle weakness or paralysis on one side of the body is common. This condition — known as hemiplegia — is often temporary, and a program of exercise and physical rehabilitation may be recommended to help patients recover.

1. **Hemorrhage** (Bleeding)

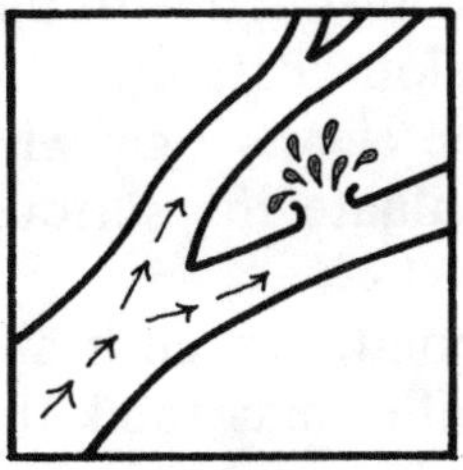

The wall of an artery of the brain may break, permitting blood to escape, reducing the oxygen supply and damaging the surrounding brain tissue.

2. **Thrombosis** (Clot formation)

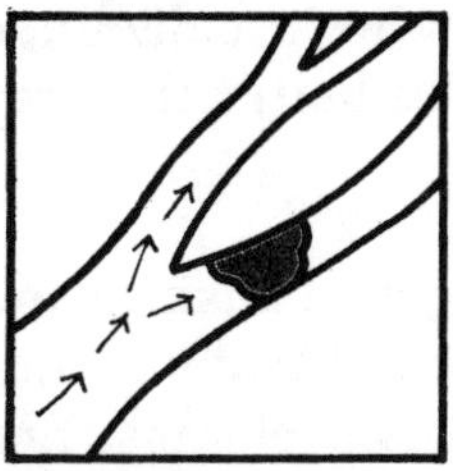

A clot of blood *may form in* an artery of the brain and thus stop the flow of blood to the part of the brain supplied by the clot-plugged artery.

3. **Embolism** (Blocking of a vessel by a clot floating in the blood stream)

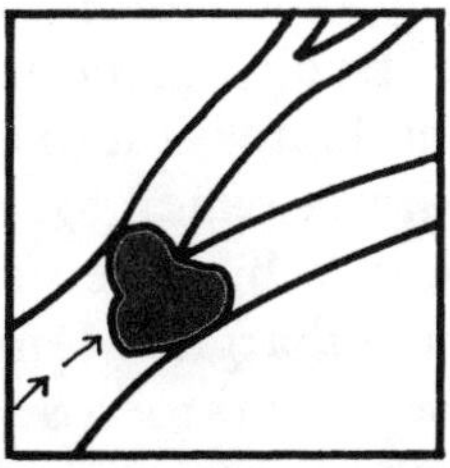

A clot from a diseased heart or, less commonly, from elsewhere in the body *may be pumped to* the brain and stop up one of the brain's arteries.

4. **Compression** (Pressure)

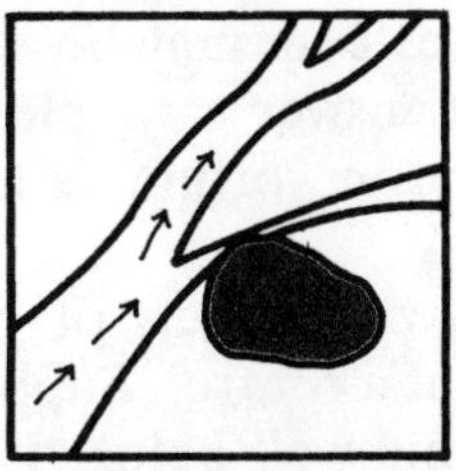

A tumor, swollen brain tissue, or a large clot from another vessel may press upon a vessel of the brain and stop its flow of blood.

5. **Spasm** (Tightening and closing down of the walls of an artery)

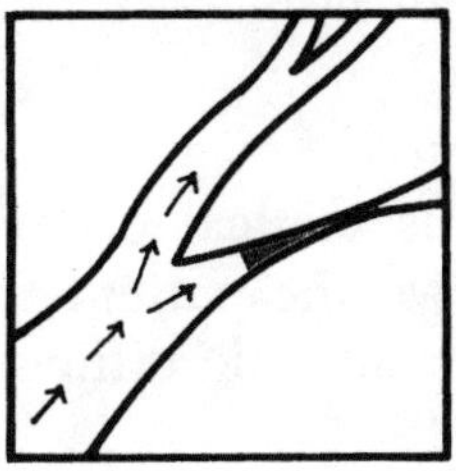

An artery of the brain may constrict and thus reduce the flow of blood to an area of the brain. If the spasm is of short duration permanent damage does not necessarily occur.

Severe headaches and seizures sometimes occur after brain damage. These can almost always be controlled with medication.

Brain damage can also affect vision. Patients may lose their peripheral vision, for example, and see clearly only what is directly in front of them. A physician can evaluate the seriousness of any such vision disturbance.

Aphasic patients often fail to respond to speech and frequently ask to have words repeated. Their families may think the problem is hearing loss, but more likely the patient is unable to understand the words he hears or to recall the words he needs for a reply. A hearing test can help resolve the question. Aphasics usually understand slow speech in single words and short phrases better than rapid speech.

Personality Changes

Most chronically ill patients occasionally feel anxious and depressed, and find relief by talking to others. The aphasic patient, however, is denied this outlet; he cannot talk out his problems. Emotions once held in abeyance now flare in behavior seldom seen before the illness. A once easy-going husband sulks because dinner is served late; a doting grandmother snaps at her grandchildren or turns them away. Tears and laughter flow more freely, sometimes without apparent cause. Moods shift quickly from depression to elation, from cooperation to defiance: the patient who is eager for therapy one morning may stubbornly refuse to get out of bed the next.

Some patients tire easily and become lethargic. Memory loss and a shortened attention span may cause them to lose interest in hobbies. Some patients no longer care about their personal appearance or tidiness, whereas others become compulsively neat and orderly. A patient's confidence or self-esteem may be eroded by an inability to perform simple tasks — to answer a simple question or talk on the telephone — and feelings of unworthiness may erupt in a tearful rage or sullen withdrawal.

Many of these behavioral changes are effects of physical and psychological stresses beyond the patient's control. Support, encouragement, and acceptance are vital to his well being. If an aphasic patient is isolated, excluded, or discouraged from participating in activities, his dignity and self-esteem will suffer.

Diagnosis and Evaluation

The first step in diagnosing aphasia is clinical observation. The physician and speech pathologist observe the patient to determine what language skills remain, to evaluate specific difficulties, and to plan the best possible program of rehabilitation. Some patients may have trouble recalling words and naming objects — a condition known as anomia. Or it may be difficult to arrange words in correct grammatical order. Other patients may pronounce words incorrectly or even speak nonsense syllables, unaware that these sounds are meaningless. For some, speech may not come at all, and for others it may come fluently but make no sense (this latter problem is called paraphasia). Still other patients may speak telegraphically without the prepositions, modifiers, and connectives that refine language.

Oral and written tests help the speech pathologist to better define the specific type and extent of language loss. The patient is asked to name objects, follow commands, and repeat words, phrases, and numbers in series. His ability to read, write, recall words, and understand speech and written material is also tested.

These tests also help to differentiate aphasia from other disorders, such as dysarthria (disturbance of the nerves and muscles involved in producing speech) and verbal dyspraxia (inability to form the mouth and tongue movements properly to pronounce a word, even though the idea of the word is clear and the muscles are normal).

Prognosis and Rehabilitation

Although the outcome of aphasia is difficult to predict, some conditions seem to favor recovery. Generally, the younger the patient the brighter the outlook. Patients with less extensive brain damage fare better. The location of the injury is also important, as some types of aphasia respond to therapy better than others. Patients with better language comprehension recover more, and expressive skills seem to improve the least.

Many stroke patients have some spontaneous recovery from aphasia within days of their stroke, and significant improvement may continue for 2 or 3 months. After 6 months, however, further progress is largely the result of language rehabilitation and speech therapy.

Therapy should begin as soon as possible — its value is greatest when started early — and should be tailored to the individual. In some severe cases, the most practical approach may be short-term therapy to improve comprehension. The more a patient understands, the less isolated he will feel, and the less apt he will be to withdraw from others and become depressed. Even aphasics who never regain speech can still participate in family affairs and enjoy social gatherings if they can understand others.

Although the results of therapy can never be predicted with absolute certainty, almost all patients benefit. A few patients will regain the same capacity for language they had before the onset of aphasia.

Rehabilitation involves intensive exercises in which the patient reads, writes, follows directions, and repeats the therapist's speech. "Cuing" techniques sometimes help patients retrieve words they seem to have lost; for example, the therapist might provide the first sound of a word (phonetic cuing), use a synonym (semantic cuing), or build a sentence around a missing word and have the patient fill in the blank (sentence completion).

Scientists have learned that patients with verbal dyspraxia benefit most from a new technique called melodic intonation therapy. Although these patients cannot coordinate their lips and tongue in the precise movements required for speech, they often have no difficulty singing. Melodic intonation therapy stresses rhythm and intonation patterns; by producing a melody while speaking, patients can more easily organize the lip and tongue movements necessary for speech.

Programmed instruction and group instruction sometimes supplement individual therapy. In programmed instruction, the patient practices one skill — such as writing a word — until he masters it, and then proceeds, step by step, to tasks of increasing difficulty.

Group instruction helps minimize feelings of isolation, intellectual deprivation, and depression that follow the sudden loss of ability to communicate. Patients in groups often support, encourage, and stimulate each other. Family members and friends can help patients achieve full potential for improvement if they, too, offer support and respect.

Current Research

The National Institute of Neurological and Communicative Disorders and Stroke (NINCDS), a part of the U.S. Government's National Institutes of Health, supports research on aphasia and other communicative disorders. With NINCDS support, scientists in Minneapolis devised a coding system for scoring the effectiveness of various treatments for aphasia. This system is being used to identify the most beneficial treatments for aphasic patients.

In a recent study of large groups of patients from several institutions, Veterans Administration scientists found that in the first 6 months after onset of aphasia, patients gain more from traditional individual speech and language therapy than they do from informal discussion groups.

NINCDS-supported scientists in Boston are developing alternate systems of communication for severely impaired aphasic adults. One system enables patients who can't talk to communicate with cards that represent objects and actions. Patients can convey thoughts by placing colored line drawings of a chair, an apple, or a bed, for example, next to cards depicting actions like sitting, eating, or sleeping.

The NINCDS also supports studies of spontaneous language recovery in the first few months of aphasia. In one such study, a multidisciplinary team of investigators is trying to find out which other regions of the brain become involved in language when the language areas have been injured.

Besides these clinical studies, basic research on language development and brain structure and function is yielding information physicians need to diagnose aphasia and other language disorders more accurately, and to devise new and better programs of rehabilitation.

Prevention

The only way to prevent aphasia is to prevent its underlying cause — brain damage. Many severe head injuries can be prevented by simple safety precautions. Motorcyclists who wear helmets, swimmers who dive only in safe areas, and careful drivers protect themselves from accidents that could lead to head wounds and aphasia.

The conquest of stroke holds the greatest hope for preventing aphasia. Research at some 14 stroke centers supported by the NINCDS focuses on the cause, prevention, and treatment of cerebral vascular disease.

Many factors contribute to strokes. Overweight, smoking, high blood pressure, blood vessel disease, excessive stress, and past history of stroke are all predisposing factors. Early detection and correction of health problems will help greatly to reduce the incidence of stroke, and thus aphasia, in this country.

Where to Get Professional Help

A neurologist will refer an aphasic patient to a speech-language pathologist for language rehabilitation. Residents new to an area who need help finding a physician may seek referral from the local medical society or from the neurology department of a nearby university or medical center. Also, the *Directory of Medical Specialists* lists board certified physicians by medical specialty and geographic location. This directory, which can be found at most neighborhood libraries, provides information on the physician's medical education and training, experience, and professional affiliations.

Several public and private organizations concerned with aphasia research and rehabilitation employ speech-language pathologists. The American Speech-Language-Hearing Association can help patients locate clinical services in their area. This association and others listed below can provide further information on aphasia and direct patients to qualified specialists:

American Speech-Language-Hearing Association
10801 Rockville Pike
Rockville, Maryland 20852

American Heart Association
7320 Greenville Avenue
Dallas, Texas 75231

The National Easter Seal Society for Crippled Children and Adults
2023 West Ogden Avenue
Chicago, Illinois 60612

Local Veterans Administration Hospitals

Chapter 4

Batten's Disease

What is Batten's disease?

What is it?

Batten's disease is an inherited disorder of the nervous system that strikes in childhood. Appearing first as vision changes or seizures, the disease causes mental impairment and progressive loss of sight and motor skills. Children with Batten's disease eventually become blind, bedridden, and demented.

These symptoms are associated with a buildup of fatty pigments in cells of the brain, the nervous system, and other parts of the body. Scientists do not know what triggers the buildup, and there is as yet no effective treatment. The disease is always fatal.

How is it inherited?

Batten's disease is an autosomal recessive disorder; that is, it occurs only when a child inherits a defective gene from both parents. Children who inherit only one defective gene are carriers: they do not have the signs and symptoms of the disorder, but they can pass the gene on to their own children. No way is yet known to identify carriers of the gene that causes Batten's disease.

Are there other disorders like Batten's disease?

Batten's disease is the most common form of a group of disorders called the neuronal ceroid lipofuscinoses. There are three childhood forms in this group. All have similar symptoms, but these symptoms become apparent at different ages and progress at different rates:

- *Infantile* (Santavuori disease) begins at about 8 months and progresses rapidly. Affected children fail to thrive and have abnormally small heads (microcephaly). Also typical are shocklike muscle contractions called myoclonic jerks. Patients usually die before age 5, although some have survived in a vegetative state a few years longer.
- *Late infantile* (Jansky-Bielschowsky disease) begins at around age 3. The typical early signs are loss of muscle coordination (ataxia) and seizures that do not respond to drugs. This form progresses rapidly and ends in death between ages 8 and 12.
- *Juvenile* (Batten's disease, Spielmeyer-Sjogren disease) infantile forms. Death usually comes in the late early twenties, but some patients have survived longer.

There are also two very rare adult forms, called Kuf's disease and Parry's disease. These are milder varieties that progress slowly and do not cause blindness.

The remainder of this fact sheet deals only with juvenile form, called Batten's disease after the British pediatrician who first described it in 1903.

How common is it?

Batten's disease is relatively rare, affecting 2 to 3 in 100,000 people. It appears to be more common in Finland, Sweden, other parts of northern Europe, and Newfoundland, Canada.

Although Batten's disease is rare, it often strikes more than one person in families that carry the defective gene.

What causes it?

The cause of Batten's disease is uncertain, but may have something to do with abnormal storage of certain fatty substances in body tissues.

In Batten's disease, substances made up of fats and proteins build up in cells of the brain and the eye as well as in skin, muscle, and many other kinds of tissue. The substances are called lipopigments — "lipo" because they contain lipids (fats) and pigments because they are colored greenish-yellow. Inside the cells, these pigments form deposits with distinctive shapes. Some look like half moons, others like fingerprints. The deposits are autofluorescent; that is, they shine in ultraviolet light under microscope. These odd-shaped, shiny deposits are what doctors look for when they examine a skin sample to diagnose Batten's disease. However, scientists do not yet know how the stored lipopigments are related to the nerve damage of Batten's disease.

What are the symptoms?

The early signs of Batten's disease may be subtle — personality and behavior changes, slow learning, clumsiness or stumbling. Sometimes the child has failing vision, followed by seizures. In other children, the seizures come first, then vision loss. As the disease advances, the child becomes progressively weak and uncoordinated. Vision and thinking ability keep getting worse, and seizures come more often. Eventually, affected children are left blind, mentally retarded, and totally disabled.

Although the course of Batten's disease can vary in different children, in general the earlier seizures begin, the faster the disease progresses.

How is it diagnosed?

Because vision loss is often an early sign, Batten's disease may be suspected first during an eye exam. An eye doctor can detect a loss of cells within the eye that occurs in Batten's as well as in some eye diseases, but cannot diagnose Batten's disease just from this sign. If there is reason to suspect Batten's, the child will be referred to a neurologist, a doctor who specializes in diseases of the brain and nervous system.

The neurologist will examine the child's blood and urine for abnormalities that may indicate Batten's disease. To help make a definite diagnosis, the doctor may examine a small piece of skin under an electron microscope. If Batten's disease is present, the typical deposits will appear inside the skin cells, especially in cells of the sweat glands.

Is there any treatment?

No treatment is yet known that can halt or reverse the symptoms of Batten's disease. Treatments with vitamins C and E and with diets low in vitamin A have reportedly stabilized some patients for a short time. However, these treatments did not change the fatal outcome of the disease.

Support and encouragement go a long way towards helping families cope with profound disability and dementia in a Batten's disease patient. Physical and occupational therapy can keep up the child's spirits, while support groups can help maintain a positive outlook. Also, seizures can be kept under control with anticonvulsant drugs, and other medical problems can be treated appropriately as they arise.

Meanwhile, scientists pursue medical research that will someday yield an effective treatment for Batten's disease.

What research is being done?

Within the federal government, the focal point for research on Batten's disease and other neurological disorders is the National Institute of Neurological and Communicative Disorders and Stroke (NINCDS). The NINCDS, a part of the National Institutes of Health, is responsible for supporting and conducting research on the brain and central nervous system.

Some scientists are working on the theory that children with Batten's disease are missing an enzyme, a natural chemical that helps the body break down substances no longer needed. Lack of such an enzyme could stop cells from breaking down fats and their associated proteins in a normal way. Some of these fats and proteins might then build up to form the lipopigments involved in Batten's disease. Investigators are searching for enzymes that might be scarce, or completely missing, in children with the disorder. Their goal is to be able to treat affected children with natural or synthetic enzymes that would replenish the missing substances in the child's body.

Other investigators are studying animals that have diseases like Batten's. At Massey University in New Zealand, an NINCDS-supported scientist is examining different kinds of tissue from sheep that have a similar disease. He is focusing on early vision changes caused by loss of retinal cells in the eye. His goal is to use what he finds for early diagnosis and for detection of carriers. Other scientists are working with English setters and Dalmatians that have diseases similar to Batten's. These animal models give scientists the chance to study Batten's disease in its early stages — a key step in devising treatment and control strategies.

By studying other inherited metabolic disorders that affect the brain, scientists can find out what goes wrong in cells that cannot break down a naturally occurring substance. To encourage an efficient approach to this problem, the NINCDS plans to fund "neurogenetic research centers" for the study of inherited brain diseases that affect infants and children. Research in these centers is expected to lead to better ways to diagnose, treat, and someday prevent Batten's disease.

How can I help research?

The National Institute of Neurological and Communicative Disorders and Stroke and the National Institute of Mental Health support two national human brain specimen banks. These banks supply investigators around the world with tissue from patients with neurological and psychiatric diseases. Both banks need brain tissue from Batten's disease patients to enable scientists to study this disorder more intensely. Prospective donors should contact:

Dr. Wallace W. Tourtellotte, Director
Human Neurospecimen Bank
VA Wadsworth Medical Center
Wilshire and Sawtelle Boulevards
Los Angeles, California 90073
Telephone: (213) 824-4307

Dr. Edward D. Bird, Director
Brain Tissue Bank, Mailman Research Center
McLean Hospital
115 Mill Street
Belmont, Massachusetts 02178
Telephone: (617) 855-2400

Is help available?

A voluntary agency actively involved in promoting research on Batten's disease and helping affected families is:

The Children's Brain Disease Foundation
350 Parnassus Avenue, Suite 900
San Francisco, California 94117
(415) 566-5402

The U.S. Government's National Center for Education in Maternal and Child Health answers inquiries on Batten's disease:

National Center for Education in Maternal and Child Health
3520 Prospect Street NW
Washington, DC 20057
(202) 625-8400

NINCDS information

For more information on research programs of National Institute of Neurological and Communicative Disorders and Stroke, contact:

Office of Scientific and Health Reports
National Institute of Neurological and Communicative Disorders and Stroke
Building 31, Room 8A-06
National Institutes of Health
Bethesda, Maryland 20892
(301) 496-5751

Chapter 5

Brain Tumors

Brain Tumors

Introduction

She was 20, an attractive English major at a Boston college, engaged to be married. Then she was diagnosed as having a brain tumor of a particularly advanced and malignant type that was invading the right frontal lobe of her brain. Marriage was definitely out, she decided, but she wasn't giving up. The surgeons removed the bulk of the tumor and followed up with radiation and chemotherapy. Now, 7 years later, there is no sign of cancer. She still rules out marriage, but she's back in college.

A 45-year-old minister and biblical scholar recently underwent his fourth operation for a meningioma, a tumor of the outer coverings of the brain. Usually a meningioma is a slow-growing tumor, often completely removable by surgery. In the minister's case, however, the tumor recurred, first after a year or so, then after only months. This time the brain surgeons planned to follow up with a new anticancer drug.

Usually. Slow-growing. Removable. Malignant. Invasive. Advanced. The words are the common jargon of the cancer expert. The words are familiar to nonexperts as well, for who among us has not been touched by the death of friend or relative who has succumbed to cancer?

When it comes to brain tumors, however, the familiar words take on new meanings. The brain is a special organ, special in the cells that compose it, in its position in the head, and in its relation to the rest of the body. When a tumor grows in the brain, doctors have to consider not only the nature of the tumor, but its relation to the brain's distinctive features.

The Nature of the Brain

First and foremost among those features is that the brain is the organ of thought, emotion, and behavior. The idea that a mass of abnormal tissue could encroach on that domain, undermining the mental faculties that make us human and ultimately threatening life itself, is what terrifies most people when they hear the words *brain tumor*. Yet some brain tumors can be removed completely at surgery leaving no neurological damage. Even advanced cancers growing deep inside the brain are being tackled today by new treatments that have saved or at least prolonged lives, while preserving the integrity of those lives.

Experts can also point to other features of the brain that offer some reason for hope. Tumors are generally classified as benign — if the tumor cells look much like ordinary cells and the tumor is confined to one place — or malignant, if the tumor cells look very disordered and the tumor can spread (metastasize) to other parts of the body. (Strictly speaking, the word *cancer* applies only to malignant growths.) Tumors that originate in the brain — primary brain tumors — may be either benign or malignant. Surprisingly, while malignant brain tumor cells can spread throughout the brain, only rarely do they spread to other parts of the body. That means that once you destroy a brain cancer, you need not worry that some cells may have escaped to seed tumors elsewhere in the body.

Another fact that startles many people is that brain tumor tissue almost never consists of the fundamental working cells of the brain — the nerve cells (neurons). Once mature, these complex nerve cells no longer divide and multiply. Instead, it is the surrounding and supporting cells of the brain that occasionally get out of control. Thus a brain tumor that is diagnosed and treated early may do little or no damage to essential brain matter — the neurons and their circuits that underlie every act of mental life and behavior.

Confusing Symptoms

There are "if's." Brain tumors are not always easy to diagnose. The symptoms can vary widely according to the brain area affected. If a tumor grows in the temporal lobe on the left side of the brain, for example, it may affect speech and memory, or alter mood and emotional state. Such symptoms might suggest mental illness or psychological problems, rather than a brain tumor. If a tumor lies near the cerebellum, an area at the back of the brain important in the control of movement, there may be early symptoms of dizziness and lack of coordination. Tumors growing on or around the major nerves supplying the ears or eyes may lead to symptoms of hearing loss, headaches, or visual problems, diverting attention from the brain as the source of trouble.

On the other hand, some brain tumors may produce few symptoms. Parts of the frontal lobes, for example, are presumed to play a role in thinking and other higher mental activities. Yet tumors can sometimes cause considerable tissue damage in these areas with little effect on a person's behavior.

Once a tumor is found, still another "if" centers on its location in relation to surrounding tissue. The brain is one of the most protected organs in the body. It is wrapped in the tough outer coverings of the meninges, bathed in shock-absorbing and nutrient liquid — the cerebrospinal fluid — and armored by the strong bones of the skull.

If a tumor lies near the skull bones or close to major blood vessels or channels circulating cerebrospinal fluid, it need not grow very large before it blocks blood or cerebrospinal fluid circulation and causes increased pressure inside the skull. Or, if the tumor is discovered deep inside the brain, surgery to remove it may be risky, with too great a chance of damaging vital brain centers. Ironically, the distinction between benign and malignant blurs in such cases. If a benign tumor is inaccessible it can be fatal. On the other hand, the young woman with the malignant tumor invading her frontal lobe had a major portion of the lobe removed and is alive and well today.

Neurosurgeons who treat brain tumor patients are well aware of the ironies of the condition. They can all tell stories of exceptional survivals as well as tragic deaths. Scientists who have made research on brain tumors their specialty are particularly concerned that the public understand the complex problems posed by brain tumors as well as the growing efforts to solve those problems.

Those investigators include scientists supported by the National Institute of Neurological and Communicative Disorders and Stroke (NINCDS) — the leading federal agency supporting research on the brain — the National Cancer Institute, and other federal health agencies. One major group effort is the clinical research program carried out by NINCDS neurosurgeons working at the Clinical Center, the research hospital of the National Institutes of Health in Bethesda, Md.

11,000 Cases a Year

The chances of developing a primary malignant brain tumor are relatively rare — about 1 in 22,000. Such cancers account for less than 2 percent of all cancers diagnosed in the United States every year. That is still an impressively large number — 11,000 brain cancers annually. At least twice as many patients have secondary brain cancers, the result of cancer metastasizing to the brain from other sites in the body, principally the breast, lung, or kidney.

Brain tumors affect children as well as adults. Indeed, primary tumors of the brain or spinal cord (the central nervous system) are the most common tumors of childhood after the leukemias. The peak for brain tumors in children is between the ages of 6 and 9. Childhood brain tumors generally differ in location and cellular makeup from adult tumors, differences thought to reflect a still growing and

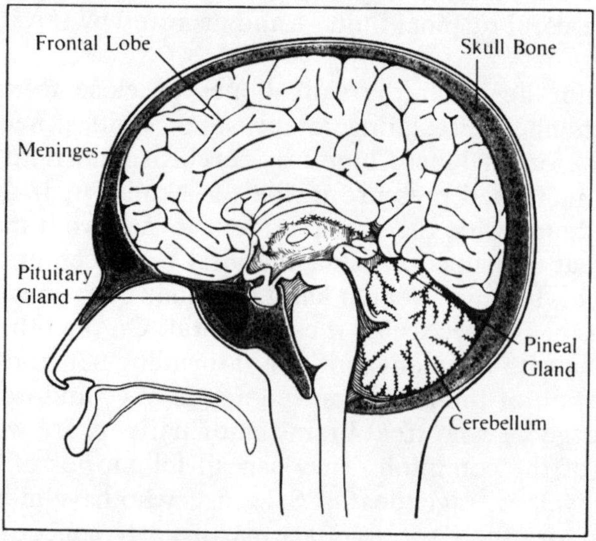

The brain, wrapped in its meningeal coverings, fits snugly against the bones of the skull.

developing nervous system. Adult brain tumors are most common between the ages of 40 and 60, with men affected slightly more than women.

Why primary brain tumors occur remains a mystery. Tumor sleuths have considered the vast array of environmental and genetic factors that have been linked to cancers in other parts of the body but, in the case of brain tumors, there are no clearcut associations. The recent finding of a slightly higher than normal occurrence of brain tumors in workers at certain petrochemical plants is interesting, but the cases are too few for scientists to come to firm conclusions. There are also a few families in the United States where cancer, including brain cancer, occurs frequently. Some genetic factor could possibly account for these families' high cancer prevalence — perhaps some defect in the body's immune system. Again, more detailed genetic and biochemical studies are needed.

Diagnosing Brain Tumors Today

Clearly not every headache, dizzy spell, or visual disturbance is a sign of brain tumor. And while symptoms can vary widely, specialists pay particular attention to certain signs:

- ***Progressive unrelenting symptoms***. Whatever they may be, the symptoms never let up and they get worse over time.

• ***Headache.*** Given the tight confines of the head, a growing tumor sooner or later will create pressure or swelling that affects tissues in the head, producing severe headache. Often the patient reports that the headache is worse upon first waking in the morning. Interestingly, brain tissue itself is normally insensitive to pain. But the meningeal layers, blood vessel walls, and the tissues lining the cavities of the brain and skull are rich in nerve endings sensitive to pain.

• ***Visual complaints.*** Double vision, blurring or other visual symptoms may occur as a result of increased pressure on the optic nerve or the blood vessels supplying the retina.

• ***Motor signs.*** Some patients report weakness or numbness in their arms and legs. Sometimes reflexes (like the familiar knee jerk reflex) are very strong. In the case of spinal cord tumors, patients may experience a growing loss of sensation below a certain level in the trunk, or increasing difficulty in moving limbs.

• ***Seizures.*** The onset of seizures or convulsions in a patient who has not been in an accident, been ill with fever, or suffered some other injury or illness is "presumptive evidence of a brain tumor until proven otherwise," says one leading authority.

To confirm the diagnosis, neurologists and neurosurgeons can conduct a battery of tests including simple X-rays of the head, standard brainwave recordings (the electroencephalogram or EEG), analysis of cerebrospinal fluid, and so on. Their principal diagnostic aid today, however, is the CT scan, the technique that produces a computerized three-dimensional X-ray image of the brain. The CT scan is highly accurate, detecting the presence of a tumor mass in 90 to 95 percent of cases — even when that mass is no larger than half an inch across.

The CT scan can not only indicate the presence of a tumor, but will pin down its location in the brain. At this point the specialist may call for an arteriogram: an X-ray that will outline the arteries supplying blood to the tumor. Some tumors are richly endowed with blood vessels; others are less so. Thus the arteriogram provides another clue to the kind of brain tumor.

The Next Step

Surgery is the first line of attack against brain tumors. How extensive the operation will be depends on the tumor size and location and whether the tumor cells are concentrated in a mass or spread throughout the brain. "Each patient's tumor is different," notes the chief of the NINCDS Surgical Neurology Branch in the NIH Clinical Center. "It is different pathologically, it behaves differently, and it grows differently."

For that reason some of the tissue removed at brain surgery is always reserved for pathological analysis. Studies of this "biopsy" material indicate whether the tumor is benign or malignant. Malignant tumor tissue removed at surgery is also being used in promising research studies aimed at improving treatment — even predicting which treatments will be successful.

Observers examining samples of brain tissue microscopically can tell what kinds of cells make up a tumor, and whether the cells are benign or malignant. Benign cells resemble normal cells of the tissue in question. Malignant cells lose more and more of their distinctive trademarks and acquire the classic characteristics of cancer: large or multiple nuclei, abnormal numbers of chromosomes, and changes in the cell's surface membrane. These changes seem to help very malignant cells to invade and take root in other tissues more easily. The extent of these changes permits classifying tumor cells by degree of malignancy from Grade I, benign, to Grade IV, the most advanced stage of malignancy.

Tumor Varieties

Most brain tumors are *gliomas*, derived from the glial cells that support the neurons of the brain. Gliomas can be either benign or malignant. Unfortunately, one of the most malignant gliomas — the *glioblastoma multiforme* — is also the most common brain tumor. In

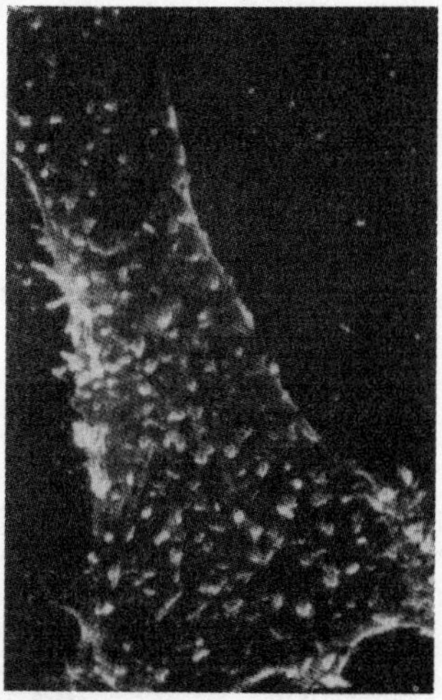

The small finger-like projections dotting the surface of this brain tumor cell are signs of malignancy.

Those bull's-eyes in the center are multiple nuclei in a single glial cell: a sign of malignancy.

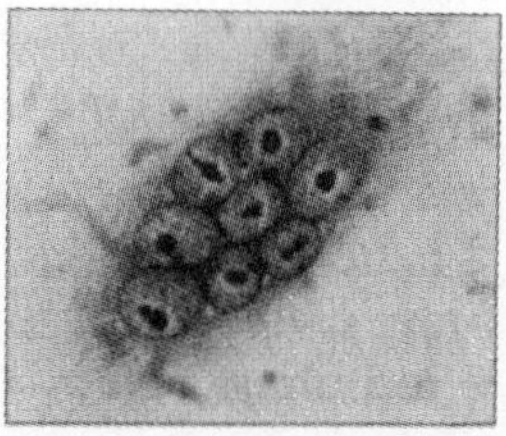

all, gliomas account for 43 percent of primary brain cancers. Glial tumors are further described in terms of the type of glial cell they contain:

• ***Astrocytomas.*** Star-shaped cells called astrocytes are the cells affected in a large subgroup of gliomas. Benign cerebellar astrocytomas are common childhood tumors. With today's tools and techniques, these tumors are often completely removable surgically. They are one of the recent success stories in tumor treatment. On the other hand, the young woman college student's frontal lobe tumor was a malignant astrocytoma. What makes her story so impressive is that it was a Grade IV malignancy — an aggressive rapidly growing tumor that is usually fatal in a year or so.

• ***Medulloblastomas.*** The root "blast" refers to a cell in an early stage of development. Medulloblasts are immature cells that may develop into either neurons or glial cells. Medulloblastomas are malignant tumors found in the rear of the brain. They typically occur in youngsters under 12 and account for a small percentage of all brain tumors.

• ***Ependymomas.*** The cells lining the hollow cavities of the brain — ependymal cells — also give rise to a small percentage of brain tumors. These "ependymomas" tend to be benign.

Other gliomas are composed of other varieties of glial cells, such as those that produce the fatty insulating material (myelin) that surrounds many nerve fibers in the brain.

The second major group of primary brain tumors are those made up of covering cells:

• ***Meningiomas.*** Tumors of the meninges (the membrane coverings of the brain and spinal cord) are usually benign, and account for some 15 percent of all brain tumors.

• ***Schwannomas.*** These tumors arise from the Schwann cells that form the fatty sheath that envelops nerve fibers in the body. One such tumor develops in relation to the nerve of hearing, the acoustic nerve. Acoustic nerve tumors, called *acoustic neuromas*, are benign tumors which, if detected early, can be completely removed without loss of hearing or other nervous system damage.

The successful removal of acoustic neuromas is a good illustration of how far neurosurgeons have advanced in techniques. During the first decade of this century the mortality rate for acoustic neuroma surgery was close to 80 percent. The tumor was deep-seated and difficult to remove because of its close relation to the brain stem, a

---

* Theodor Schwann, German naturalist.

core of brain tissue that contains vital nerve centers such as those controlling breathing. By 1917, however, the doctor considered to be the father of neurosurgery, Harvey Cushing, demonstrated a new technique for acoustic neuroma removal which reduced mortality to 20 percent. With more experience, Cushing was able to reduce mortality to below 10 percent. Today the mortality rate for acoustic neuroma is down to 1 percent.

Other kinds of tumor may involve cells in or near the pituitary gland at the base of the brain, or the pineal gland, deep in the center of the brain. In rare instances a brain tumor will develop from types of nerve cells.

Surgery Plus...

In the case of a benign accessible brain tumor, surgery may be the beginning and end of treatment: The tumor is completely removed and the patient resumes activities with little likelihood of recurrence. If the tumor is malignant, it may not be possible to remove it completely. In that case, or if a tumor is large or difficult to reach, treatment will include radiation and chemotherapy. Radiation is sometimes used before surgery in the hope of reducing tumor size.

Today, an increasing number of tumors formerly considered inoperable can be tackled surgically. Microsurgery — the use of an operating microscope — has played an important role in that development. But often it is a combination of great technical skill

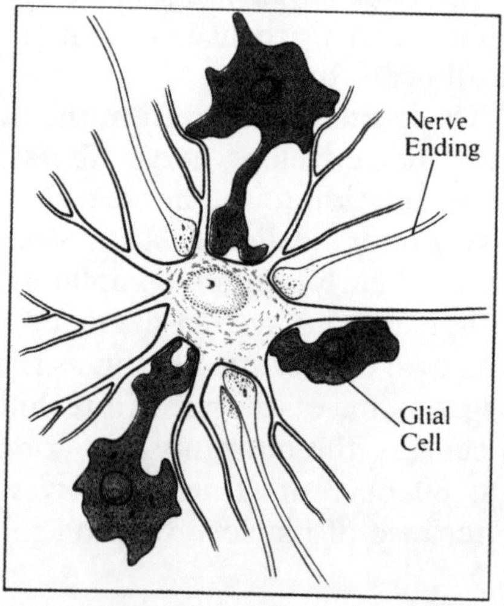

A typical nerve cell in the brain surrounded by glial cells and nerve endings.

and an ingenious strategy for getting at the tumor that has led to surgical success.

A few neurosurgeons are currently using high frequency sound waves (ultrasound) and laser beams to destroy brain tumors. In one laser technique, for example, the surgeon uses an operating microscope and aims the laser beam at the center of the tumor, using the high intensity rays to burn out the tissue. The exact position of the tumor is calculated by a computer that translates CT scan images into a set of coordinates referable to a framework set up around the patient's head. Time will tell whether such techniques will improve the success rate for tumor treatment.

Radiation usually begins within a week or two after surgery and continues for 6 weeks. Among recent refinements in radiation therapy are the use of drugs that make tumor tissue more sensitive to radioactive bombardment, and new radioactive sources that provide more powerful rays or charged particles that can be sharply focused on the tumor.

Chemotherapy, the other major weapon in the attack on brain tumors, has also benefited from refinements and advances. The principal brain tumor-killing drugs in use today go by the initials BCNU and CCNU, both chemically known as nitrosoureas. These drugs pass readily into the brain when given by mouth or injected into the bloodstream. Many drugs are prevented from reaching brain cells by an elaborate meshwork of fine blood vessels and cells — the blood-brain barrier — that filters blood reaching the brain.

The combined treatment of brain cancers with better drugs and radiotherapy, along with surgical techniques aimed at removing as much tumor tissue as possible, has meant longer survival times and richer lives for brain cancer patients. Further improvements in these traditional forms of treatment can be expected in the years ahead. In addition, scientists are developing new therapies based on promising laboratory studies.

The New Research

If a single word could describe the aim of much current research on malignant brain tumors it might be the word *fingerprint*. Scientists want to characterize tumor tissue in ways that make the tissue as unique to the patient as his or her fingerprints. Armed with that information, the hope is that doctors can design more effective treatments — with added confidence that those treatments will work.

The impetus for this research comes first from the need to determine what kinds of cells are found in the tumor and their degree of malignancy. Second, there is a strong suspicion that the reason that those tumor cells are there to begin with is that the body's immune system is deficient in some way.

Normally, the immune system seeks out and destroys invading organisms or foreign tissue. These defense mechanisms are called into play because foreign tissue is studded with telltale surface proteins — antigens — that differ from the surface antigens normally found on body cells. The immune system recognizes the foreign tissue and is stimulated to make a variety of cells — scavengers, "killer" cells, and others — as well as the protein compounds called antibodies — all specifically designed to fight that particular foreign invader. When the body's *own* cells become cancerous, their surface antigens also change. They, too, should appear foreign. By rights, a person's immune system ought to attack the cancer and destroy it.

There is evidence that the immune system tries to do just that. Investigators have been able to take samples of brain tumor tissue removed during surgery and grow the cells in tissue culture. When the scientists later expose the cultured cells to blood serum from the patient who provided the cells, they find that the serum contains antibodies that attack the tumor cells. The ammunition is there; it is just not powerful enough.

Scientists at NINCDS and elsewhere are exploring ways to boost patients' immune responses so that they can successfully fight their brain tumors or any remnants of tumor tissue not removed during surgery. One way is through *immune stimulation*. The idea is to use the patient's own tumor cells as the stimulating material. The cells are grown in tissue culture and then irradiated to prevent them from reproducing. The cells still contain their surface antigens, however, and so when injected back into the patient's body, they should provoke a strong response — both cells and antibodies — from the immune system. Currently NINCDS investigators are conducting such experimental treatments in selected patients with highly malignant astrocytomas.

The ability to grow human brain cancer cells in tissue culture has paid off in other ways as well. Tumor samples from a patient can be grown on separate culture plates and subjected to a variety of tests. Some tests are used to determine the degree of malignancy of tumor cells, a necessary step in planning treatment. One way to measure malignancy is to observe how rapidly the cells multiply and fill the culture plate. Investigators can also expose the cells to a fine-holed filter and see how aggressively the cells try to penetrate the openings.

Scientists can also transplant human brain tumor cells to laboratory animals to see if the human tumor will take root in the animal's body. The animals used are mice with a hereditary defect that renders them hairless as well as lacking the thymus, an organ important in the immune system. The immune system defect makes these "nude mice" less likely than normal animals to reject foreign tissue. The ability to grow a human cancer in a living animal is in itself of great importance: Scientists can observe how the tumor behaves at all stages of growth, as well as experiment with new therapies.

Tailor-made Treatments

Provided with samples of a patient's tumor cells in tissue culture, investigators can also test the effectiveness of antitumor drugs. There appears to be a correlation between the way tumor cells respond to drugs in the laboratory dish and the way they respond in the brain. Thus if the lab studies show that BCNU and CCNU have little or no effect on cells grown in culture, there is little likelihood that these drugs will benefit the patient. For these "nonresponders," investigators may try other tactics, such as the use of new antitumor drugs still in the experimental stage. (The biblical scholar will receive such an experimental drug.)

With continued experience and refinements in culturing techniques, it may be possible to custom design brain tumor treatment programs, selecting the right drug at the right dosage and initiating treatment quickly, without having to go through a lengthy trial and error period. Such tactics not only save precious time, they also spare the patient the futility of ineffective treatments and may also reduce side effects.

Tissue culture techniques may also make it easier to diagnose a brain tumor early — when physicians may suspect that a tumor is present, but nothing is detectable on a CT scan. NINCDS scientists and others have taken blood samples from patients with suspected malignancies and added the serum to established laboratory cultures of human brain tumor cells. If the patient has a brain tumor, there is a high probability that the blood serum will contain antitumor antibodies that will react with the tumor cells on the laboratory plate.

Alternative Treatments

The tissue culture and immunotherapy techniques are among the most promising and exciting lines of investigation being explored in brain tumor research today. There are others as well. Radiologists continue to seek out more effective methods of irradiating tumor tissue in the brain without jeopardizing surrounding tissue. Likewise, pharmacologists search for better antitumor drugs and ways of delivering those drugs to the brain. The use of a type of sugar called mannitol, for example, can disrupt the blood-brain barrier for a brief period of time and allow chemicals access to brain tissue. However, specialists have noted that the blood-brain barrier does not appear to be as intact around tumor tissue, so the need to circumvent it may not be so crucial.

Scientists are also exploring the use of agents that can cause malignant cells to become more like normal cells again. Such a transformation may be effective in halting tumor growth or in enhancing sensitivity to other forms of treatment. The advantage of this technique — called *biological modification* — is that the substances used are nontoxic compounds that are normally produced in the body.

Professional journals as well as popular magazines and newspapers report a steady stream of promising new treatments for cancer. One reads, for example, of heat produced by microwaves being used to kill brain tumors. Some investigators are also experimenting with raising body temperature on the theory that an artificial fever will provoke the immune system into action. Another well-publicized potential cure for cancer is interferon, the substance body cells produce naturally to fight infection. These new therapies may prove to be important, but as yet there is not enough evidence to establish their roles as therapeutic agents. All new approaches to treating

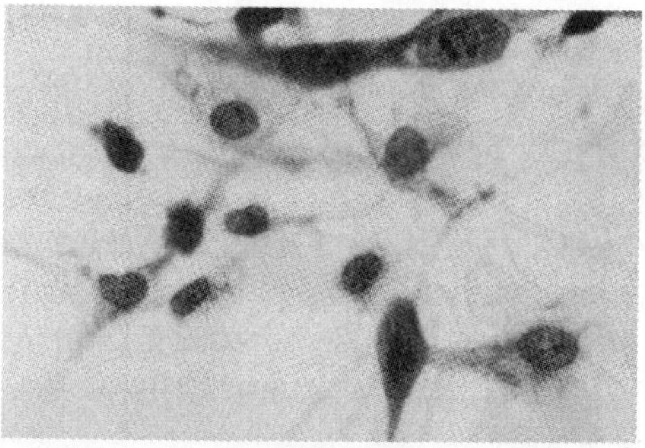

These benign cells from an acoustic neuroma were grown in tissue culture. If diagnosed early, acoustic neuromas can be removed completely with no neurological damage.

brain tumors must stand the test of well-designed, carefully controlled clinical tests and long-term follow-up before any conclusions can be drawn about the safety or the effectiveness of treatments.

Watching The Brain In Action

Aiding and abetting follow-up of new treatments for brain tumors, as well as providing a versatile research tool in many basic and clinical studies, is a new form of brain scanning called positron emission tomography (PET). PET scans of the brain show which brain cells are most active metabolically. An aggressively growing tumor, for example, might show up on a PET scan as an area lighter or brighter than surrounding tissue, indicating higher metabolic activity. A tumor that is dying, however, might be correspondingly lower in activity and, over time, shrink in size.

The PET technique depends on the fact that metabolically active cells absorb nutrients at a high rate. The bloodstream of a patient or an experimental animal is injected with a nutrient like sugar that is labeled with a radioactive compound. As the blood circulates in the brain, the most active cells will take up more of the labeled sugar and then broadcast their location by virtue of their radioactivity. Detectors placed around the head pick up the radioactivity, and with the aid of a computer, translate the readings into a brain image. PET scans can be color-coded to make the differences in cell uptake of nutrient stand out better. PET studies are being used to compare the healthy brain with the tumorous brain, and to observe changes in brain metabolism at all stages of disease.

When Brain Tumor Strikes

It is especially important to have a clear idea of the facts, should you or someone close to you be diagnosed as having a brain tumor. The news inevitably comes as a shock, so much so that much of what the specialist may say by way of explanation may be lost in the immediate emotional reaction to the news. Most patients and their families are caught up in a turmoil of feelings which may range from disbelief to paralyzing grief at the thought of impending death. Yet it is precisely at this point that hard decisions have to be made about the course of treatment and about family affairs. During this time you may find it helpful to turn to the larger family, friends, and outside resources such as clergymen or hospital counselors. Such people may assist you with many of the practical arrangements that may have to be made, as well as provide psychological and moral support.

What you should also do is inform yourself about the tried and true treatments as well as the highly regarded clinical research and treatment programs available in major medical centers in the United States. You should also seek treatment by physicians who are experienced in tumor therapy. Because brain tumors are relatively rare, many physicians see only a few brain tumor patients a year. There are others, however, who have made brain tumors their specialty.

Psychologically, the brain tumor patient and the family need to adapt to the situation. No one says that this is easy, and it is expected that there may be stages of anger or indignation (Why me?), denial, frustration, sadness, and depression. Some parents have seen a child die from a brain tumor and have written books about their experience, as John Gunther did in *Death Be Not Proud*. Knowing that others experience grief and tragedy, reading their stories, or sharing accounts can help in working through the emotional upheaval. In this regard the Association for Brain Tumor Research, a voluntary health organization formed by individuals concerned about brain tumors — usually because of personal experience — can be a valuable source of information and help. NINCDS, the National Cancer Institute, groups like the American Cancer Society, and major treatment centers like New York's Memorial Sloan-Kettering Center for Cancer Research and Houston's M.D. Anderson Hospital and Tumor Institute are other useful sources of information.

Probably one of the most unsettling aspects of the diagnosis and treatment of brain tumors is the uncertainty with which you have to live. In some cases of secondary brain tumors or advanced primary malignancies, death may be imminent. As we have seen, however, the combination of new and improved therapies have added months or even years to life, while preserving its quality.

As more and more brain tumors come to treatment earlier, and the treatments themselves prove more effective, there will still be worrisome wait-and-see problems. Will the tumor recur? Is a minor memory lapse or mood change an omen of cancer's return? Those questions and fears are not helped when brain tumor patients experience episodes of brain swelling, fever, or headache as a result of treatment. Needless to say checkups can allay such fears, and there are medications that can relieve brain swelling or other side effects of treatment.

In the end, how well patients, friends, and family members adapt to the experience of a brain tumor depends on their understanding of the problem and the inner resources and personality traits they bring to bear on it. For a 27-year-old college student in Boston, it has paid to be an optimist.

Voluntary Health Organizations

The Association for Brain Tumor Research supports research on brain tumors and provides information to the general public through brochures and newsletters.

Association for Brain Tumor Research
6232 N. Pulaski Road, Suite 200
Chicago, Ill. 60646
(312)286-5571

The Acoustic Neuroma Association is a new organization for patients, families, and medical personnel concerned with tumors of the acoustic nerve as well as other cranial nerves.

Acoustic Neuroma Association
240 Mooreland Avenue
Carlisle, Pa. 17013
(717) 249-2973

The Candlelighters is an organization for parents of children with cancer. The group publishes a newsletter and promotes the establishment of self-help chapters throughout the country.

The Candlelighters Foundation
2025 I Street, N.W.
Washington, D.C. 20006
(202) 659-5136

The American Cancer Society is a source of information on all varieties of cancer. The society has divisions in many cities in the United States and headquarters in New York.

American Cancer Society
777 3rd Avenue
New York, N.Y. 10017
(212) 371-2900

National Institutes of Health

For additional information on brain tumor research and clinical treatment programs contact:

Office of Scientific and Health Reports
National Institute of Neurological and Communicative Disorders and Stroke
Building 31, Room 8A06
National Institutes of Health
Bethesda, Md. 20205
(301) 496-5751

Office of Cancer Communications National Cancer Institute
Building 31, Room 10A29
National Institutes of Health
Bethesda, Md. 20205
(301) 496-6631

Chapter 6

Cerebral Palsy

Cerebral Palsy

A child is born. And it is only natural to want that child to be normal and healthy. But complications can arise throughout pregnancy and birth. Certain infections in a mother-to-be can seriously harm her unborn child. Cigarette smoking, excessive use of alcohol, and a variety of drugs can also impair a baby's growth and development. Labor and delivery are sometimes long and difficult. Birth may be premature, or result in a full-term infant of low birth weight. Each of these possibilities is known to increase the risk of injury to the baby — a risk that is especially high for the baby's rapidly developing brain. If the injury affects the brain areas vital in the control of movement — the motor systems — the baby may develop cerebral palsy.

Cerebral refers to the two large wrinkled hemispheres that dominate any picture of the human brain. *Palsy* means paralysis, but frequently is used to refer to problems in the control of nerves and muscles that make voluntary movements difficult or impossible. The words are broad enough in meaning to allow the term *cerebral palsy* to cover a large group of movement disorders of varying symptoms and severity. A child with mild cerebral palsy may be a little awkward. A child with more severe cerebral palsy may be mentally retarded or subject to convulsions, as well as physically handicapped. For a disorder to be classified as cerebral palsy, not only must there be a problem with movement or posture, but the problem must also occur early in development, during the time of the brain's most rapid growth. (By age 5 the brain will have reached 90 percent of its adult weight.) Doctors can't always pinpoint the precise cause of brain injury, but agree that sometimes it is the end result of a shortage of oxygen to brain cells, possibly combined with a diminished blood supply. Since the brain makes a high demand on blood-borne oxygen and nutrients, periods of deprivation can have devastating effects.

In many cases of cerebral palsy, the movement disorder may be accompanied by mental or emotional impairment, convulsive seizures (epilepsy), or losses in hearing, vision, or the other senses. Some of these associated conditions can be treated successfully, and some kinds of movement disturbance may improve in time. However, nerve cells are extremely limited in their powers of repair and regeneration, and even in cases where a child appears to recover full control over the limbs, mental or emotional deficits may remain.

On the other hand, the brain damage doesn't get worse over time: cerebral palsy is a nonprogressive disorder (although symptoms may change as a child matures). Cerebral palsy is not contagious, either, and only rarely are the symptoms associated with a hereditary disorder. Close to 90 percent of the time, the brain damage happens in pregnancy, often around the time of birth (the perinatal period). The condition is then called *congenital* cerebral palsy. Head injuries, infections such as meningitis, and other forms of brain damage (including injury from child abuse) occurring in the first months or years of life are the main causes of acquired cerebral palsy.

The words "may" and "can" used to describe the mishaps of pregnancy and early life are important. Not every infection or trauma of pregnancy harms the unborn child (the fetus). Not every fetus is equally vulnerable: many newborns endure long complicated deliveries with no lasting effects. Some low birth weight babies — today even babies under 2 pounds — may spend months in a newborn (neonatal) intensive care unit and emerge with all systems intact. Indeed, advances in neonatal care have been so impressive that babies are surviving today for whom there would have been no hope a decade ago.

At the same time, research has progressed in identifying some of the leading causes of cerebral palsy and finding means of prevention and treatment. One of the largest, most comprehensive research projects ever undertaken was the Collaborative Perinatal Project sponsored by the National Institute of Neurological and Communicative Disorders and Stroke (NINCDS). The project entailed following 55,000 women through pregnancy and delivery, and periodically examining their offspring from birth to age 7. The results of the study, still being analyzed, have already revealed a variety of environmental factors and events in pregnancy that increase the risk that a child will develop cerebral palsy or other serious nervous system disorders, and have helped focus attention on what can be done about these problems.

Meanwhile, other researchers have found ways to prevent or treat several well-known causes of cerebral palsy. There is now a vaccine for German measles (rubella), a virus disease notorious for its destructive effects on the fetal nervous system. Mothers-to-be are now urged to seek prenatal care early, eat wisely, and avoid the use of any nonessential drugs, including alcohol and nicotine. (One finding confirmed by the Collaborative Perinatal Project was that women who smoke during pregnancy tend to produce babies of lower than normal weight.)

Preventive methods as well as treatments are now available for a number of blood disorders, such as Rh incompatibility, in which antibodies in the mother's bloodstream attack fetal red blood cells — the very cells that carry oxygen and nutrients to all parts of the baby's body. Usually a mother's first child is not affected, but the first born's red blood cells may sensitize the mother, causing her body to manufacture antibodies that will attack the fetus in the next pregnancy. A mother with Rh incompatibility can be injected with a special serum shortly after her first child's birth to prevent the unwanted antibody production. Babies born with the Rh blood disorder can be treated with exchange transfusions in which a large volume of the baby's blood is removed and replaced with normal blood.

Treatments are also available for jaundice of the newborn, a blood disorder associated with Rh incompatibility, but one that can arise independently. In this condition there is a buildup of bile pigments in the baby's bloodstream (hyperbilirubinemia) which, if unrelieved, can destroy brain cells. As a result of Collaborative Perinatal Project findings, it now appears that even moderate hyperbilirubinemia in the newborn can be toxic to the brain and should be treated accordingly. Thus some major causes of cerebral palsy can now be eliminated.

"But none of those things happened to my child . . ."

Still cerebral palsy occurs. The majority of cases (58 percent in the Collaborative Perinatal Project study) develop in babies born at full term and full weight. Exact figures for the United States population are not available because doctors are not obliged to report cases of cerebral palsy to state health boards. The estimate of the United Cerebral Palsy Associations, the major voluntary health organization concerned with this problem, is that between 1 and 3 infants out of every thousand live-born develop cerebral palsy — about 9,000 new cases a year. At present, the association estimates there are 750,000 Americans alive with the condition. The most severely handicapped usually do not survive infancy, but most patients will reach maturity and many will attain a normal life span.

While better prenatal and obstetric care and new treatments are undoubtedly preventing some cases of cerebral palsy, it is not clear whether the number of new cases each year has significantly decreased. Moreover, the premature and very frail infants who are able to survive today thanks to the new intensive care technology do not always escape damage to the nervous system. Sadly, too, there are still some babies whose deliveries are uncomplicated, who appear normal at birth, yet later show signs of cerebral palsy.

Complicating the search for a cause of cerebral palsy in cases where no obvious mishap is implicated, is the fact that the brain is one of the most inaccessible organs in the body to study. Doctors cannot conveniently sample brain tissue or fluids the way they can blood or urine. This situation has improved greatly in the last decade with the development of new safe diagnostic tools such as computerized tomography — the CT scan — which produces a computer-drawn X-ray image of the brain, and ultrasound, which uses the echoes from high-frequency sound waves to detect brain abnormalities. These methods can sometimes reveal treatable cases of brain swelling or show up a small blood clot or hemorrhage — a stroke — not otherwise evident in an infant with cerebral palsy. But many times brain abnormality eludes detection.

A delay in development

Generally the diagnosis of cerebral palsy is made on the basis of symptoms that develop over the first or second year of life. Cerebral palsy is frequently not evident at birth because newborns have very little voluntary control over their bodies. They depend on reflexes — automatic responses built into the nervous system. Reflexes serve to protect and preserve the baby. For example, if you thump the mattress sharply on either side of a newborn lying flat on its back in a crib, the baby will react by throwing its arms around in an embrace-like gesture called the Moro reflex. Or if you touch a nipple to the baby's mouth, it will automatically pucker its lips in the sucking reflex. As development unfolds, a normal infant gradually loses the more primitive reflexes (which often involve movement of major parts of the body) and gains increasingly fine control over the body's separate parts.

In contrast, an infant with cerebral palsy usually shows a delay in development. Often the primitive reflexes remain and may dominate behavior so that the child has difficulty mastering such familiar landmarks of growth as rolling over, sitting, crawling, smiling, or making speech sounds. Sometimes an infant will favor a particular side of the body or assume an unusual posture. In other instances the major symptom may be an overall muscle weakness or decreased muscle tone (hypotonia): the baby is as floppy as a Raggedy Ann doll and even some of the primitive reflexes may be weak or absent.

Alert parents are often the first to note signs of developmental delay or abnormality. In other cases the family doctor may be suspicious and refer the parents to a neurologist, a specialist in nervous system disorders. The neurological examination is important because it will be on the basis of the findings that the specialist will decide whether the child has cerebral palsy and will discuss treatment. Corrective measures including orthopedic surgery, drugs, the use of casts, braces, hearing aids and other devices, as well as an overall program of education, psychological support, and rehabilitation can then be initiated. These measures are aimed at relieving symptoms and increasing the mobility, confidence, and independence of the child. At the same time they can forestall serious secondary changes in muscles, joints, and bones, such as curvature of the spine or hip dislocation, that can result from abnormal postures. Early detection of hearing loss is especially important since the development of speech is so crucially linked to a child's ability to hear.

Many symptoms and mixed varieties

Doctors classify cerebral palsy according to the quality of the movement disturbance and the limbs affected. If the legs are primarily affected, the condition is called *diplegia*. If both the arm and leg on one side are affected, it is a case of *hemiplegia* or *hemiparesis*. If both arms and legs are affected, the term is *quadriplegia* or *quadriparesis*. (The ending "plegia" means paralysis and "paresis" means weakness; while both terms are used, "paresis" is more accurate since cerebral palsy rarely leads to total paralysis.)

Spastic cerebral palsy. Spastic muscles are tense and contracted, resistant to movement. When reflexes are tested they may be very

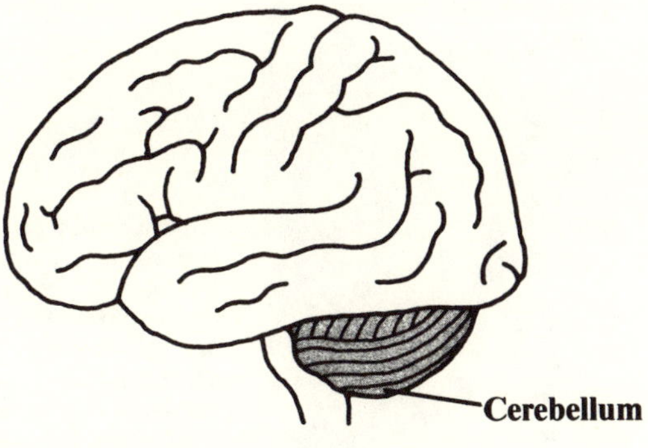

The brain grows rapidly during pregnancy. At 9 months the wrinkles of the cerebral hemispheres are already present.

brisk, resulting in repeated contractions: clonus. If a child with spastic diplegia is supported under the arms, the legs often hang straight down, unable to flex at the knees. The lower legs may turn in and cross at the ankle. The movements of the legs are stiff and resemble the crossed blades of a pair of scissors, hence the term "scissors" gait. This condition can sometimes be corrected by surgery to release tight hip muscles. Sometimes the leg muscles are so tightly contracted the child's heels do not touch the floor, so the child walks on tiptoe. Physical therapy, plaster casts, or, if necessary, orthopedic surgery to release the heel tendons can permit more normal walking.

Spasticity is the most common abnormality in cerebral palsy. Spastic diplegia is also the characteristic form of cerebral palsy seen in either premature or low birth weight infants, as revealed in the Collaborative Perinatal Project and other studies.

***Athetoid cerebral palsy*.** A second common form of cerebral palsy is characterized by involuntary writhing movements of the parts of the body affected. This incessant, slow activity is called athetosis. The hands may turn and twist and often there is facial grimacing, tonguing, and drooling. Another form of involuntary movement, sometimes occurring with athetosis, involves abrupt flailing or jerky motions of the body, described as *chorea*, from the Greek word for dance. Many cases of athetoid or choreic cerebral palsy involve damage to motor centers only. To the uninformed, however, the unnatural movements and facial expressions of such patients are often taken as signs of mental or emotional disturbance — a tragic compounding of the patient's problems.

***Ataxic cerebral palsy*.** In some cases of cerebral palsy the principal movement disturbance is a lack of balance and coordination described as ataxia. Persons with ataxic cerebral palsy may sway when

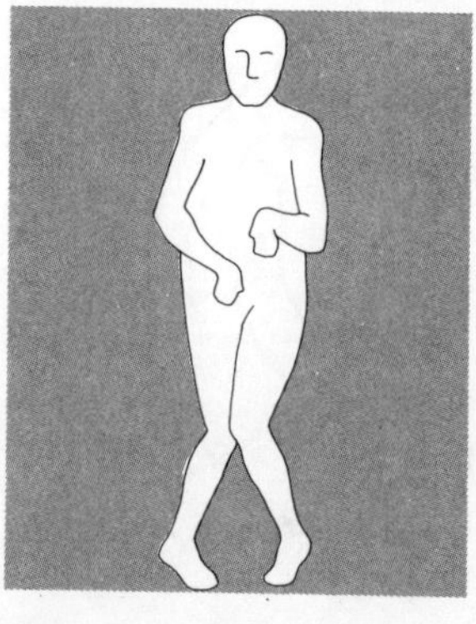

A person with spastic diplegia may stand with arms bent and legs stiff, turned in at the knees. Physical therapy, bracing, and surgery are among the ways used to correct posture and make walking more normal.

standing, have trouble maintaining balance, and may walk with feet spread wide apart to avoid falling. The motor centers involved lie in the cerebellum, a large white globe of tissue at the back of the brain tucked under the cerebral hemispheres.

Mixed cases. When several motor centers are affected, the symptoms of cerebral palsy are mixed. The doctor's lengthy description may be spastic diplegia with athetosis of the upper limbs (tense, contracted leg muscles with writhing arms); right hemiparesis with rigidity (stiff muscles in right arm and leg), diplegia with hypotonia (floppy muscles in both legs) and so on.

Other symptoms. In addition to the major limb disturbances, cerebral palsy patients sometimes have hand tremors, making fine movements difficult. They may have problems in speaking, chewing, or swallowing, maintaining visual focus, or following a moving target. There may also be drooling, a cooler surface temperature over affected parts of the body, or the loss of bowel or bladder control.

The common associated problems of convulsive seizures, mental or emotional impairments, hearing, visual, or other sensory handicaps, such as the loss of the ability to identify objects by touch, add to the difficulties faced by many cerebral palsy patients and their families. In such complex cases it is particularly important to distinguish true intellectual deficits from problems in language, learning, and attention that may be due to severe speech and sensory handicaps.

"Will my child ever walk?"

The diagnosis of cerebral palsy is always upsetting and parents are inevitably anxious and concerned over the future? Will the child ever talk? Walk? Go to college? Be able to work? In mild cases the doctor can usually be reassuring. But often there are no simple answers. Every individual with cerebral palsy presents a unique set of symptoms along with a unique capacity and potential for coping. A lot may depend on rehabilitation and education programs; a lot on the cooperation and positive but realistic attitudes of all concerned. Some physicians generalize that if a child can sit up unsupported by the end of the second year, or stand by age 3, the chances for independent walking are good. But there are always exceptions. Sometimes orthopedic surgery may be necessary. Almost always there will be a need for a coordinated treatment program provided by a team of skilled professionals. Still, not all children may respond.

Coordinated programs are available through the physical medicine or rehabilitation departments of hospitals, state crippled children's programs, and a variety of clinics or centers for the handicapped financed by public or private agencies. Both the United Cerebral Palsy Associations, Inc., and the National Easter Seal Society, Inc., have local chapters and clinics throughout the country. In addition, special programs are available to assure that no handicapped person is denied free public education.

At the same time, it is important to maintain a stable and reassuring home environment. The presence of a handicapped child is hard on all members of the family. Parents may quarrel or feel guilty, and occasionally experience such strain that the marriage is threatened. Parents are sometimes overprotective and pampering, creating serious personality and behavioral problems for the child, and leading brothers and sisters to feel denied attention and love. In a few instances parents may be rejecting or show indifference to the handicapped child. Excellent advice comes from the mother of a child with cerebral palsy: "If the parents accept the child, the child will then accept himself." Many agencies and clinics providing treatment for individuals with cerebral palsy include social workers or psychologists skilled in family counseling, or else can refer families to appropriate professionals to guide families through the initial adjustment and as problems arise.

The combined education and rehabilitation programs currently available will enable some children to progress to excellent control over their bodies and a nearly normal life. Those with more severe handicaps may be able to move from bed to wheelchair or from wheelchair to braces or other mechanical aids. Most authorities agree that progress in overcoming handicaps is harder if there are mental impairments.

Treatments old and new

Physical therapy. An integral part of rehabilitation is physical therapy, a program of exercises and activities supervised by a professional therapist. The program is designed to make the most of the individual's potential and to recruit whatever reserves the nervous system may have for learning new skills.

Some physical therapy programs popular today follow specific principles of nervous system development. The Bobath technique, for example, pioneered by a husband-wife team in England, is based on the idea that the primitive reflexes exhibited by many children with cerebral palsy are major impediments to learning voluntary control. The reflexes also give rise to abnormal sensations: the child's muscles always feel very tense or very loose. The therapist tries to break down the reflexes by deliberately positioning the child in opposing postures. If an arm had been extended it is now flexed, and so on.

Gradually, some children are able to maintain the new "reflex inhibiting postures" and begin to experience more normal muscle tone. As therapy proceeds, the child gradually is able to extend his repertoire of voluntary movements. Some therapists report that the combination of relaxation and success achieved with limb muscles helps the child with speech problems, enabling real progress in learning how to talk.

Other innovations in physical therapy make use of the psychological principles of behavior modification in which the individual is rewarded ("positively reinforced") for certain behavior. Thus, a child who habitually turns his head to one side in a primitive neck reflex may learn to turn it to the opposite side if rewarded by the sight of a toy, the sound of a music box, or other pleasant surprises.

Many therapists stress the importance of providing a varied and stimulating environment for the physically handicapped child. This constitutes "treatment" that can be as valuable as more formal therapies. Children normally learn by active exploration of their world — think of the toddler crawling to reach a block or ball, or turning to listen to his mother and look at her face. All the more reason to make sure that the child who is limited in exploration is not additionally deprived of the richness of sights, sounds, and other pleasurable experiences of life.

Biofeedback. One of the latest methods of treatment of cerebral palsy combines behavior modification with the techniques of biofeedback. In biofeedback, an individual is supplied with information — usually in the form of vivid visual or auditory signals — about the functioning of a particular part of the body. Heart rate, for example, may be translated into a musical tone which rises and falls according to whether heart rate goes up or down. The individual is told to alter the rate — usually lower it — by concentrating on making the musical tone fall. Surprisingly, many people are able to do this, how they do it is not clear.

Now, investigators whose research is supported by NINCDS have been able to train some youngsters with cerebral palsy to lower the tension of their muscles by lowering the pitch of muscle "sounds." The sounds correspond to the electrical activity generated whenever muscles contract; the greater the tension, the higher the voltage (and the musical pitch). Concentrating on one muscle at a time, and rewarding each little step in the right direction, scientists at Johns Hopkins Hospital in Baltimore have trained children to drink from a cup and to control their bowels and bladder. One 7-year-old boy with severe athetoid cerebral palsy was able to keep his arm muscles relaxed for some time even after the training sessions were over. In some cases the investigators have observed a transfer phenomenon:

a child trained to relax one group of muscles is able to lower the tension in other groups.

Similar studies of the use of biofeedback to control spastic muscles are being supported by NINCDS at Emory University in Atlanta, Ga. Further research is needed to explore what nervous system activities are involved, specify which patients are most likely to benefit, and evaluate long-term results.

Occupational therapy. The urge for independence is universal. Occupational therapy teaches the practical skills that enable a person to say, "I can do it myself." For handicapped children, occupational therapy means learning how to dress, comb hair, clean teeth, hold a cup or a pen or pencil. For older people, occupational therapy may mean vocational training or learning how to shop, cook, or keep house. Today there are a growing number of safe and ingeniously designed gadgets and aids to make the handicapped more self-sufficient, ranging from shoes with laces that can be tied with one hand to elaborate voice synthesizers or pint-sized portable typewriters that enable patients with speech and hearing impairments to communicate. For children, there are learning toys like illuminated pens to facilitate eye-hand coordination. A number of these devices are the by-products of engineering research supported by the United Cerebral Palsy Associations and other groups.

In discussing cerebral palsy the focus is so often on children that it is easy to forget that children with cerebral palsy grow up to be adults with cerebral palsy. Some are bright college students who may go on to professional careers; others may learn skilled or semiskilled jobs and be financially independent; for still others, the handicaps are so extensive, so unresponsive to treatment — or the condition so neglected — that they face life in an institution.

Rehabilitation may still be possible, however, as was recently demonstrated in a group of patients long confined to state mental institutions or homes for the retarded. The patients were established in a cerebral palsy clinic, weaned off all medication, and provided with therapists who worked with individuals on a nearly one-to-one basis. Within a year or two of the start of the program some patients were able to find jobs and live in halfway houses; others were developing new social and practical skills and working in a sheltered workshop.

Drugs. Certain drugs are important in the treatment of cerebral palsy. If epilepsy is a complication, for example, anticonvulsant drugs are usually prescribed and are very effective in preventing seizures in many patients. Diazepam (Valium®) and other muscle-relaxant drugs can sometimes help to relieve the tension of spastic muscles. Other nervous system drugs may also enable a child who is restless, easily distracted, or has other behavior problems to relax and concentrate in school. However, the chronic use of any drugs in children must be watched carefully. There may be unwanted side effects, and the long-term effects on the developing nervous system are largely unknown.

Surgery. Over the years there have been attempts to modify the symptoms of cerebral palsy through surgery to destroy the brain sites assumed to be responsible for involuntary movements. More recently, surgery has been performed to implant electrodes in the brain. The electrodes can be activated by a transmitter to stimulate nerves important in motor coordination and control. These techniques are

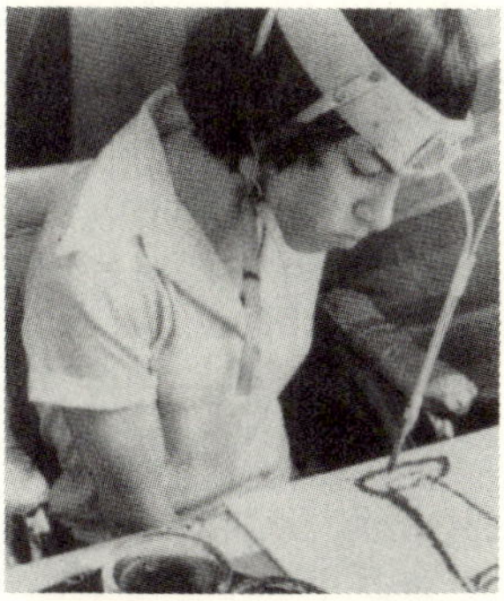

Occupational therapy for cerebral palsy patients can mean learning to paint with a head stick equipped with a brush.

The foot pedal arrangement allows this man with cerebral palsy to be fully employed as a drill press operator.

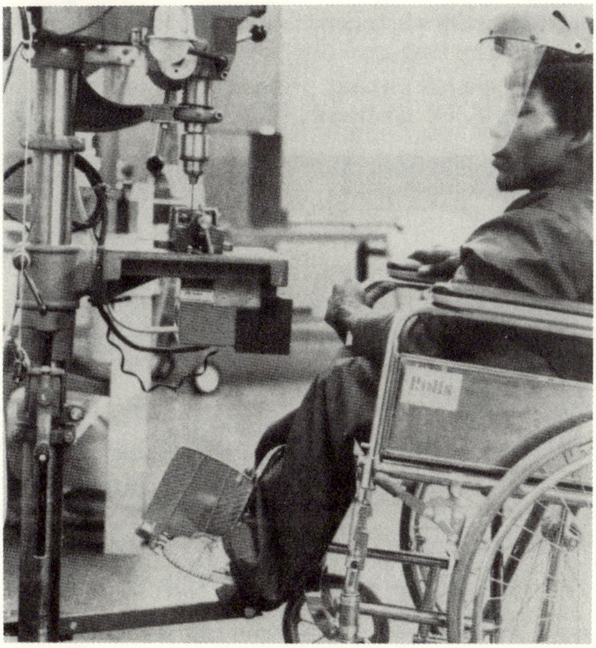

experimental and very controversial; they involve some risk to the patient, and the results have been mixed: some patients report improvements, others none at all.

Electrical stimulation. An alternative technique that involves far less risk to the patient than implanting electrodes in the brain is the use of electrical stimulating devices applied locally to nerves in affected limbs. NINCDS is currently encouraging research on the development of such devices to control spasticity.

There have been no carefully controlled studies to determine if any one treatment or combination of treatments for cerebral palsy is superior to any other. Such studies require the careful matching of patient groups by age, symptoms, and so on — a requirement difficult to achieve in a disorder as varied and complex in symptoms as cerebral palsy. The studies might also entail withholding treatment from one group of patients, which would be undesirable. In addition, there have been no objective measurements or scales of motor performance in cerebral palsy patients which could be used to assess progress or change. To address that need, NINCDS is currently supporting research at Rush-Presbyterian-St. Luke's Medical Center in Chicago, where an investigator is developing standard measures of spasticity in patients with cerebral palsy and other forms of brain damage.

Working toward prevention

Much of the research on cerebral palsy supported by NINCDS and other federal agencies, such as the National Institute of Child Health and Human Development, the National Heart, Lung, and Blood Institute, and the National Institute of Allergy and Infectious Diseases, as well as by private voluntary agencies, is aimed at eliminating known risks and threats:

Breathing and circulation problems. The Collaborative Perinatal Project confirmed the greater risk for cerebral palsy — especially spastic diplegia — associated with premature and low birth weight infants. The risk in relation to weight was highest for babies weighing under 3.3 pounds at birth (no matter how many weeks of gestation). Very immature babies often have serious breathing and circulatory problems which constitute a threat to the brain. Current research is focusing on lung development in prematurely delivered experimental animals, with emphasis on finding ways to prevent or treat respiratory disease.

Other investigators are studying the flow of blood through the immature brain. Brain hemorrhage — especially bleeding into the fluid-filled spaces of the brain (the ventricles) — is a major cause of death or neurological handicap in low birth weight infants. But little is understood of how such intraventricular hemorrhage occurs. Possibly breathing problems lead to an oxygen shortage (hypoxia), which causes changes in blood pressure and acidity, along with other metabolic alterations. In turn, these changes may cause the very tiny blood vessels in the infant's brain to distend and rupture. Fortunately, better and safer means of measuring blood gases and careful monitoring of the brain using ultrasound or CT scanning are helping to identify the problem and evaluate complicating factors.

The NINCDS is currently supporting research at Pennsylvania State University to study the effects of hypoxia on the brains of fetal, newborn, and adult rats. In particular, the researchers are concerned with how oxygen deprivation affects the ability of nerve cells to transmit impulses from one to another.

At NINCDS, scientists have found that a partial cutoff of oxygen may cause the immature brain to swell. This sets up a vicious cycle in which the swelling compresses brain blood vessels, further limiting oxygen to brain cells, and ultimately leading to their death. Armed with this knowledge, neonatal specialists are developing better methods of monitoring circulation to prevent brain swelling; they are also developing treatments for brain swelling, should it occur.

Low birth weight. There is also growing interest in the problem of low birth weight itself. In spite of improvements in maternal care, the number of babies born weighing under 5.5 pounds has remained stable in America at about 7½ percent of all births each year. Poor nutrition, illness, accidents, and psychological stress during pregnancy are contributing factors, certainly, and some women may also be genetically predisposed to premature labor and delivery. Scientists currently investigating the problem are particularly interested in the hormonal and other chemical changes that occur in pregnancy. In research supported by the United Cerebral Palsy Research and Education Foundation, for example, investigators are studying the role of relaxin, a hormone produced in pregnancy which may prevent premature contractions of the uterus as well as prepare the cervix for birth.

Seizures. Collaborative Perinatal Project data showed that convulsive seizures in the first months of life were serious events associated with a relatively high rate of death. Seizures in the newborn — not always obvious because they may not look like seizures in older infants — were also found to be a major marker for subsequent neurological problems, including cerebral palsy. In every case, the examining physician will try to determine the underlying cause of the seizures, such as infection, hemorrhage, or oxygen shortage, and correct it if possible. Control of the seizures themselves may be important because very lengthy or repeated seizures in early life may, in themselves, cause damage to the developing brain.

Infections. While vaccines to prevent German measles have greatly reduced the hazard to the fetus from this infection, not all women have been immunized. An estimated 15-20 percent of women now entering childbearing age are at risk for German measles. These women, who were already in school in the late 1960s when immunization programs were begun for preschoolers, have not acquired natural immunity because there have been no epidemics in their lifetimes. It is important that all women know their immunological status and are vaccinated *before* becoming pregnant.

Several major infectious diseases for which there are no vaccines and no treatments remain serious threats to the fetus or newborn. Again, the nervous system is particularly vulnerable to these infectious agents, which, while not as well known as the rubella virus, are no less destructive.

Toxoplasmosis, a disease caused by a parasite that infects cats, other domestic animals, and food sources, produces few or no symptoms in most adults but may be highly damaging to the fetus. Infection is common in adults and increases with age: between one-third and one-half of women of childbearing age have been infected. The danger to the fetus occurs if a woman acquires toxoplasmosis while pregnant.

Also highly prevalent is cytomegalovirus, estimated to infect 3 percent of all pregnant women. The virus causes few or no symptoms in a woman, although it infects a variety of body organs, including the cervix. It is estimated that 1 out of every 100 infants born in the United States is infected with cytomegalovirus, while half of those infants exposed prenatally but not infected at birth will become infected through breast milk or handling in the first months of life. Some babies will be severely damaged and may die. Between 5 and 10 percent of those remaining will later show signs of hearing loss, especially for high tones, and have I.Q.s less than 80. Research under way at NINCDS laboratories in Bethesda, Md., and elsewhere is aimed at developing an animal model for the human disease, a key step in evaluating vaccines and effective treatments.

Cytomegalovirus is one of the viruses of the herpes group. These agents include the virus that causes cold sores, and, of more consequence to the newborn, the type II herpes virus which infects the genital tract and is usually transmitted sexually. The infection is particularly painful in women, and often recurs after initial infection. The virus lies dormant in the nervous system, but periodically may descend to the genital tract to cause an acute attack. Babies can acquire infection during passage through the birth canal. Physicians attempt to prevent this infection by recognizing the disease in the mothers and delivering the child by cesarean section to avoid exposure to the virus. Investigators at NINCDS are working on new methods for the rapid viral diagnosis of genital herpes to aid physicians in selecting patients for cesarean section. As with the cytomegalovirus, research is also directed toward developing safe and effective vaccines, as well as treatment for those already infected.

A "cure" for cerebral palsy?

While research goes on to eliminate known risks and find more effective treatments for cerebral palsy, the disorder has also inspired research on the most basic questions of nervous system operation: How does the nervous system develop? Is it true that the nervous system cannot recover from major damage? Why are the motor systems so often vulnerable in pregnancy? Why should spastic diplegia be the prevalent form of cerebral palsey.

Years ago, scientists lacked the tools and techniques to tackle these questions and were generally pessimistic about the potential of the nervous system for healing itself once damaged. Nowadays, not only are they more hopeful, they have also developed extraordinarily powerful methods for studying the nervous system. The result is a far more detailed picture of nerve cell behavior. Scientists know, for example, that when nerve cells fire off nerve impulses — tiny bursts of electrical energy — to neighboring cells, a minute amount of a chemical — a neurotransmitter — is usually released. That transmitter allows the nerve impulse to cross the gap between cells. Scientists know, too, that certain chemicals called growth factors are important in the development of nerve cells, guiding nerve fibers to their proper connections in the system, and playing a role in nervous system maintenance and repair.

This kind of information is leading some researchers interested in cerebral palsy to examine the chemicals involved in muscle movements. For example, one researcher at the University of Michigan is studying the neurotransmitters used by small nerve cells in the spinal cord of rats. The rat develops spasticity after its spinal cord is severed, and the investigator is studying the chemical changes that then occur in nerve cells below the level of injury. Other researchers are studying the effects of drugs on motor centers of the brain. Certain drugs injected into the brains of pregnant rabbits are able to cross the placenta and damage motor centers in the fetal brain, producing a movement disorder similar to cerebral palsy. Such neurochemical research might some day lead to new drug treatments for cerebral palsy in which the drug would restore the balance of neurotransmitters needed for normal muscle coordination and control.

A window on the living brain

Equally exciting in terms of research potential is the recent advance in brain scanning techniques: positron emission transverse tomography (PETT). Development of PETT's potential is now being supported by NINCDS at over half a dozen universities throughout the United States. When a patient or an experimental animal is supplied with a radioactive form of a natural nutrient used by the brain (like sugar) bursts of energy are generated and recorded by the equipment. The cells that are most active in taking up the radioactive substance will show the greatest concentrations of energy on the PETT scan. Thus, investigators can actually observe the living brain in action. They can note exactly which parts of the brain are working when you plan and execute a muscle movement, for example, or do a problem in mental arithmetic. With such a dynamic window into the brain, scientists can determine more precisely what goes wrong in the brain of a child with cerebral palsy — and, ultimately, find out what can be done to make things go right.

National voluntary agencies

Two national voluntary agencies support research and provide services to patients. For information about their programs, and listings of their local chapters and clinics, write to:

United Cerebral Palsy Associations, Inc.
66 East 34th Street
New York, N. Y. 10016
(212)481-6300

The National Easter Seal Society, Inc.
2023 West Ogden Avenue
Chicago, Ill. 60612
(312)243-8400

Tissue Banks

The study of brain and other tissue from persons with neurological disorders is invaluable to research, especially in disorders like cerebral palsy where the causes and associated changes in the brain are complex. NINCDS supports two national human specimen banks, one in Los Angeles, Calif., and one near Boston, Mass. For information about tissue donation collection write:

Dr. Wallace W. Tourtellotte, Director
Human Neurospecimen Bank
VA Wadsworth Hospital Center
Los Angeles, Calif. 90073

Dr. Edward D. Bird, Director
Brain Tissue Bank
Mailman Research Center
McLean Hospital
Belmont, Mass. 02178

Chapter 7

Chronic Pain

Chronic Pain

What was the worst pain you can remember? Was it the time you scratched the cornea of your eye? Was it a kidney stone? Childbirth? Rare is the person who has not experienced some beyond-belief episode of pain and misery. Mercifully, relief finally came. Your eye healed, the stone was passed, the baby born. In each of those cases, pain flared up in response to a known cause. With treatment, or with the body's healing powers alone, you got better and the pain went away. Doctors call that kind of pain *acute* pain. It is a normal sensation triggered in the nervous system to alert you to possible injury and the need to take care of yourself.

Chronic pain is different. Chronic pain persists. Fiendishly, uselessly, pain signals keep firing in the nervous system for weeks, months, even years. There may have been an initial mishap — a sprained back, a serious infection — from which you've long since recovered. There may be an ongoing cause of pain — arthritis, cancer, ear infection. But some people suffer chronic pain in the absence of any past injury or evidence of body damage. Whatever the matter may be, chronic pain is real, unremitting, and demoralizing — the kind of pain New England poet Emily Dickinson had in mind when she wrote:

Pain — has an Element of Blank —
It cannot recollect
When it begun — or if there were
A time when it was not

The terrible triad

Pain of such proportions overwhelms all other symptoms and becomes *the* problem. People so afflicted often cannot work. Their appetite falls off. Physical activity of any kind is exhausting and may aggravate the pain. Soon the person becomes the victim of a vicious circle in which total preoccupation with pain leads to irritability and depression. The sufferer can't sleep at night and the next day's weariness compounds the problem — leading to more irritability, depression, and pain. Specialists call that unhappy state the "terrible triad" of suffering, sleeplessness, and sadness, a calamity that is as hard on the family as it is on the victim. The urge to do something

— anything — to stop the pain makes some patients drug dependent, drives others to undergo repeated operations, or worse, resort to questionable practitioners who promise quick and permanent "cures."

"Chronic pain is the most costly health problem in America," says one of the world's authorities on pain. He and others estimate annual costs, including direct medical expenses, lost income, lost productivity, compensation payments and legal charges, at close to $50 billion. Here's how that adds up:

- *Headache*. At least 40 million Americans suffer chronic recurrent headaches and spend $4 billion a year on medications. Migraine sufferers alone account for 65 million workdays lost annually.
- *Low back pain*. Fifteen percent of the adult U.S. population have had persistent low back pain at some time in their lives. Five million Americans are partially disabled by back problems, and another 2 million are so severely disabled they cannot work. Low back pain accounts for 93 million workdays lost every year and costs over $5 billion in health care.
- *Cancer pain*. The majority of patients in intermediate or advanced stages of cancer suffer moderate to severe pain. More than 800,000 new cases of cancer are diagnosed each year in the U.S., and some 430,000 people die.
- *Arthritis pain*. The great crippler affects 20 million Americans and costs over $4 billion in lost income, productivity and health care.

Other pain disorders like the neuralgias and neuropathies that affect nerves throughout the body, pain due to damage to the central nervous system (the brain and spinal cord), as well as pain where no physical cause can be found — psychogenic pain — swell the total to that $50 billion figure.

Many chronic pain conditions affect older adults. Arthritis, cancer, angina — the chest-binding, breath-catching spasms of pain associated with coronary artery disease — commonly take their greatest toll among the middle-aged and elderly. Tic douloureux (trigeminal neuralgia) is a recurrent, stabbing facial pain that is rare among young adults. But ask any resident of housing for retired persons if there are any tic sufferers around and you are sure to hear of cases. So the fact that Americans are living longer contributes to a widespread and growing concern about pain.

Neuroscientists share that concern. At a time when people are living longer and painful conditions abound, the scientists who study the brain have made landmark discoveries that are leading to a better understanding of pain and more effective treatments.

In the forefront of pain research are scientists supported by the National Institute of Neurological and Communicative Disorders and

Stroke (NINCDS), the leading federal agency supporting research on pain. Other federal agencies important in pain research include the National Institute of Mental Health (NIMH), the National Institute of Dental Research (NIDR) and the National Cancer Institute (NCI). Within the last decade, both the International Association for the Study of Pain and the American Pain Society have been established and grown into flourishing professional organizations attracting young as well as established research investigators and practicing physicians.

Sounding the pain alarm

Part of the inspiration for the new groups has come from a deeper understanding of pain made possible by advances in research techniques. Not long ago, neuroscientists debated whether pain was a separate sense at all, supplied with its own nerve cells and brain centers like the senses of hearing or taste or touch. Maybe you hurt, the scientists reasoned, because nerve endings sensitive to touch are pressed very hard. To some extent, that is true: Some nerve fibers in your skin will be stimulated by a painful pinch as well as a gentle touch. But neuroscientists now know that there are many small nerve cells with extremely fine nerve fibers that are excited exclusively by intense, potentially harmful stimulation. Scientists call the nerve cells *nociceptors*, from the word noxious, meaning physically harmful or destructive.

Some nociceptors sound off to several kinds of painful stimulation — a hammer blow that hits your thumb instead of a nail; a drop of acid; a flaming match. Other nociceptors are more selective. They are excited by a pinprick but ignore painful heat or chemical stimulation. It's as though nature had sprinkled your skin and your insides with a variety of pain-sensitive cells, not only to report what kind of damage you're experiencing, but to make sure the message gets through on at least one channel.

Broadcasting the news

That same dispersion of forces continues once pain messages reach the central nervous system. Suppose you touch a hot stove. Some incoming pain signals are immediately routed to nerve cells that signal muscles to contract, so you pull your hand back. That streamlined pathway is a reflex, one of many protective circuits wired into your nervous system at birth.

Meanwhile, the message informing you that you've touched the stove travels along other pathways to higher centers in the brain. One path is an express route that reports the facts: where it hurts; how bad it is; whether the pain is sharp or burning. Other pain pathways plod along more slowly, the nerve fibers branching to make connections with many nerve cells (neurons) en route. Scientists think that these more meandering pathways act as warning systems alerting you of impending damage and in other ways filling out the pain picture. All the pathways combined contribute to the emotional impact of pain — whether you feel frightened, anxious, angry, annoyed. Experts called those feelings the "suffering" component of pain.

Still other branches of the pain news network are alerting another major division of the nervous system, the *autonomic nervous system*. That division handles the body's vital functions like breathing, blood flow, pulse rate, digestion, elimination. Pain can sound a general alarm in that system, causing you to sweat or stop digesting your food, increasing your pulse rate and blood pressure, dilating the pupils of your eye, and signaling the release of hormones like epinephrine (adrenaline). Epinephrine aids and abets all those responses as well as triggering the release of sugar stored in the liver to provide an extra boost of energy in an emergency.

Censoring the news

Obviously, not every source of pain creates a full-blown emergency with adrenaline-surging, sweat-pouring, pulse-racing responses. Moreover, observers are well aware of times and places when excruciating pain is ignored. Think of the quarterback's ability to finish a game oblivious of a torn ligament, or a fakir sitting on a bed of

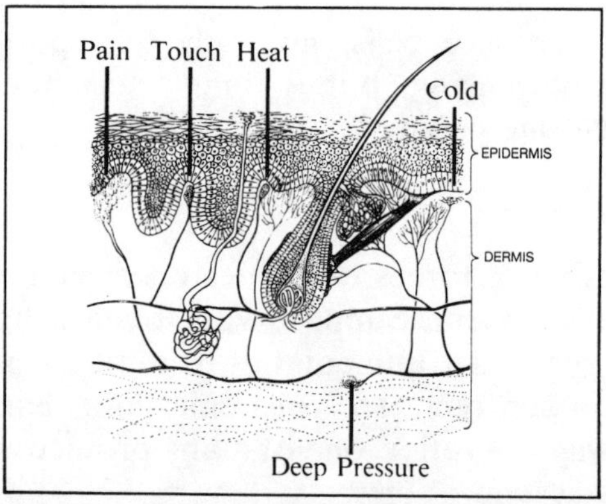

Your skin is supplied with a variety of nerve endings sensitive to touch, pressure, heat, cold—and pain. The pain fibers are extremely fine in diameter, branching to form bare nerve endings.

spikes. One of the foremost pioneers in pain research adds his personal tale, too, of the time he landed a salmon after a long and hearty struggle, only then to discover the deep blood-dripping gash on his leg.

Acknowledging such events, neuroscientists have long suspected that there are built-in nervous system mechanisms that can block pain messages.

Now it seems that just as there is more than one way to spread the news of pain, there is more than one way to censor the news. These control systems involve pathways that come down from the brain to prevent pain signals from getting through.

The gate theory of pain

Interestingly, a pair of Canadian and English investigators speculated that such pain-suppressing pathways must exist when they devised a new "gate theory of pain" in the mid-sixties. Their idea was that when pain signals first reach the nervous system they excite activity in a group of small neurons that form a kind of pain "pool." When the total activity of these neurons reaches a certain minimal level, a hypothetical "gate" opens up that allows the pain signals to be sent to higher brain centers. But nearby neurons in contact with the pain cells can suppress activity in the pain pool so that the gate stays closed. The gate-closing cells include large neurons that are stimulated by nonpainful touching or pressing of your skin. The gate could also be closed from above, by brain cells activating a descending pathway to block pain.

The theory explained such everyday behavior as scratching a scab, or rubbing a sprained ankle: the scratching and rubbing excite just those nerve cells sensitive to touch and pressure that can suppress the pain pool cells. The scientists conjectured that brain-based pain control systems were activated when people behaved heroically — ignoring pain to finish a football game, or to help a more severely wounded soldier on the battlefield.

The gate theory aroused both interest and controversy when it was first announced. Most importantly, it stimulated research to find the conjectured pathways and mechanisms. Pain studies got an added boost when investigators made the surprising discovery that the brain itself produces chemicals that can control pain.

The landmark discovery of the pain-suppressing chemicals came about because scientists in Aberdeen, Scotland, and at the Johns Hopkins University Hospital in Baltimore were curious about how morphine and other opium-derived painkillers, or analgesics, work.

For some time, neuroscientists had known that chemicals were important in conducting nerve signals (small bursts of electric current) from cell to cell. In order for the signal from one cell to reach the next in line, the first cell secretes a chemical "neurotransmitter" from the tip of a long fiber that extends from the cell body. The transmitter molecules cross the gap separating the two cells and attach to special receptor sites on the neighboring cell surface. Some neurotransmitters *excite* the second cell — allowing it to generate an electrical signal. Others *inhibit* the second cell — preventing it from generating a signal.

When investigators in Scotland and at Johns Hopkins injected morphine into experimental animals, they found that the morphine molecules fitted snugly into receptors on certain brain and spinal cord neurons. Why, the scientists wondered, should the human brain — the product of millions of years of evolution — come equipped with receptors for a man-made drug? Perhaps there were naturally occurring brain chemicals that behaved exactly like morphine.

The brain's own opiates

Both groups of scientists found not just one pain-suppressing chemical in the brain, but a whole family of such proteins. The Aberdeen investigators called the smaller members of the family *enkephalins* (meaning "in the head"). In time, the larger proteins were isolated and called *endorphins*, meaning the "morphine within." The term *endorphins* is now often used to describe the group as a whole.

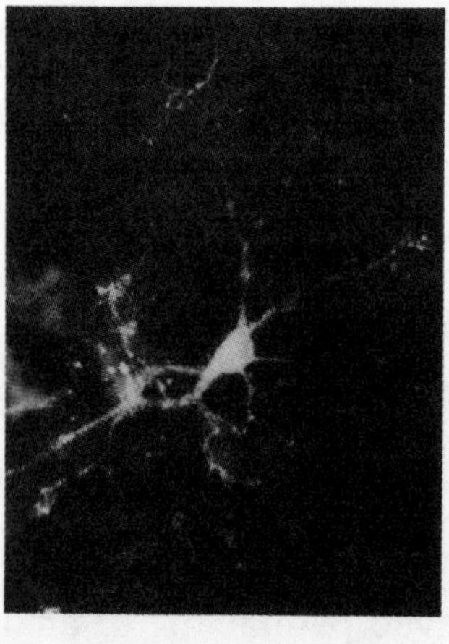

Enkephalin fills the cell body and branches of this mouse spinal cord nerve cell grown in tissue culture by an NINCDS scientist. The mouse cells are stained with a fluorescent dye that reacts with enkephalin.

The discovery of the endorphins lent weight to the general concept of the gate theory. Endorphins released from brain nerve cells might inhibit spinal cord pain cells through pathways descending from the brain to the spinal cord. Endorphins might also be activated when you rub or scratch your itching skin or aching joints. Laboratory experiments subsequently confirmed that painful stimulation led to the release of endorphins from nerve cells. Some of these chemicals then turned up in cerebrospinal fluid, the liquid that circulates in the spinal cord and brain. Laced with endorphins, the fluid could bring a soothing balm to quiet nerve cells.

A new look at pain treatments

Further evidence that endorphins figure importantly in pain control comes from a new look at some of the oldest and newest pain treatments. The new look frequently involves the use of a drug that prevents endorphins and morphine from working. Injections of this drug, naloxone, can result in a return of pain which had been relieved by morphine and certain other treatments. But, interestingly, some pain treatments are not affected by naloxone: Their success in controlling pain apparently does not depend on endorphins. Thus nature has provided us with more than one means of achieving pain relief.

• *Acupuncture.* Probably no therapy for pain has stirred more controversy in recent years than acupuncture, the 2,000-year-old Chinese technique of inserting fine needles under the skin at selected points in the body. The needles are agitated by the practitioner to produce pain relief which some individuals report lasts for hours, or even days. Does acupuncture really work? Opinion is divided. Many specialists agree that patients report benefit when the needles are placed near where it hurts, not at the body points indicated on traditional Chinese acupuncture charts. The case for acupuncture has been made by investigators who argue that local needling of the skin excites endorphin systems of pain control. Wiring the needles to stimulate nerve endings electrically (electroacupuncture) also activates endorphin systems, they believe. Further, some experiments have shown that there are higher levels of endorphins in cerebrospinal fluid following acupuncture.

Those same investigators note that naloxone injections can block pain relief produced by acupuncture. Others have not been able to repeat those findings. Skeptics also cite long-term studies of chronic pain patients that showed no lasting benefit from acupuncture treatments. Current opinion is that more controlled trials are needed to define which pain conditions might be helped by acupuncture and which patients are most likely to benefit.

- ***Local electrical stimulation.*** Applying brief pulses of electricity to nerve endings under the skin, a procedure called transcutaneous electrical nerve stimulation (TENS), yields excellent pain relief in some chronic pain patients. The stimulation works best when applied to the skin near where the pain is felt and where other sensibilities like touch or pressure have not been damaged. Both the frequency and voltage of the electrical stimulation are important in obtaining pain relief.
- ***Brain stimulation.*** Another electrical method for controlling pain, especially the widespread and severe pain of advanced cancer, is through surgically implanted electrodes in the brain. The patient determines when and how much stimulation is needed by operating an external transmitter that beams electronic signals to a receiver under the skin that is connected to the electrodes. The brain sites where the electrodes are placed are areas known to be rich in opiate receptors and in endorphin-containing cells or fibers. Stimulation-produced analgesia (SPA) is a costly procedure that involves the risk of brain surgery. However, patients who have used this technique report that their pain "seems to melt away." The pain relief is also remarkably specific: The other senses remain intact, and there is no mental confusion or cloudiness as with opiate drugs. NINCDS is currently supporting research on how SPA works and is also investigating problems of tolerance: Pain may return after repeated stimulation.
- ***Placebo effects.*** For years, doctors have known that a harmless sugar pill or an injection of salt water can make many a patient feel better — even after major surgery. The placebo effect, as it has been called, has been thought to be due to suggestion, distraction, the patient's optimism that something is being done, or the desire to please the doctor (*placebo* means "I will please" in Latin).

Now experiments suggest that the placebo effect may be neurochemical, and that people who respond to a placebo for pain relief — a remarkably consistent 35 percent in any experiment using placebos — are able to tap into their brain's endorphin systems. To evaluate it, two NINCDS- and NIDR-supported investigators at the University of California at San Francisco designed an ingenious experiment. They asked adults scheduled for wisdom teeth removal to volunteer in a pain experiment. Following surgery, some patients were given morphine, some naloxone, and some a placebo. As expected, about a third of those given the placebo reported pain relief. The investigators then gave these people naloxone. All reported a return of pain.

How people who benefit from placebos gain access to pain control systems in the brain is not known. Scientists cannot even predict whether someone who responds to a placebo in one situation will respond in another. The San Francisco investigators suspect that stress may be a factor. Patients who are very anxious or under stress are more likely to react to a placebo for pain than those who are more calm, cool, and collected. But dental surgery itself may be sufficiently stressful to trigger the release of endorphins — with or without the effects of placebo. For that reason, many specialists believe further studies are indicated to analyze the placebo effect.

As research continues to reveal the role of endorphins in the brain, neuroscientists have been able to draw more detailed brain

X-ray showing implanted electrodes for stimulating the cells that produce pain relievers. The patient controls the stimulation by operating an external transmitter.

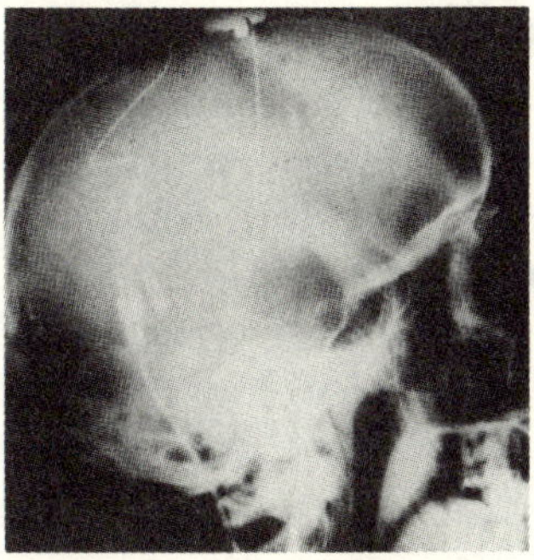

Electrostimulator used by patient with chronic pain. The small electrical impulses stimulate the brain to produce naturally occurring pain-relieving substances.

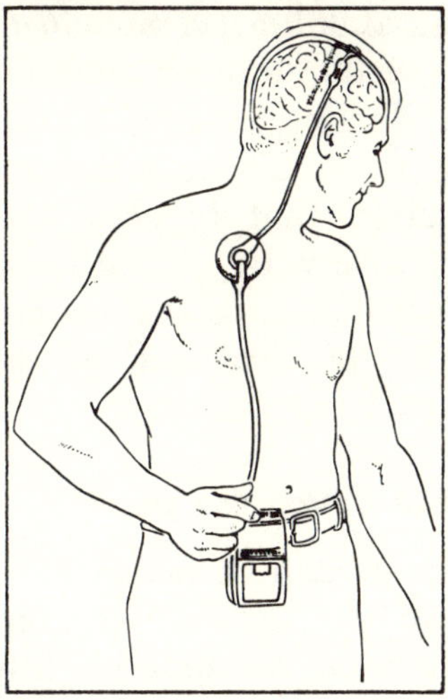

maps of the areas and pathways important in pain perception and control. They have even found new members of the endorphin family: Dynorphin, the newest endorphin, is reported to be 10 times more potent a painkiller than morphine.

At the same time, clinical investigators have tested chronic pain patients and found that they often have lower-than-normal levels of endorphins in their spinal fluid. If you could just boost their stores with manmade endorphins, perhaps the problems of chronic pain patients could be solved.

Not so easy. Some endorphins are quickly broken down after release from nerve cells. Other endorphins are longer lasting, but there are problems in manufacturing the compounds in quantity and getting them into the right places in the brain or spinal cord. In a few promising studies, clinical investigators have injected an endorphin called beta-endorphin under the membranes surrounding the spinal cord. Patients reported excellent pain relief lasting for many hours. Morphine compounds injected in the same area are similarly effective in producing long-lasting pain relief.

But spinal cord injections or other techniques designed to raise the level of endorphins circulating in the brain require surgery and hospitalization. And even if less drastic means of getting endorphins into the nervous system could be found, they are probably not the ideal answer to chronic pain. Endorphins are also involved in other nervous system activities such as controlling blood flow. Increasing the amount of endorphins might have undesirable effects on these other body activities. Endorphins also appear to share with morphine a potential for addiction or tolerance.

Meanwhile, chemists are synthesizing new analgesics and discovering painkilling virtues in drugs not normally prescribed for pain. Much of the drug research is aimed at developing nonnarcotic painkillers. The motivation for the research is not only to avoid introducing potentially addictive drugs on the market, but is based on the observation that narcotic drugs are simply not effective in treating a variety of chronic pain conditions. Developments in nondrug treatments are also progressing, ranging from new surgical techniques to physical and psychological therapies like exercise, hypnosis, and biofeedback.

New and old drugs for pain

When you complain of headache or low back pain and the doctor says take two aspirins every 4 hours and stay in bed, you may think your pain is being dismissed lightly. Not at all. Aspirin, one of the most universally used medications is an excellent painkiller. Scientists still cannot explain all the ways aspirin works, but they do know that it interferes with pain signals where they usually originate, at the nociceptive nerve endings outside the brain and spinal cord: peripheral nerves. Aspirin also inhibits the production of chemicals manufactured in the blood to promote blood clotting and wound healing: prostaglandins. Unfortunately, prostaglandins, released from cells at the site of injury, are pain-*causing* substances. They actually sensitize nerve endings, making them — and you — feel more pain. Along with increasing the blood supply to the area, the chemicals contribute to inflammation — the pain, heat, redness and swelling of tissue damage.

Some investigators now think that the continued release of pain-causing substances in chronic pain conditions may lead to long-term nervous system changes in some patients that make them hypersensitive to pain. People suffering such *hyperalgesia* can cry out in pain at the gentlest touch, or even when a soft breeze blows over the affected area. In addition to the prostaglandins, blister fluid and certain insect and snake venoms also contain pain-causing substances. Presumably these chemicals alert you to the need for care — a fine reaction in an emergency, but not in chronic pain.

There are several prescription drugs that usually can provide stronger pain relief than aspirin. These include a newly approved nonopiate drug, zomepirac (Zomax®)* as well as the opiate-related compounds codeine, propoxyphene (Darvon®), morphine, and meperidine (Demerol®). All these drugs have some potential for abuse, and may have unpleasant and even harmful side effects. In combination with other medications or alcohol, some can be dangerous. Used wisely, however, they are important recruits in the chemical fight against pain.

In the search for effective analgesics, physicians have discovered pain-relieving benefits from drugs not normally prescribed for pain. Certain antidepressants as well as antiepileptic drugs are used to treat several particularly severe pain conditions, notably the pain of shingles and of facial neuralgias like tic douloureux.

---

* The prescription drug Zomax has been temporarily withdrawn from the market by its manufacturer, McNeil Pharmaceutical. The drug's withdrawal was prompted by reports of allergic reactions — some quite severe — and several deaths.
The Food and Drug Administration and McNeil Pharmaceutical are developing new prescription guidelines for Zomax that will impose tighter restrictions on the use of the drug.

Interestingly, pain patients who benefit from antidepressants report pain relief before any uplift in mood. Pain specialists think that the antidepressant works because it increases the supply of a naturally produced neurotransmitter, serotonin. (Doctors have long associated decreased amounts of serotonin with severe depression.) But now scientists have evidence that cells using serotonin are also an integral part of a pain-controlling pathway that starts with endorphin-rich nerve cells high up in the brain and ends with inhibition of pain-conducting nerve cells lower in the brain or spinal cord. Antidepressant drugs have been used successfully in treating the excruciating pain that can follow an attack of shingles.

Antiepileptic drugs have been used successfully in treating tic douloureux, the riveting attacks of facial pain that affect older adults. The rationale for the use of the antiepileptic drugs (principally carbamazepine — Tegretol®) does not involve the endorphin system. It is based on the theory that a healthy nervous system depends on a proper balance of incoming and outgoing nerve signals. Tic and other facial pains or neuralgias are thought to result from damage to facial nerves. That means that the normal flow of messages to and from the brain is disturbed. The nervous system may react by becoming hypersensitive: It may create its own powerful discharge of nerve signals, as though screaming to the outside world "Why aren't you contacting me?" Antiepileptic drugs — used to quiet the excessive brain discharges associated with epileptic seizures — quiet the distress signals associated with tic and may relieve pain that way.

Psychological methods

Psychological treatment for pain can range from psychoanalysis and other forms of psychotherapy to relaxation training, meditation, hypnosis, biofeedback, or behavior modification. The philosophy common to all these varied approaches is the belief that patients can do something on their own to control their pain. That something may mean changing attitudes, feelings, or behaviors associated with pain, or understanding how unconscious forces and past events have contributed to the present painful predicament.

- *Psychotherapy*. Freud was celebrated for demonstrating that, for some individuals, physical pain symbolizes real or imagined emotional hurts. He also noted that some individuals develop pain or paralysis as a form of self-punishment for what they consider to be past sins or bad behavior. Sometimes, too, pain may be a way of punishing others. This doesn't mean that the pain is any less real; it does mean that some pain patients may benefit from psychoanalysis or individual or group psychotherapy to gain insights into the meaning of their pain.

• ***Relaxation and meditation therapies.*** These forms of training enable people to relax tense muscles, reduce anxiety, and alter mental state. Both physical and mental tension can make any pain worse, and in conditions such as headache or back pain, tension may be at the root of the problem. Meditation, which aims at producing a state of relaxed but alert awareness, is sometimes combined with therapies that encourage people to think of pain as something remote and apart from them. The methods promote a sense of detachment so that the patient thinks of the pain as confined to a particular body part over which he or she has marvelous control. The approach may be particularly helpful when pain is associated with fear and dread, as in cancer.

• ***Hypnosis.*** No longer considered magic, hypnosis is a technique in which an individual's susceptibility to suggestion is heightened. Normal volunteers who prove to be excellent subjects for hypnosis often report a marked reduction or obliteration of experimentally induced pain, such as that produced by a mild electric shock. The hypnotic state does not lower the volunteer's heart rate, respiration, or other autonomic responses. These physical reactions show the expected increases normally associated with painful stimulation.

The role of hypnosis in treating chronic pain patients is uncertain. Some studies have shown that 15 to 20 percent of hypnotizable patients with moderate to severe pain can achieve total relief with hypnosis. Other studies report that hypnosis reduces anxiety and depression. By lowering the burden of emotional suffering, pain may become more bearable.

• ***Biofeedback.*** Some individuals can learn voluntary control over certain body activities if they are provided with information about how the system is working — how fast their heart is beating, how tense are their head or neck muscles, how cold are their hands. The information is usually supplied through visual or auditory cues that code the body activity in some obvious way — a louder sound meaning an increase in muscle tension, for example. How people use this "biofeedback" to learn control is not understood, but some masters of the art report that imagery helps: They may think of a warm tropical beach, for example, when they want to raise the temperature of their hands. Biofeedback may be a logical approach in pain conditions that involve tense muscles, like tension headache or low back pain. But results are mixed.

• ***Behavior modification.*** This psychological technique (sometimes called operant conditioning) is aimed at changing habits, behaviors, and attitudes that can develop in chronic pain patients. Some patients become dependent, anxious, and homebound — if not bedridden. For some, too, chronic pain may be a welcome friend, relieving them of the boredom of a dull job or the burden of family responsibilities. These psychological rewards — sometimes combined with financial gains from compensation payments or insurance — work against improvements in the patient's condition, and can encourage increased drug dependency, repeated surgery, and multiple doctor and clinic visits.

There is no question that the patient feels pain. The hope of behavior modification is that pain relief can be obtained from a program aimed at changing the individual's lifestyle. The program begins with a complete assessment of the painful condition and a thorough explanation of how the program works. It is essential to enlist the full cooperation of both the patient and family members. The treatment is aimed at reducing pain medication and increasing mobility and independence through a graduated program of exercise, diet, and other activities. The patient is rewarded for positive efforts with praise and attention. Rewards are withheld when the patient retreats into negative attitudes or demanding and dependent behavior.

How effective are any of these psychological treatments? Are some superior to others? Who is most likely to benefit? Do the benefits last? The answers are not yet in hand. Patient selection and patient cooperation are all-important. Analysis of individuals who have improved dramatically with one or another of these approaches is helping to pinpoint what factors are likely to lead to successful treatment.

Surgery to relieve pain

Surgery is often considered the court of last resort for pain: When all else fails, cut the nerve endings. Surgery can bring about instant, almost magical release from pain. But surgery may also destroy other sensations as well, or, inadvertently, become the source of new pain. Further, relief is not necessarily permanent. After 6 months or a year, pain may return.

For all those reasons, the decision for surgery must always involve a careful weighing of the patient's condition and the outlook for the future. If surgery can mean the difference between a pain-wrecked existence ending in death, versus a pain-free time in which to compose one's life and see friends and family, then surgery is clearly a humane and compassionate choice.

There are a variety of operations to relieve pain. The most common is cordotomy: severing the nerve fibers on one or both sides of the spinal cord that travel the express routes to the brain. Cordotomy affects the sense of temperature as well as pain, since the fibers travel together in the express route.

Besides cordotomy, surgery within the brain or spinal cord to relieve pain includes severing connections at major junctions in pain pathways, such as at the places where pain fibers cross from one side of the cord to the other, or destroying parts of important relay stations in the brain like the thalamus, an egg-shaped cluster of nerve cells near the center of the brain.

In addition, surgeons sometimes can relieve pain by destroying nerve fibers or their parent cell bodies outside the brain or spinal cord. A case in point is the destruction of sympathetic nerves (a part of the autonomic nervous system) to relieve the severe pain that sometimes follows a penetrating wound from a sharp instrument or bullet.

When pain affects the upper extremities, or is widespread, the surgeon has fewer options and surgery may not be as effective. Still,

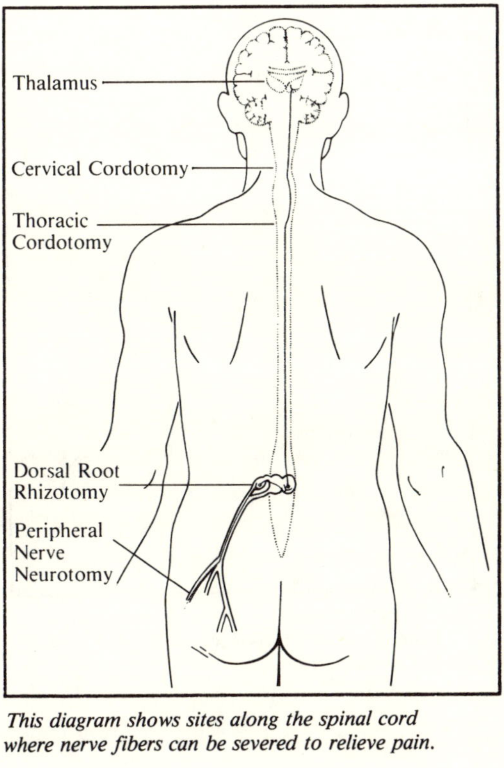

This diagram shows sites along the spinal cord where nerve fibers can be severed to relieve pain.

skilled neurosurgeons have achieved excellent results with upper spinal cord or brain surgery to treat severe intractable pain. These procedures may employ chemicals or use heat or freezing treatments to destroy tissue, as well as the more traditional use of the scalpel.

Recently, Harvard Medical School surgeons reported success with a new brain operation called cingulotomy to relieve intractable pain in patients with severe psychiatric problems. The nerve fibers destroyed are part of a pathway important in emotions and motivation. The surgery appears to eliminate the discomfort and suffering the patient feels, but does not interfere with other mental faculties such as thinking and memory.

Prior to operating, physicians can often test the effectiveness of surgery by using anesthetic drugs to block nerves temporarily. In some chronic pain conditions — like the pain from a penetrating wound — these temporary blocks can in themselves be beneficial, promoting repair of nerve damage.

How do these current treatments apply to the more common chronic pain conditions? What follows is a brief survey of major pain disorders and the treatments most in use today.

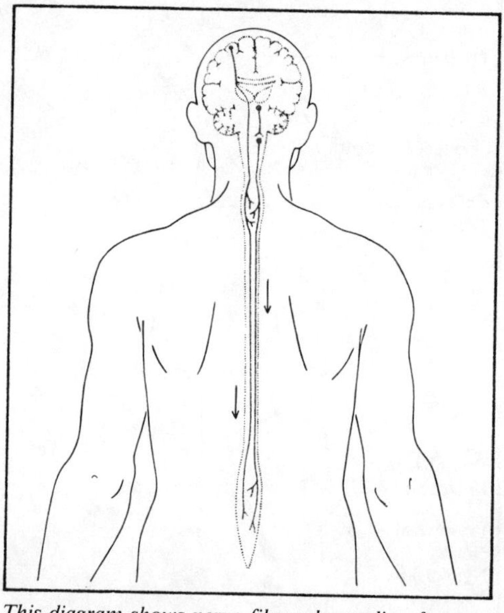

This diagram shows nerve fibers descending from the brain to the spinal cord where they can inhibit pain in various areas.

The major pains

• *Headache*. Tension headache, involving continued contractions of head and neck muscles, is one of the most common forms of headache. The other common variety is the vascular headache involving changes in the pressure of blood vessels serving the head. Migraine headaches are of the vascular type, associated with throbbing pain on one side of the head. Genetic factors play a role in determining who will be a victim of migraine, but many other factors are important as well. A major difficulty in treating migraine headache is that changes occur throughout the course of the headache. Blood vessels may first constrict and then dilate. Changing levels of neurotransmitters have also been noted. While a number of drugs can relieve migraine pain, their usefulness often depends on when they are taken. Some are only effective if taken at the onset.

Drugs are also the most common treatment for tension headache, although attempts to use biofeedback to control muscle tension have had some success. Physical methods such as heat or cold applications often provide additional if only temporary relief.

• *Low back pain*. The combination of aspirin, bed rest, and modest amounts of a muscle relaxant are usually prescribed for the first-time low back pain patient. At the initial examination, the physician will also note if the patient is overweight or works at an occupation such as truck-driving or a desk job that offers little opportunity for exercise. Some authorities believe that low back pain is particularly prevalent in Western society because of the combination of overweight, bad posture (made worse if there is added weight up front), and infrequent exercise. Not surprisingly, then, when the patient begins to feel better, the suggestion is made to take off pounds and take on physical exercise. In some cases, a full neurological examination may be necessary, including an x-ray of the spinal cord called a myelogram, to see if there may be a ruptured disc or other source of pressure on the cord or nerve roots.

Sometimes x-rays will show a disc problem which can be helped by surgery. But neither the myelogram nor disc surgery is foolproof. Milder analgesics (aspirin or stronger nonnarcotic medications) and electrical stimulation — using TENS or implanted brain electrodes — can be very effective. What is *not* effective is long-term use of the muscle-relaxant tranquilizers. Many specialists are convinced that chronic use of these drugs is detrimental to the back patient, adding to depression and increasing pain. Massage or manipulative therapy are used by some clinicians but, other than individual patient reports, their usefulness is still undocumented.

• *Cancer pain.* The pain of cancer can result from the pressure of a growing tumor or the infiltration of tumor cells into other organs. Or the pain can come about as the result of radiation or chemotherapy. These treatments can cause fluid accumulation and swelling (edema), irritate or destroy healthy tissue causing pain and inflammation, and possibly sensitize nerve endings. Ideally, the treatment for cancer pain is to remove the cancerous tissue. When that is not possible, pain can be treated by any or all of the currently available therapies: electrical stimulation, psychological methods, surgery, and strong painkillers.

• *Arthritis pain.* Arthritis is a general descriptive term meaning an affliction of the joints. The two most common forms are *osteoarthritis* that typically affects the fingers and may spread to important weight-bearing joints in the spine or hips, and *rheumatoid arthritis*, an inflammatory joint disease associated with swelling, congestion, and thickening of the soft tissue around joints. Recently, a distinguished panel of pain experts commenting on arthritis reported that "in all probability aspirin remains the most widely used . . . and important drug . . . although it may cause serious side effects." In the 1950s the steroid drugs were introduced and hailed as lifesavers — important anti-inflammatory agents modeled after the body's own chemicals produced in the adrenal glands. But the long-term use of steroids has serious consequences, among them the lowering of resistance to infection, hemorrhaging, and facial puffiness — producing the so-called "moonface."

Besides aspirin, current treatments for arthritis include several nonsteroid anti-inflammatory drugs like indomethacin and ibuprofen. But these drugs, too, may have serious side effects. TENS and acupuncture have been tried with mixed results. In cases where tissue has been destroyed, surgery to replace a diseased joint with an artificial part has been very successful. The "total hip replacement" operation is an example.

Arthritis is best treated early, say the experts. A modest program of drugs combined with exercise can do much to restore full function and forestall long-term degenerative changes. Exercise in warm water is especially good since the water is both relaxing and provides buoyancy that makes exercises easier to perform. Physical treatments with warm or cold compresses are helpful sources of temporary pain relief.

• *Neurogenic pain.* The most difficult pains to treat are those that result from damage to the peripheral nerves or to the central nervous system itself. We have mentioned tic douloureux and shingles as examples of extraordinarily searing pain, along with several drugs that can help. In addition, tic sufferers can benefit from surgery to destroy the nerve cells that supply pain-sensation fibers to the face. "Thermocoagulation" — which uses heat supplied by an electrical current to destroy nerve cells — has the advantage that pain fibers are more sensitive to the treatment, resulting in less destruction of other sensations (touch and temperature).

Sometimes specialists treating tic find that certain blood vessels in the brain lie near the group of nerve cells supplying sensory fibers to the face, exerting pressure that causes pain. The surgical insertion of a small sponge between the blood vessels and the nerve cells can relieve the pressure and eliminate pain.

Among other notoriously painful neurogenic disorders is pain from an amputated or paralyzed limb — so called "phantom" pain — that affects up to 10 percent of amputees and paraplegia patients. Various combinations of antidepressants and weak narcotics like Darvon® are sometimes effective. Surgery, too, is occasionally successful. Many experts now think that the electrical stimulating techniques hold the greatest promise for relieving these pains.

- ***Psychogenic pain.*** Some cases of pain are not due to past disease or injury, nor is there any detectable sign of damage inside or outside the nervous system. Such pain may benefit from any of the psychological pain therapies listed earlier. It is also possible that some new methods used to diagnose pain may be useful. One method gaining in popularity is thermography, which measures the temperature of surface tissue as a reflection of blood flow. A color-coded "thermogram" of a person with a headache or other painful condition often shows an altered blood supply to the painful area, appearing as a darker or lighter shade than the surrounding areas or the corresponding part on the other side of the body. Thus, an abnormal thermogram in a patient who complains of pain in the absence of any other evidence may provide a valuable clue that can lead to a diagnosis and treatment.

Where to go for help

People with chronic pain have usually seen a family doctor and several other specialists as well. Eventually they are referred to neurologists, orthopedists, or neurosurgeons. The patient/doctor relationship is extremely important in dealing with chronic pain. Both patients and family members should seek out knowledgeable specialists who neither dismiss nor indulge the patient — physicians who understand full well how pain has come to dominate the patient's life and the lives of everyone else in the family.

Many specialists today refer chronic pain patients to pain clinics for treatment. Over 800 such clinics have opened their doors in the United States since a world leader in pain therapy established a pain clinic at the University of Washington in Seattle in 1960.

Pain clinics differ in their approaches. Generally speaking, clinics employ a group of specialists who review each patient's medical history and conduct further tests when necessary. If the applicant is admitted, the clinic staff designs a personal treatment program that may include individual and group psychotherapy, exercise, diet, ice massage for pain (especially before bedtime), electrical stimulation techniques, and the use of a variety of analgesic, but nonnarcotic, drugs. The aim is to reduce pain medication and so improve the patient's pain problem that when he or she leaves the hospital it is with the prospect of resuming more normal activities with a minimal requirement for analgesics and a positive self-image.

Contrary to what many people think, pain clinic patients are not malingerers or hypochondriacs. They are men and women of all ages, education, and social background, suffering a wide variety of painful conditions. Patients with low back pain are frequent, and so are people with the complications of diabetes, stroke, brain trauma, headache, arthritis, or any of the rarer pain conditions. The majority of patients participate for 2 or 3 weeks and usually report substantial improvement at discharge. One young man who had suffered painful chest injury as a result of a factory accident said he literally "felt taller" after his pain clinic experience. Followup at 3- and 6-month intervals, and at lengthier intervals thereafter, is an essential part of the program, both to evaluate the long-term effectiveness of treatment and to initiate a further course of treatment or counseling if necessary.

Pain clinics have the virtue that they bring together people with pain problems that have left them feeling isolated, helpless, and hopeless. But not everyone with a pain problem may need the support of a group or residence in a hospital. The important factors are that the pain patient — and the family — understand all the ramifications of pain, and the many and varied steps that can now be taken to undo what chronic pain has done. As a result of the strides neuroscience has made in tracking down pain in the brain — and in the mind — we can expect more and better treatments in the years to come. The days when patients were told "I'm sorry, but you'll have to learn to live with the pain" will be gone forever.

Voluntary health organizations

Two lay organizations are concerned directly with pain problems. The National Migraine Foundation supports research and education on migraine headaches. The National Committee on the Treatment of Intractable Pain was started several years ago to stimulate attention and research on the prevention and treatment of severe pain that may accompany advanced cancer and other terminal or intractable conditions. In addition, many organizations concerned with specific diseases, such as arthritis or heart disease, provide information and advice about attendant pain problems.

National Migraine Foundation
5252 N. Western Avenue
Chicago, Ill. 60625
(312) 878-7715

National Committee on the Treatment of Intractable Pain
P.O. Box 9553 (Friendship Station)
Washington, D.C. 20006
(301)983-1710

Pain clinics

While there is no official certifying agency accrediting pain clinics throughout the country, there are many excellent clinics, often affiliated with university-associated medical centers. Your family doctor or university medical center may be able to refer you to reputable clinics nearby. If not, physicians can write to the American Society of Anesthesiologists, 515 Busse Highway, Park Ridge, Ill. 60068, which publishes a worldwide pain clinic directory.

NINCDS information

For additional information concerning NINCDS research on pain write:

Office of Scientific and Health Reports
National Institute of Neurological and
Communicative Disorders and Stroke
Building 31, Room 8A06
National Institutes of Health
9000 Rockville Pike
Bethesda, Md. 20205
(301)496-5751

Chapter 8

Creutzfeldt-Jakob Disease

Creutzfeldt-Jakob Disease

What is Creutzfeldt-Jakob disease?

Creutzfeldt-Jakob disease is a rare, fatal brain disorder caused by an unknown organism — possibly a virus — that can be transmitted from patients to animals and from one animal to another. The disease causes mental deterioration and a variety of neurological symptoms, and usually leads to death within a year of onset.

How does it affect the patient?

In early stages of the disease, patients may have failing memory, changes in behavior, lack of coordination, or visual disturbances. As the illness progresses, mental deterioration becomes pronounced, involuntary movements (especially muscle jerks) appear, and the patient may become blind, develop weakness in the arms or legs, and ultimately lapse into coma. Death is usually due to infections in the bedridden, unconscious patient.

Symptoms of Creutzfeldt-Jakob disease can be similar to those seen in other progressive neurological disorders such as Alzheimer's disease and other dementias. However, Creutzfeldt-Jakob disease causes unique changes in brain tissue that at this time can be detected only by surgical biopsy or at autopsy.

Who gets Creutzfeldt-Jakob disease?

Anybody can get Creutzfeldt-Jakob disease. Since the disease was identified by Dr. Alfons Maria Jakob in the 1920s, over 3,000 cases have been reported worldwide. The disease afflicts both men and women, and most often appears in people ages 50 to 75 years.

Internationally, there is one Creutzfeldt-Jakob death per year for every million people. Certain areas, such as rural Slovakia and Chile show much higher rates. In Israel, there are considerably higher rates in Libyan-born Jews. Genetic factors appear to be important in the disease's occurrence in relatively isolated rural areas of the world.

An estimated 200 Americans die each year with Creutzfeldt-Jakob disease. Many Americans first heard of the disease in 1983, when they learned it had claimed the life of New York City Ballet choreographer George Balanchine. Between 10 and 15 percent of persons afflicted in the U.S. have a family history of presenile dementia.

What causes the disease?

Scientists agree that a transmissible agent causes Cruetzfeldt-Jakob disease, but this agent has not yet been fully identified. The agent has been classified as a "slow" and "unconventional" virus: slow, because there is a long incubation period — up to 3 years, or longer — before symptoms appear; and unconventional, because a core of nucleic acids commonly seen in other viruses has not been identified. (Nucleic acids contain a cell's genetic material.) The agent is also unusual because it has not been recognized with the electron microscope, conventional laboratory methods fail to destroy or completely inactivate it, and it elicits no detectable immune response.

The unusual characteristics of the Creutzfeldt-Jakob agent are similar to the characteristics of the agent that causes scrapie, a disease of sheep and goats. Animals with scrapie undergo neurologic and behavioral changes like those found in Creutzfeldt-Jakob disease. Although Creutzfeldt-Jakob disease sometimes occurs in people living where scrapie is found, there is no strong evidence that scrapie has a role in the human disease.

Is the disease contagious?

The low incidence of Creutzfeldt-Jakob disease indicates that person-to-person transmission is rare. Spouses of patients and other household members have no higher risk of contracting the disorder than the general population.

There is evidence, however, that the transmissible agent has been introduced into the nervous system of healthy persons during certain medical procedures. One such tragic case occurred when a cornea was transplanted from an organ donor who at autopsy was discovered to have had Creutzfeldt-Jakob disease. The patient who received the cornea showed symptoms within 18 months, and died of Creutzfeldt-Jakob disease 6 months after symptoms first appeared. Animal studies later confirmed that the disease can be transmitted through transplanted corneas.

Creutzfeldt-Jacob disease has also been accidentally transmitted through implantation of contaminated electrodes in the brain. Also, clusters of Creutzfeldt-Jakob cases have been documented among patients undergoing neurosurgery at a few medical facilities; however, no such case has occurred since the mid 1970s.

In 1984 and 1985, at least four patients who had received natural human growth hormone to correct growth deficiencies died from Creutzfeldt-Jakob disease. Scientists suspect that several batches of the hormone, derived from human pituitary tissue, were contaminated by the Creutzfeldt-Jakob agent. The use of natural human growth hormone has been discontinued in the U.S. and Great Britain, and drug companies are now marketing a synthetic form of the hormone to avoid any possibility of such contamination.

Are health professionals at risk of contracting the disease?

In a few instances, Creutzfeldt-Jakob disease has occurred among physicians, dentists, and other health workers, possibly after having been exposed to the agent in the course of their work. Health-care professionals would be wise to take precautions when handling blood and spinal fluid samples taken from patients with Creutzfeldt-Jakob disease. Scientists recommend that health workers:

- Be careful not to cut or puncture themselves when using instruments contaminated by a patient's blood or spinal fluid.
- Wear gloves when handling a patient's tissues and fluids.
- Sterilize equipment that comes into contact with a patient's tissues. The most effective method of sterilization is to place instruments in a steam autoclave for at least 1 hour at 132 degrees Centigrade.

Is there any treatment?

No effective treatment for Creutzfeldt-Jakob disease is known. Drugs are now being evaluated against the laboratory-induced disease in rodents and nonhuman primates, but none has shown evidence of lasting benefit.

Current clinical studies include tests of antiviral drugs such as amantadine, a compound useful in parkinsonism. Some patients taking these drugs have experienced brief periods of improvement and treatment has not proven harmful. But, to date, drugs have neither controlled nor cured the disease.

What is research achieving?

Within the federal government, the focal point for research on Creutzfeldt-Jakob disease is the National Institute of Neurological and Communicative Disorders and Stroke (NINCDS). The NINCDS is a unit of the National Institutes of Health, and is responsible for basic and clinical investigation on the brain and central nervous system.

In 1968, NINCDS scientists first transmitted Creutzfeldt-Jakob disease to nonhuman primates. This animal model was produced by inoculating human Creutzfeldt-Jakob brain tissue directly into the brains of chimpanzees and monkeys. The resulting disease appeared identical to the human disease, with a long symptom-free phase followed by progressive behavioral and physical deterioration leading to death.

More practical models of Creutzfeldt-Jakob disease appeared in 1975, when NINCDS grantees at Yale University transmitted the disorder to guinea pigs and later to mice and hamsters. These animal models are providing investigators with a wealth of Creutzfeldt-Jakob tissue for more detailed studies of the development and progression of the disease, as well as purification of the agent. The Yale scientists are now cooperating with other NIH grantees in evaluating a series of antiviral compounds in the rodent models.

At the University of California at San Francisco, an NINCDS grantee has reported discovering a protein-containing particle which he proposes is the Creutzfeldt-Jakob agent. He believes the particle (which he calls "prion") represents an entirely new class of disease-causing agents. Unlike most viruses, prions contain no apparent genetic material; the gene for this protein is contained in normal cells.

For scientists studying Creutzfeldt-Jakob disease, the chief obstacle to development of a treatment has been locating and purifying the transmissible agent itself. This difficulty persists, despite the fact that brain tissue from Creutzfeldt-Jakob disease patients contains up to a million or more lethal doses of the agent per gram.

How can I help research?

Scientists are conducting biochemical analyses of brain tissue, blood, and serum in hope of determining the nature of the transmissible agent or agents causing Creutzfeldt-Jakob disease. To help with this research, the scientists are seeking biopsy and autopsy tissue, blood, and cerebrospinal fluid from patients with Creutzfeldt-Jakob and related diseases. The following investigators have expressed an interest in receiving such material:

Dr. Stephen DeArmond/Dr. Stanley Prusiner
Department of Pathology/Neuropathology Unit
HSW 430
University of California
San Francisco, California 94143
Telephone: (415) 476-5236

Dr. Clarence J. Gibbs/Dr. D. Carleton Gajdusek
National Institute of Neurological and Communicative Disorders and Stroke
Laboratory of Central Nervous System Studies
Building 36, Room 4A-15
National Institutes of Health
Bethesda, Maryland 20892
Telephone: (301) 496-4821 (Call collect)

Dr. Elias Manuelidis
Yale University School of Medicine
Section of Neuropathology
333 Cedar Street
New Haven, Connecticut 06510
Telephone: (203) 785-4442

How can I cope?

Those who cope best with a fatal disease usually face life one day at a time, accepting each day's challenges with as much courage as they can summon. Some have achieved a measure of peace and relief with the following approach recommended by the chief of psychiatry consultation, Clinical Center, National Institutes of Health:

- Remember that disease strikes randomly, affecting persons in all walks of life.
- Seek emotional and other support from family, friends, social service workers, and members of the clergy.
- Express any feelings of fear and anger in your discussions with a trained counselor. Fears and concerns should also be communicated

to your spouse or the person who is closest to you. Such feelings are natural, and often need to be shared with others.
- Extend love and understanding to everyone within your circle of loved ones.

These guidelines may also be helpful to families of patients with Creutzfeldt-Jakob disease. Relatives should realize that the patient is generally not in pain and usually becomes unaware of his or her surroundings long before the last stages of the disease. Family members may wish to discuss their concerns with a counselor.

Where can I get help?

No voluntary organization has yet been established expressly for Creutzfeldt-Jakob disease patients and their families. However, the National Organization for Rare Disorders will put families affected by Creutzfeldt-Jakob disease (or any other rare disorder) in touch with each other. For information about this group's networking service and other educational and outreach activities, contact:

National Organization for Rare Disorders
P.O. Box 8923
New Fairfield, Connecticut 06812
(203) 746-6518

In addition, the Alzheimer's Disease and Related Disorders Association offers publications and support to Creutzfeldt-Jakob disease patients and their families. For more information about the association's services, write:

Alzheimer's Disease and Related Disorders Association
70 East Lake Street
Chicago, Illinois 60601
(312) 853-3060

Family members might also want to consider contacting a local hospice program. Hospices help terminally ill patients and their families arrange for medical supplies and home-based nursing care, and also offer emotional support and advice on daily living. The National Hospice Organization refers patients to programs in their area. For more information, write:

National Hospice Organization
Suite 902
1901 N. Fort Myer Drive
Arlington, Virginia 22209
(703) 243-5900

NINCDS information

For more information about the research activities of the National Institute of Neurological and Communicative Disorders and Stroke, contact:

Office of Scientific and Health Reports
National Institute of Neurological and
Communicative Disorders and Stroke
Building 31, Room 8A-06
National Institutes of Health
Bethesda, Maryland 20892
(301) 496-5751

Chapter 9

Dementias

The Dementias

> . . . the major diseases of human beings have become approachable biological puzzles ultimately solvable. Stroke and senile dementia . . . are not natural aspects of the human condition, and we ought to rid ourselves of such impediments as quickly as we can.
>
> — Lewis Thomas, *The Medusa and the Snail*

What is the look of dementia? Is there a glazed stare or strange smile that signals that this man or that woman is fast losing the power to remember or reason, reckon or plan? No. There is no telltale look. Yet the very word *dementia* conjures up nightmare pictures of patients numb to the world and immobile, or else shuffling about, babbling incoherently. Such images color our fears and heighten anxiety, for the thought of ourselves — or someone close — becoming demented, is terrifying.

There is some reason for fear. Dementia — more accurately, the dementias — are brain diseases that result in the progressive loss of mental faculties, often beginning with memory, learning, attention, and judgment. While some types of dementia are curable, the most common dementing illnesses are not. In time, an unrelenting dementia will erode all aspects of thought, feeling, and behavior, and lead to death.

It is important to realize that demented persons are not insane in the sense of suffering a psychiatric disorder. They become — as the word *dementia* literally means — *deprived* of mind, deprived of the use of parts of the brain associated with a range of intellectual skills and activities unique to human beings.

There is also good reason not to be afraid. Contrary to what many people think, dementing disorders are not the fate that awaits us all with aging. An estimated 5 percent of the U.S. population 65 or over is severely demented. Another 10 percent may be mildly to moderately impaired. That means that 85 percent of the elderly are *not* demented.

But there is an association of dementia with aging, and because Americans are living longer, the numbers affected will grow. There are now 1 million people in the U.S. 65 or over who are severely impaired intellectually; 2 million more are moderately impaired.

Still another smaller group of adults succumbs to dementing

illnesses earlier in life. Over half of these *presenile* dementias are due to Alzheimer's disease, a progressive dementia named for Alois Alzheimer, the German doctor who described the disorder in 1907. Neurologists now agree that over half the dementias occurring among the elderly — disorders called *senile dementia*, or *chronic organic brain syndrome* — are actually cases of disease of the Alzheimer type, but beginning at a later stage of life.

The power of words

Words like *presenile, senile,* and *senility* help perpetuate the myth that aging means mental decline: The words are derived from a Latin root that simply means "to grow old." In Greek and Roman times, people so dreaded the infirmities of old age that they regarded aging itself as a disease. Too many people today still hold such beliefs, and it is only as the proportion of older people in the population has risen — and become more vocal — that the myths are beginning to fade. Today, neuroscientists know there are age-related changes in the brain, but the changes do not seriously affect mental vigor. Moreover, there are so many examples of intelligence and creativity among the elderly — think of Picasso and Toscanini — but think, too, of friends, neighbors, and relatives — that the belief that getting old means getting senile is simply not true.

Negative feelings about aging, compounded with the fear and shame so often associated with brain disease, have made it difficult for laymen and health professionals to deal with problems posed by the dementias.

That situation is changing now as a result of major developments in the neurosciences and a new concern for the process — and problems — of aging. Two components of the National Institutes of Health are vitally involved: the National Institute of Neurological and Communicative Disorders and Stroke (NINCDS), the leading federal agency that supports neurological research; and the National Institute on Aging (NIA), the agency concerned with all aspects of aging, psychological and sociological, as well as biological.

Both institutes work closely with other federal agencies and with voluntary health organizations concerned with the dementias. These groups of dedicated people have faced dementing illness in their families and have come together in a national organization, the Alzheimer's Disease and Related Disorders Association, to urge education and research on the dementias.

The need is particularly poignant in classic (early onset) Alzheimer's disease. Not only do the symptoms appear in the prime of midlife — the forties and fifties — but the downhill course of the disease may extend over 10 years or so before death intervenes. In comparison, older patients with dementia of the Alzheimer type may survive only a few years. Often the cause of death is pneumonia or other infection. But Alzheimer's disease patients are also prone to accidents, stroke, and certain cancers. Indeed, the high mortality rate and the large numbers affected make Alzheimer's disease a major killer in America today: It is ranked as the fourth or fifth leading cause of death. Yet the death certificate may list only the immediate cause of death — pneumonia or stroke — rather than Alzheimer's disease*.

The signs of Alzheimer's

A woman in the early stages of Alzheimer's disease was recently seen by NINCDS neurologists at the Clinical Center, the research hospital of the National Institutes of Health in Bethesda, Md. She was an attractive, well-dressed, and pleasant-voiced woman of 50, a former music teacher and pianist, whose memory problems had progressed to the point where she was no longer able to read music at sight. Her family acknowledged that for some time the woman also had had trouble taking telephone messages and recognizing faces. She could no longer do the family accounts, and more than once she had become lost while driving. The woman was aware of her memory

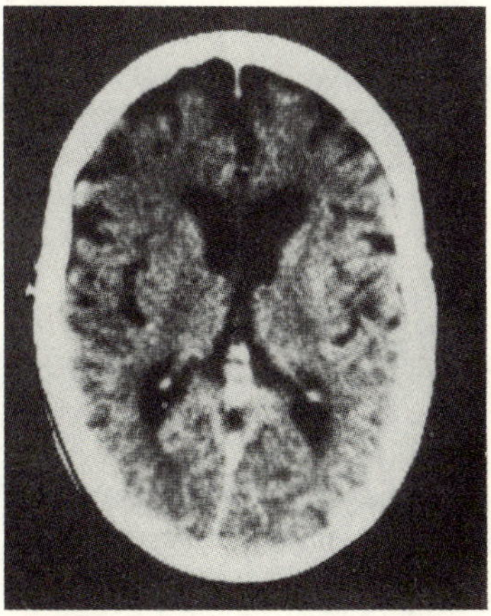

CT scan shows atrophy: Dark upper central areas are enlarged fluid-filled spaces; dark indents at border are enlarged spaces between brain convolutions.

---

* see chapter, "Alzheimer's Disease"

problems, but when she was asked about her life she was generally alert and articulate.

The neurologist then asked a few everyday questions: "Who is the president of the United States?" "Reagan," she replied. "What is today's date?" She scratched her head and smiled embarrassedly, "Don't know." "The month?" " . . . maybe April?" [It was June.] "What year?" "19 . . . something," she said. And so it went. At one point the specialist asked her to memorize three short phrases: *red shoes, black box, 300 Broadway*. She repeated the phrases and the specialist went on to ask her to spell some common words like *world* and *home* forwards and backwards, and to count down from 100 to 80. She had problems with all these tasks. Then the doctor asked her to repeat the phrases she had just learned. "Red . . ." she said, but could remember nothing else.

Until her failings on that typical "mental status" exam — a rapid test of a person's orientation and mental competence — there was nothing in the woman's appearance, mood, or behavior to suggest that she might be suffering a serious brain disease. Furthermore, her medical history and the results of extensive physical and laboratory tests were largely negative.

Her brain X-rays were suggestive, however. Using computerized tomography — the technique that produces the computer-drawn X-ray images of the brain known as CT scans — neurologists noted widespread loss of nerve tissue in the cortex. (The cortex is the outer gray covering of the brain associated with higher mental faculties.) The channels that circulate cerebral spinal fluid in the brain were

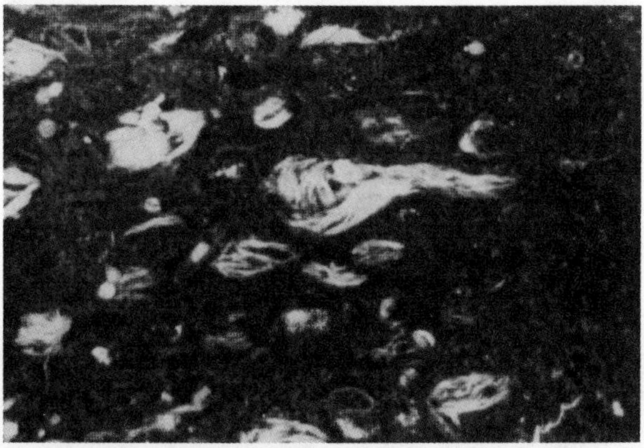

Tangles are well named. The white areas that look like twisted bits of yarn are neurofibrillary tangles, magnified in this view of the cortex of a patient with Alzheimer's disease.

also enlarged, another indication that brain substance has been lost and fluid has filled in the gap.

Certainly finding such extensive brain shrinkage in a middle-aged woman would be cause for alarm. Surprisingly, however, this brain atrophy is not always obvious in Alzheimer's disease, especially in elderly patients. And when there is atrophy, the amount is not always matched with the severity of symptoms. Neurologists suspect that in addition to the nerve cells (neurons) that die in Alzheimer's disease, many other neurons are sick: They do not die and drop out, but they may stop working. The disease process may also lead to new growth of supporting brain tissue. Thus, an Alzheimer-diseased brain may not differ much in size or weight from the brain of a normal person matched in age and sex.

But brain cells in normal people also wear out and die (without replacement) over the course of a lifetime. Some experts estimate that the loss may be as high as 50 percent in some parts of the brain. Overall, the brain may shrink in size by as much as 20 to 30 percent between ages 25 and 70. Thus, the brain of a mentally alert 70-year-old may look distinctly atrophied.

Specific brain changes associated with Alzheimer's disease are visible under the microscope, however. The most prominent are *neurofibrillary tangles* and *neuritic plaques*. The tangles are pairs of fine nerve fibers twisted around each other and lying in the cell

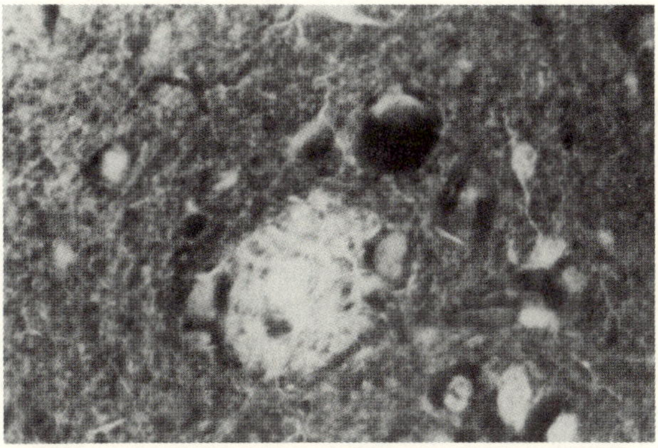

A single neuritic plaque is shown at the center of this magnified view of the cortex of an Alzheimer's disease brain. The dense white area in the center is the core of the plaque, composed of amyloid. Surrounding the core are wisps of amyloid material and degenerating bits of nerve fibers. Two neurofibrillary tangles can also be seen: one at center top; the other at the upper right.

bodies of neurons. The plaques are degenerating bits of nerve cells surrounding a core of fibrous material called amyloid. Plaques are found outside nerve cells.

Interestingly, some plaques are seen in the normal human brain in aging, as well as in the brains of older mammals. Tangles, too, are sometimes found in normal human brains in age, but they have not been seen in any other species. In any case, many more plaques and tangles are seen in the brains of patients with Alzheimer's disease, and here a correlation holds: The more plaques and tangles, the more severe the patient's symptoms.

Normally, doctors don't get a chance to sample brain tissue in living patients and examine it microscopically. That means that, at present, the diagnosis of Alzheimer's disease can only be confirmed at death. Investigators hope that new diagnostic tools under development, and the CT scan, already invaluable in detecting such brain abnormalities as tumors or cysts, may some day be subtle enough to detect the changes seen in Alzheimer's disease. Meanwhile, neurologists seeing patients with suspected dementia work by a process of elimination: They review all the ailments that can masquerade as dementia ("pseudodementias") as well as the roster of true dementing disorders.

The pseudodementias

- *Depression*. High among the disorders than can simulate dementia are depression and manic-depression. Depressed individuals are frequently passive and unresponsive. They may appear confused, slow, and forgetful. In manic-depression, the individual may experience mood swings between depression and mania — the latter an excited state in which a person feels powerful and often acts recklessly or foolishly.

People experiencing a dementing illness may also act irrationally and appear excited. They may also be depressed — either as part of the disease process itself or as a reaction to their failing mental powers.

In sorting out depression from dementia the physician may find that depressed individuals have had earlier bouts of depression along with symptoms of insomnia, fatigue, or loss of appetite. In contrast, a person in the early stages of dementia often singles out a memory problem, or difficulties in arithmetic, as the trouble. The onset of a progressive dementia like Alzheimer's disease is also likely to be slow and insidious, while depressions usually develop more quickly.

Sometimes an older person who appears passive, slow, or confused may have recently lost a spouse or close friend and is suffering what is called a reactive depression. It is not unusual for the mourner to seem distracted, speaking and acting as if the dead person were still alive, for example.

In other cases, a person who appears withdrawn or absent-minded may be reacting to the diminished circumstances of life, the loss of income and influence, for example. Loneliness and a disappointment with fate or with the state of society may be added burdens. Such a person's prevailing mood has been described as "existential sadness" — a mood that might benefit from sensitive human contact and rewarding activity, but not one that should be considered either mental or physical illness.

• ***Drugs***. Rivaling depression as a major factor complicating the diagnosis of dementia are reactions to drugs. One 66-year-old public speaking instructor was given a drug to control high blood pressure and chest pain due to angina. Within 24 hours he became disoriented, denied he had any health problems, suffered memory lapses and speech difficulties. Stopping the medication reversed all the dementing symptoms. In that instance, a single drug was the culprit. Often — especially in older adults — people are taking more than one drug for chronic conditions: "water" pills (diuretics) to control high blood pressure, sedatives for sleeplessness, tranquilizers for "nerves" — in addition to aspirin, laxatives, other over-the-counter drugs, and alcohol.

It is wise to assume that all drugs are powerful; all drugs have side effects, and most drugs interact: In combination, two or more drugs may be more powerful than each taken alone. One physician who was being treated for manic-depressive illness developed a hand tremor that was thought to be an early sign of Parkinson's disease. His blood pressure was also found to be high. The doctor ended up taking a variety of nervous system drugs as well as blood pressure medication. He became so disoriented he was unable to recognize his wife, sign his name. or hold a drinking glass. Again, there was a dramatic change for the better once the medications were stopped.

What makes drug use a particularly vexing problem in older people are age-related changes in metabolism. Both the liver and the kidney may be less efficient in clearing the body of drugs and, along with a general slowing of metabolism, a drug may persist in the body longer than in a younger person. Often, too, the dosage appropriate for a 25-year-old is much too strong for a 60-year-old. Some physicians routinely wean a patient off all medications when confronted with mental symptoms.

- *Chemical imbalances*. The brain makes a high demand on nutrients, and poor eating habits or problems in food absorption can seriously affect the brain. Again the problems can be worse in older people who may be inactive, have little appetite, and often skimp on food. Interestingly, mental symptoms may appear before physical ones. Pernicious anemia, for example, is a blood disorder caused by impaired ability to use one of the B vitamins. In older people, the first symptoms may be irritability or depression. Inadequate thyroid hormone can result in apathy, depression, or dementia. Hypoglycemia — a condition in which there is not enough sugar in the bloodstream — can give rise to confusion or personality change. Too little or too much sodium or calcium can also trigger disturbing mental changes. Tests can determine whether any of these imbalances are present.
- *Heart and lung problems*. Just as the brain demands high-quality nutrition, it also requires a high level of oxygen. Chronic lung disease can lead to an oxygen shortage that can starve brain cells and lead to the symptoms of dementia. If the heart is not pumping efficiently, if there are disturbances in heart rhythm, malfunctioning heart valves, or other indications of heart disease, the brain may suffer.

All of these "pseudodementias" are treatable, and if the brain has not suffered permanent damage, the dementing symptoms should abate. Other potentially reversible dementias may be caused by brain swelling (hydrocephalus), meningitis, brain tumor, head injury, certain hereditary disorders, and poisoning by lead, mercury, or by exposure to carbon monoxide, some pesticides, and industrial pollutants. Chronic alcoholism can also seriously impair mental faculties, notably memory for recent events. Some investigators think that alcohol in itself may cause irreparable brain damage, but the memory deficit appears to be related to the chronic drinker's inadequate diet — specifically, thiamine (vitamin B_1) deficiency.

The true dementias

Once the pseudodementias have been eliminated, the physician faced with a patient with failing mental powers will suspect circulatory problems or primary brain disease to be the cause. Next to Alzheimer's disease, the leading cause of dementia in aging is obstruction to blood flow in the brain. Most commonly, a blood clot will clog a blood vessel, or a vessel may burst, hemorrhaging into a part of the brain. If a major vessel is involved, the symptoms are sudden, dramatic, and sometimes fatal — the consequences of a major stroke. A small stroke may go unnoticed, however, or result in specific symptoms — a slurring of speech, perhaps, or a numbness in one hand. The evidence of a brain blood vessel (cerebrovascular) accident shows up as a small mass of coagulating blood and dead tissue called an infarct. If the number of infarcts increases over time, the chances are that the individual will experience progressive mental and physical decline.

Multi-infarct dementia is now the preferred term for mental deterioration due to blood vessel disease in the brain. It replaces the old-fashioned and inaccurate "hardening of the arteries of the brain." Multi-infarct dementia is now thought to account for between 12 and 20 percent of dementia in the elderly; another 16 to 20 percent of dementia patients have both infarcts and Alzheimer's disease.

It is usually not difficult to distinguish between the two most common dementias. Persons with infarct dementia often have a history of high blood pressure, vascular disease, or previous stroke. Infarcts are also the result of events that may occur months or years apart. Thus, the dementia progresses in stepwise fashion, in contrast to the steady decline seen in Alzheimer's disease. Since the infarct is usually limited to one part of the brain, the symptoms, too, are limited; they may affect only one side of the body or involve a specific faculty like language. Neurologists call these "local" or "focal" symptoms, as opposed to the "global" symptoms seen in Alzheimer's disease.

The remaining causes of progressive dementia are less-usual nervous system diseases. While each disorder alone affects a relatively small number of people, the group as a whole accounts for over a million patients with progressive and dementing brain disease in America today:

- ***Multiple sclerosis***. Among the better known neurological diseases is multiple sclerosis, a disorder characterized by destruction of the insulating material covering nerve fibers. Usually the disease progresses through a series of acute episodes and partial recoveries. In time, both mental and physical deterioration can occur.
- ***Parkinson's disease***. Tremor and difficulty in originating voluntary movements are the hallmarks of Parkinson's disease, a disorder which strikes older adults. Drugs can relieve symptoms, but do not halt the progression of the disease. Symptoms of dementia may appear in severe or advanced cases.
- ***Huntington's disease***. Children with a parent who has Huntington's disease stand a 50 percent chance of inheriting this relentless dementing disease. Symptoms usually appear in early middle age and can include personality change, mental decline, psychotic symptoms, and a movement disturbance. Restlessness and facial tics may

progress to severe uncontrollable flailing of head, limbs, and trunk. At the same time, mental capacity can deteriorate to dementia.

- *Pick's disease*. Symptoms of Pick's disease are very similar to those of Alzheimer's disease, but the disease is associated with different changes in brain tissue.
- *Creutzfeldt-Jakob disease*. Infectious agents are recognized as the culprits in a growing number of progressive dementias. In Creutzfeldt-Jakob disease, the infectious agent is an unusual virus that may lie dormant in the body for years (hence it is called a *slow* virus). When activated, the virus produces a rapidly progressive dementia along with muscle spasms and changes in gait.

Each of these "true" dementias has inspired new research into causes and cures. In each case, too, active voluntary organizations have mobilized efforts to educate the public and come to the aid of patients and families (see p. 156).

From the neuroscientist's point of view, the neurological disorders that cause dementia belong to a "classic" group of brain diseases that share certain features: In every case, the disease involves the accelerated death of nerve cells. Sometimes the cell death is widespread. More often, the death is selective: The disease strikes a particular kind of nerve cell, or it affects several types of cell confined to a specific area of the nervous system. The clue to understanding these diseases is to find out why certain neurons — or certain brain sites — are chosen for death, and what can be done to prevent or halt the destructive process.

Years ago, neurologists despaired of finding answers to such questions. Today they take them as a challenge. Neuroscientists now have vastly improved tools and techniques for exploring the nervous system. They can observe nerve cells in development, maturity, and old age. They can tease out individual neurons and grow them in tissue culture, or they can observe interactions between whole clusters of nerve cells in the living brain. If a cell is doomed to die, scientists can seek out the cause — chemical, toxic, infectious, immunological, genetic — that could bring on destruction.

This kind of research is vigorously encouraged and supported by the National Institute of Neurological and Communicative Disorders and Stroke. In some cases the research has taken investigators to such remote parts of the world as northern New Guinea, the Orkney Islands, Guam, and rural lake villages in Venezuela. Those areas are intriguing because they are places where the incidence of a rare dementing disease is uncommonly high. It was field work in New Guinea, for example, that provided an NINCDS scientist with the

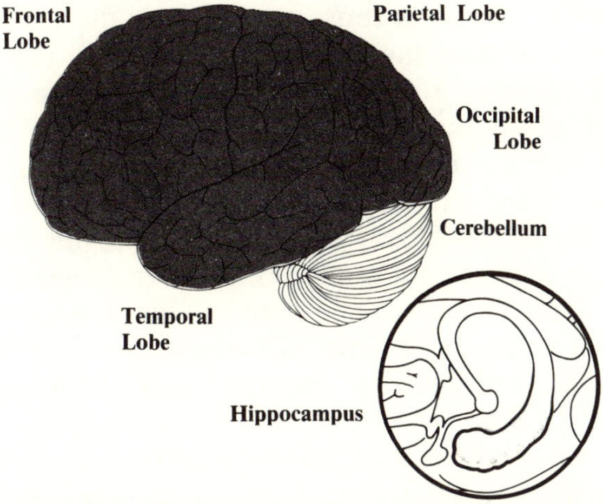

The gray and wrinkled outer covering of the brain is the cerebral cortex, associated with thought, language, memory and other uniquely human faculties. The detail shows the inner surface of one-half of the brain containing a small mass of nerve cells—the hippocampus—important in memory.

first clues that dementia could be caused by an unusual virus — studies for which he was awarded the Nobel prize.

Some scientists believe that an infectious agent may be involved in Alzheimer's disease, but it is only one of several possible causes currently being explored:

• ***Neurochemical changes***. One of the most fruitful findings in the past several decades has been the discovery that nerve cells secrete chemicals — neurotransmitters — that enable nerve signals to move from one nerve cell to another. A major discovery in Alzheimer's disease is that an enzyme needed to manufacture acetylcholine, an important neurotransmitter, is in short supply. Neurons using this transmitter are especially prominent in the hippocampus, a small cluster of brain cells important in memory. Hippocampal neurons are among the earliest and hardest hit in the disease.

NINCDS- and NIA-supported scientists at Albert Einstein College of Medicine in the Bronx, New York, are among those who have measured enzyme changes and cell losses in Alzheimer's disease. Using an automated cell counter, they examine cross sections of brain tissue and count which cells look normal, which are affected by disease.

• ***Metal deposits***. Aluminum has been found in suspiciously large amounts in the brains of some Alzheimer's disease patients. The metal shows up in cells that also contain neurofibrillary tangles. Whether aluminum deposits cause Alzheimer's disease by acting as a toxin, or whether the metal accumulates as a result of other changes associated with Alzheimer's disease is not known. Investigators in the U.S. and Canada are exploring both possibilities.

Other metals such as manganese have also been implicated in dementia. One reason NINCDS has established a research center on Guam is that the native Chamorro Indians are highly susceptible to several brain diseases, including a Parkinson-like dementia. Important clues to these disorders may lie hidden in Guamanian soil, which is unusually rich in both manganese and aluminum.

NINCDS plans a long-range study of Guam natives who develop dementia. The patients will be examined periodically; after their death, attempts will be made to correlate symptoms with changes in their brains. For comparison, investigators will examine tissue from natives who die from other causes.

Measurements of trace elements in the brain are also being conducted by an NINCDS grantee at the University of Kentucky, and an NIA grantee at the University of Vermont. One aim of this research is to define normal levels of trace elements throughout life, and check whether the levels go up as a consequence of normal aging.

• *Genetic factors*. Alzheimer's disease sometimes runs in families. An adult's chances of developing Alzheimer's disease are about 1 in 100, but the odds increase fourfold or more if a close relative is affected. Because there is no clear-cut pattern of inheritance, geneticists suspect that there is a genetic "component" in Alzheimer's disease: Probably several genes are involved, and these in turn must interact with environmental factors for the disease to develop.

Abnormalities in chromosomes — the larger structures that house genes in body cells — are also seen in Alzheimer's disease. Normally there are 23 pairs of chromosomes in human cells. But a higher than normal percentage of cells from Alzheimer's disease patients shows up with too many or too few chromosomes. Defective chromosomes are found as well. Alzheimer's disease has also been linked with Down syndrome (mongolism), the birth disorder in which there is an extra 21st chromosome. Not only do the two conditions sometimes show up in the same family, but individuals with Down syndrome frequently develop Alzheimer's disease.

Several other chromosomes are of interest because they contain genes which govern the production of certain proteins. These proteins are found in increased amounts in the blood of Alzheimer's disease patients. While these studies are interesting in their own right, the discovery that a particular gene often occurs in association with a particular disease means that the gene can act as a "marker": An individual who carries that gene may be susceptible to the disease in question.

• *Infectious agents.* Pairs of twisted nerve fibers — similar to those seen in neurofibrillary tangles — have appeared in cultures of human brain tissue exposed to extracts of Alzheimer's-disease brains. Investigators have also seen typical neuritic plaques develop in the brains of mice inoculated with a virus that causes brain degeneration in sheep. These observations are stimulating further study.

• *Immunological defects.* When a disease carries such distinctive trademarks as the plaques and tangles of Alzheimer's disease — trademarks whose frequency matches the severity of symptoms — investigators rightly turn to them for closer scrutiny. Scientists who have analyzed the amyloid core of neuritic plaques find that it is composed of fibers of an abnormal protein. The fibers may be signs of a defect in the body's immune system. Normally, the system attacks and destroys foreign tissue such as bacteria. Occasionally — possibly as a result of aging — the immune system may turn against the body's own tissue. If the native tissue consists of brain cells, the immune system may manufacture antibodies and launch scavenger cells that seek out brain neurons and destroy them. In the course of the attack, the abnormal plaque material may accumulate outside cells like so much trash in corridors.

Other investigators have looked at the twisted fibers that make up neurofibrillary tangles. The fibers are also abnormal proteins, but similar to the proteins that make up normal neurofilaments found in nerve cells. Since genes control the manufacture of proteins, the abnormal filaments could reflect the working of a defective gene. The abnormal filaments might also be the result of viral damage to the genetic material in nerve cells. Still another possibility is one based on a general theory of aging: The theory proposes that certain genes that control the repair of minor damage to chromosomes become less efficient in age. In this way, "errors" could creep into the genetic code, leading to defective gene products — abnormal proteins — or perhaps to defects in the body's immune system.

NINCDS- and NIA-supported investigators at Albert Einstein College of Medicine, as well as NINCDS grantees at the Institute for Basic Research in Mental Retardation in Staten Island, New York, are comparing normal neurofilaments with those seen in Alzheimer's disease and those formed in the brains of animals injected with aluminum compounds. An NINCDS-supported neuroscientist at New York University in New York City is classifying the many fibrous proteins found in the brain, while grantees of both institutes at McLean Hospital in Belmont, Mass., are focusing on the role fibrous proteins play throughout life. One important question raised is why abnormal fibers accumulate in the brains of many normal older people.

A casual reading of the many causes suggested for Alzheimer's disease should make it clear that neurochemical, toxic, genetic, viral, and immunological factors are not as distinct and separate as they appear to be: Whatever triggers the onset of Alzheimer's disease may result in a chain of destruction that upsets the nervous system's inherent ability to sustain, repair, and defend itself.

The urgency of treatment

Ideally, the successful treatment of disease follows from an understanding of the cause. But sometimes useful treatments are found long before the cause is known. Quinine was used to treat malaria before the malarial parasite was discovered. Even more to the point is the case of Parkinson's disease. The cause of the disease is unknown, but scientists know that there is a deficit in an important neurotransmitter, dopamine. Nowadays, Parkinson's patients can be treated with the drug L-dopa, which can be used in the brain to manufacture dopamine. While the drug does not cure the disease, it has greatly relieved symptoms in many patients. Treatments proposed for Alzheimer's disease and other dementias are based on similar lines of reasoning.

• *Nutrition.* The finding that the enzyme needed to produce acetylcholine is in short supply in Alzheimer's disease has prompted diet therapy: Patients are given foods rich in the raw materials that make up acetylcholine. The results have been inconclusive.

Because diet therapy may not work, some investigators are testing drugs. The drug physostigmine, for example, prevents the rapid breakdown of acetylcholine after it is released from nerve cells. Thus, the transmitter is coaxed into working harder and longer. There is some evidence that physostigmine helps Alzheimer's disease patients, but side effects may be severe.

Many scientists think the ideal treatment for Alzheimer's disease would be a drug that perfectly mimics acetylcholine. Such a drug, called an "agonist," would not have to be processed by the acetylcholine enzyme; it would work directly at the nerve cell junction. Unfortunately, the few acetylcholine agonists that have been found so far are either too short-lived or have bad side effects.

• ***Memory enhancers.*** Another approach to drug therapy in Alzheimer's disease and other dementias is the use of chemicals to improve memory. Some years ago, Dutch investigators began working with the hormone vasopressin, produced by the pituitary gland. Like most hormones, vasopressin exerts multiple effects in the body.

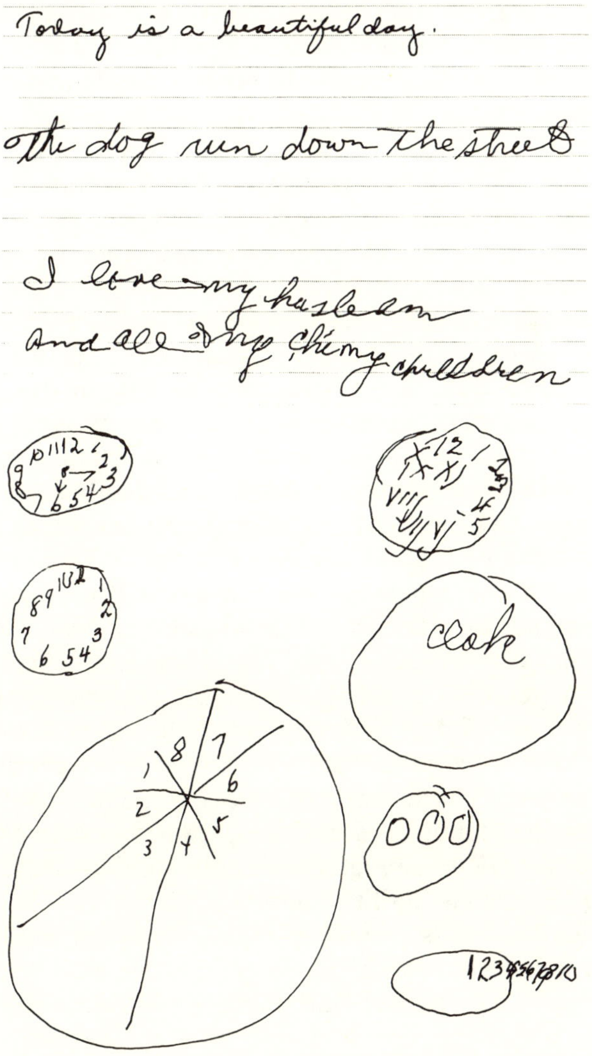

The relentless progression of dementia can be charted in the handwriting and drawings of Alzheimer's disease patients at various stages of disease. Patients were asked to write a sentence and to draw a clock with hours on it and time set at 3:30.

The Dutch investigators used vasopressin in learning experiments with rats. The rats received a mild electric shock if they made the wrong turn in a simple T-shaped maze. If the rats were given vasopressin either before or shortly after they explored the maze, their memories improved. Many rats avoided shock when retested up to 48 or 72 hours after their first trial. (Untreated rats usually forget which side is associated with shock after 24 hours.)

In the animal studies, vasopressin improved the process by which memories are stored in the brain; recall also improved. Since the rats were normal, scientists believe the drug may act as a general memory tonic: It might improve memory in normal adults as well as enhance the remaining capacity of patients with brain disease.

At present, vasopressin is being tested on patients with Alzheimer's disease at the NIH Clinical Center. The hormone is administered as an inhalant because there is some evidence that nerve endings sensitive to smell may pick up vasopressin and transport it to the brain.

• *Chelating agents*. Following up on the aluminum hypothesis, a number of investigators are experimentally treating Alzheimer's disease patients with drugs that bind aluminum, the first step in eliminating the metal from the body. Treatment using such "chelating" agents is currently being tried at a clinical research unit associated with Ohio State University in Columbus.

From time to time there are reports of new drugs that improve learning or memory: Some supposedly act as brain "stimulators," some as general rejuvenators — "Fountain of Youth" potions. Often, the first time such chemicals are used, patients report extraordinary benefits. This may be due to the placebo effect: The patient's high hopes, the stimulation of being a subject in an experiment, the desire to please the investigator and, possibly, body changes associated with the patient's positive mood can sometimes bring about measurable improvements in the patient's condition. Repeated trials of any drug under controlled conditions, and long-term followup of patients are always necessary before judgments can be made — and this is where many drug "bonanzas" fail the test.

• *Patient studies*. It is important that scientists study dementing diseases in living patients. Most dementias are slow and insidious in onset, difficult to diagnose. Had doctors a better idea of what signs to look for, they might come up with better diagnostic tests and be able to identify risk factors. For example, one NINCDS grantee working at the University of California, Irvine, is developing new psychological tests to aid in the diagnosis of Alzheimer's disease.

Other research studies are tracing blood flow in the brain, using improved CT scanning techniques. These studies are important in understanding multi-infarct dementia as well as other neurological disorders.

Among the newest research tools is an even more advanced method of recording brain images called positron emission tomography (PET), a process allowing investigators to observe what parts of the brain are active during particular mental activities. The positron emission technique may be able to identify parts of the brain used in thought and memory, for example, and compare the metabolism of the normal brain with the brain of a patient with dementing illness.

Still other approaches involve screening patients who volunteer for study. At Albert Einstein College of Medicine, New York City, for example, two programs are aimed at identifying risk factors for Alzheimer's disease and other dementias.

In one study, patients judged to have Alzheimer's disease will be compared to a matched control group. In addition to a detailed medical history and examination, special immunological tests, blood analyses, and hormone measurements will be made.

A second study is aimed at determining risk factors for multi-infarct dementia. A group of 500, 75-year-olds without dementia, will be followed for 5 years. During that time an estimated 20 percent of the group will develop some type of dementia. Among the variables to be assessed are stress, personal habits, and nutrition.

Scientists studying neurological diseases know they are dealing with distinctively *human* afflictions of the *human* brain. They are limited in what they can learn from other animal species. Ultimately, they rely on detailed analysis of the brain and other tissue from patients who have died with dementing disease.

Most of what has been learned to date about the dementias has come from postmortem study of brain tissue. NINCDS supports two brain banks for the study of Huntington's disease, Alzheimer's disease, and related disorders. The banks work closely with voluntary health organizations and have set up simple procedures to make it easy for families to donate tissue. (See p.156).

Sensitive caring

From the moment of diagnosis of dementia to the end of life, patients and families are subjected to pressures and strains that rarely let up. If there is a genetic component, the effect of the doctor's pronouncement of the diagnosis can be even more devastating. Sons and daughters, sisters and brothers, fear they themselves may one day succumb to the same remorseless symptoms.

In conditions like Alzheimer's disease, it is often the spouse alone who is left to do the caring — at a time of life when he or she may be elderly and in diminished health. The role is truly exhausting: "It's like a 36-hour day," as one man described it.

More often than not, the husband or wife of a patient will have assumed the burden of responsibility before the patient was diagnosed, quietly covering up for mental failings. After the diagnosis is made, there may be a period in which the loyal spouse and other family members deny the severity of the symptoms. The patient is really not so bad, they say, not as bad as someone else with a similar disorder.

Increasingly, health care professionals are acknowledging that all dementing diseases are family afflictions; patients need family support and flexibility in care — at home, in the community, and finally, if necessary, in a hospital or nursing facility. The voluntary health organizations concerned with dementing disorders understand this, and through their programs of advice and information come to the psychological and practical aid of families. Often they catalogue community resources, offer nursing care tips, and direct families to programs designed for patients with chronic neurological disorders.

A program at the Long Term Care Gerontology Center of Albert Einstein College of Medicine may be typical of new directions in the care of the aging and neurologically ill. The idea is to provide weekly sessions when Alzheimer's disease patients can meet in a small group with mental health workers, while family members meet with other professionals. The relatives have a chance to air their feelings and discuss problems. Meanwhile, the patients enjoy a social occasion that is also therapeutic. Gently, patiently, the patients are encouraged to learn to help themselves. Their attention is directed to a "reality board," a large display with the day and the date, and other relevant information. They are guided in relearning everyday activities — making sandwiches, setting the table, writing postcards, playing bingo. In the early stages of Alzheimer's disease and other dementias, individual symptoms vary: Some people may retain arithmetic skills, others remain fluent in speech, and so on. Often, well-learned skills like driving a car or carpentry may persist. So it was not surprising that at the end of one session a man with Alzheimer's disease entertained the group by playing the viola.

Such programs are medically beneficial. By stimulating the patient and encouraging independence, they can forestall the rapid decline that all too often occurs when patients are neglected, hospitalized too soon, or overprotected to the point of "infantilization." A well-meaning spouse — or an impatient one — often finds that it is easier to do everything for the patient just as a mother might do for an infant — thereby unwittingly hastening the patient's decline.

While it is important for patients with dementia to relearn old skills and to socialize, it is equally important that family members have time off — respite from around-the-clock nursing demands. Most families want to keep their ailing relatives at home as long as possible. But they need the support of community resources to provide respite facilities — places where a patient can go for brief stays. And they need practical guidance in caring for the patient at home.

An excellent manual for families has been prepared by the Dementia Research Program group at Burke Rehabilitation Center (see bibliography at the end of the chapter). The manual describes the typical phases that mark the progression of Alzheimer's disease and related disorders. It also offers ways to make the home safe and to encourage patients to care for themselves. Simple reminders like a calendar with the days ticked off, a bulletin board with menus posted, or signs in the bathroom (*flush*, over the toilet), help orient the patient and make the daily routine run smoothly. The manual covers such subjects as bathing, smoking, driving a car, using the telephone, losing things, medications, safety, sexual behavior, and depression.

Among new facilities offering diagnostic services and research programs for dementia are a memory disorder clinic at the New England Medical Center in Boston, and a Center for the Study of Dementia at the Johns Hopkins University School of Medicine in Baltimore. Johns Hopkins is also the site of one of two new Centers Without Walls — an NINCDS-sponsored research project for the study of Huntington's disease and other degenerative neurological disorders. The idea of this center — and a comparable one at Massachusetts General Hospital in Boston — is to provide a focus for research that will attract investigators from many different departments of a hospital, or from a variety of universities or hospitals. The multidisciplinary approach, combined with access to patients who volunteer for study, can lead to rapid advances in understanding and treatment.

These are signs of the times. Americans are increasingly concerned that the final turns in the cycle of life be rich and rewarding. For people faced with catastrophic dementing disease — disease that saps the very core of life — everything should be done that can be done. Answers to Alzheimer's disease, or any dementia, may not come for those presently afflicted, but in a society that no longer accepts these diseases as "natural aspects of the human condition," the answers will come.

Voluntary health organizations

The Alzheimer's Disease and Related Disorders Association represents seven independent organizations concerned with research, care, and treatment of Alzheimer's disease and related disorders. For information about the association's programs, publications, or referrals to local affiliates, write:

Alzheimer's Disease and Related Disorders Association
360 Michigan Avenue
Chicago, Illinois 60601
(312) 853-3060

The names and addresses of the many voluntary health organizations dealing with stroke, Parkinson's disease, Huntington's disease, and other neurological orders that can lead to dementia are listed in a directory, *Voluntary Health Agencies Working to Combat Neurological and Communicative Disorders*, NIH Publication No. 81-74. Single copies are available free by writing:

Office of Scientific and Health Reports
National Institute of Neurological and
Communicative Disorders and Stroke
National Institutes of Health
Building 31, Room 8A-06
Bethesda, Md. 20205.

Human tissue banks

The study of brain and other tissue from persons with neurological disorders is invaluable to research, especially in dementing conditions where the cause remains elusive and animal models are inadequate. NINCDS supports two national human specimen banks, one in Los Angeles and one near Boston. For information about tissue donation and collection write:

Dr. Wallace W. Tourtellotte, Director
Human Neurospecimen Bank
VA Wadsworth Hospital Center
Los Angeles, Calif. 90073

Dr. Edward D. Bird, Director
Brain Tissue Bank, Mailman Research Center
McLean Hospital
115 Mill Street
Belmont, Mass. 02178

Bibliography

Burke Rehabilitation Institute has published an excellent practical guide to care of patients with dementing disorders:
Managing the Person with Intellectual Loss (Dementia or Alzheimer's Disease) at Home.
Copies are available at $1.50 through the Women's Auxiliary, Burke Rehabilitation Center, 785 Mamaroneck Ave., White Plains, N.Y. 10605.

A family guidebook for patients with Alzheimer's and related disorders is available from:

The Johns Hopkins University Press
34th and Charles Streets
Baltimore, Md. 21218.

Many of the publications listed include names of voluntary organizations, publications, or other resources of value to concerned individuals. Specific inquiries concerning programs on the dementias may also be directed to:

NINCDS Office of Scientific and Health Reports
Bldg. 31, Room 8A-06
National Institutes of Health
Bethesda, Md. 20205

or to:

Information Office
National Institute on Aging
Bldg. 31, Room 5C-36
National Institutes of Health
Bethesda, Md. 20205.

Chapter 10

Dizziness

Dizziness

Most of us can remember feeling dizzy — after a roller coaster ride, maybe, or when looking down from a tall building, or when, as children, we would step off a spinning merry-go-round. Even superbly conditioned astronauts have had temporary trouble with dizziness while in space. In these situations, dizziness arises naturally from unusual changes that disrupt our normal feeling of stability.

But dizziness can also be a sign that there is a disturbance or a disease in the system that helps people maintain balance. This system is coordinated by the brain, which reacts to nerve impulses from the ears, the eyes, the neck and limb muscles, and the joints of the arms and legs. If any of these areas fail to function normally, or if the brain fails to coordinate the many nerve impulses it receives, a person may feel dizzy. The feeling of dizziness varies from person to person and, to some extent, according to its cause; it can include a feeling of unsteadiness, imbalance, or even spinning.

Disease-related dizziness, whether it takes the form of unsteadiness or spinning, is fairly common in the older population. Today, both older and younger people with serious dizziness problems can be helped by a variety of techniques — from medication to surgery to balancing exercises. Such techniques have been developed and improved by scientists studying dizziness.

Much of today's research on dizziness is supported by the National Institute of Neurological and Communicative Disorders and Stroke (NINCDS). This institute is a unit of the National Institutes of Health. It is the focal point within the federal government for research on the brain and central nervous system, including studies of the senses through which we interact with our surroundings.

With NINCDS support, scientists are searching for better ways to diagnose and treat dizziness, and are investigating the mechanisms that help us maintain our normal sense of balance. These studies, along with basic research on how the ear, the brain, and the nerves work, hold the best hope for relief for dizziness sufferers.

A delicate balancing act

To understand what goes wrong when we feel dizzy, we need to know about the vestibular system by which we keep a sense of balance amid all our daily twisting and turning, starting and stopping, jumping, falling, rolling, and bending.

The vestibular system is located in the inner ear, and contains the following structures: vestibular labyrinth, semicircular canals, vestibule, utricle, and saccule. These structures work in tandem with the vestibular areas of the brain to help us maintain balance.

The vestibular labyrinth is located behind the eardrum. The labyrinth's most striking feature is a group of three semicircular canals or tubes that arise from a common base. At the base of the canals is a rounded chamber called the vestibule. The three canals and the vestibule are hollow and contain a fluid called endolymph, which moves in response to head movement.

Within the vestibule and the semicircular canals are patches of special nerve cells called hair cells. Hair cells are also found in two fluid-filled sacs, the utricle and saccule, located within the vestibule. These cells are aptly named: rows of thin, flexible, hairlike fibers project from them into the endolymph.

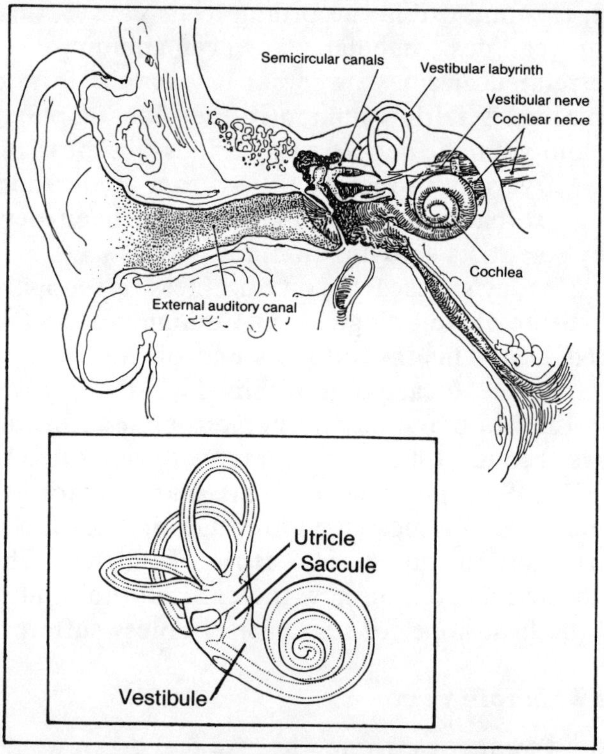

The semicircular canals and vestibule of the inner ear contain a fluid called endolymph that moves in response to head movement.

Also located in the inner ear are tiny calcium stones called otoconia. When you move your head or stand up, the hair cells are bent by the weight of the otoconia or movement of the endolymph. The bending of the hair cells transmits an electrical signal about head movement to the brain. This signal travels from the inner ear to the brain along the eighth cranial nerve — the nerve involved in balance and hearing. The brain recognizes the signal as a particular movement of the head and is able to use this information to help maintain balance.

The senses are also important in determining balance. Sensory input from the eyes as well as from the muscles and joints is sent to the brain, alerting us that the path we are following bends to the right or that our head is tilted as we bend to pick up a dime. The brain interprets this information — along with cues from the vestibular system — and adjusts the muscles so that balance is maintained.

Dizziness can occur when sensory information is distorted. Some people feel dizzy at great heights, for instance, partly because they cannot focus on nearby objects to stabilize themselves. When one is on the ground it is normal to sway slightly while standing. A person maintains balance by adjusting the body's position to something close

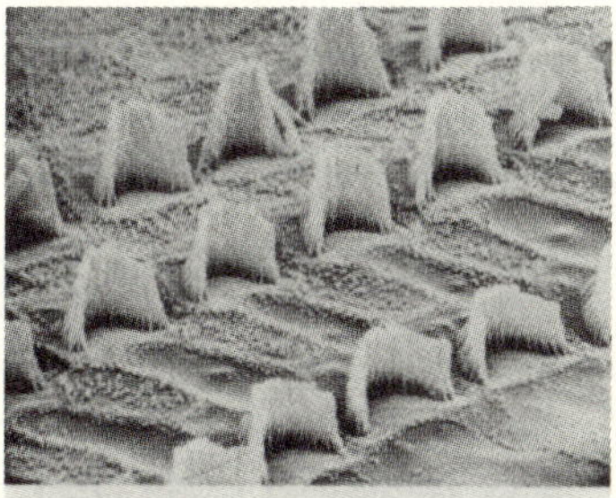

In the inner ear, rows of hairlike fibers project from tiny patches of nerve cells called hair cells.

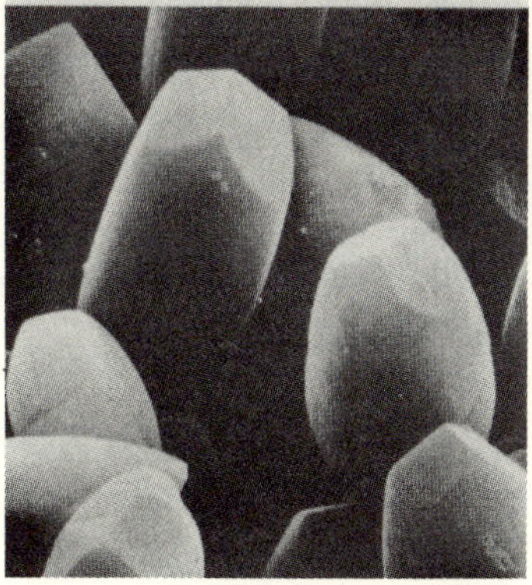

These tiny calcium stones called otoconia are part of the inner ear's balance system.

by. But when someone is standing high up, objects are too far away to use to adjust balance. The result can be confusion, insecurity, and dizziness which is sometimes resolved by sitting down.

Some scientists believe that motion sickness, a malady that affects sea, car, and even space travelers, occur when the brain receives conflicting sensory information about the body's motion and position. For example, when someone reads while riding in a car, the inner ear senses the movement of the vehicle, but the eyes gaze steadily on the book that is not moving. The resulting sensory conflict may lead to the typical symptoms of motion sickness: dizziness, nausea, vomiting, and sweating.

Another form of dizziness occurs when we turn around in a circle quickly several times and then stop suddenly. Turning moves the endolymph. The moving endolymph tells us we are still rotating but our other senses say we've stopped. We feel dizzy.

Diagnosing the problem

The dizziness one feels after spinning around in a circle usually goes away quickly and does not require a medical evaluation. But when symptoms appear to be caused by an underlying physical problem, the prudent person will see a physician for diagnostic tests. According to a study supported by the National Institute of Neurological and Communicative Disorders and Stroke, a thorough examination can reveal the underlying cause of dizziness in about 90 percent of cases.

A person experiencing dizziness may first go to a general practitioner or family physician: between 5 and 10 percent of initial visits to these physicians involve a complaint of dizziness. The patient may then be referred either to an ear specialist (otologist) or a nervous system specialist (neurologist).

The patient will be asked to describe the exact nature of the dizziness, to give a complete history of its occurrence, and to list any other symptoms or medical problems. Patients give many descriptions of dizziness — depending to some extent on its cause. Common complaints are light-headedness, a feeling of impending faint, a hallucination of movement or motion, or a loss of balance without any strange feelings in the head. Some people also report they have vertigo — a form of dizziness in which one's surroundings appear to be spinning uncontrollably or one feels the sensation of spinning.

The physician will try to determine what components of a patient's nervous system are out of kilter, looking first for changes in blood pressure, heart rhythm, or vision — all of which may contribute to the complaints. Sometimes dizziness is associated with an ear disorder. The patient may have loss of hearing, discomfort from loud sounds, or constant noise in the ear, a disorder known as *tinnitus*. The physician will also look for other neurological symptoms: difficulty in swallowing or talking, for example, or double vision.

Tests and scans

After the initial history-taking and physical examination, the physician may deliberately try to make the patient feel dizzy. The patient may be asked to repeat actions or movements that generally cause dizziness: to walk in one direction and then turn quickly in the opposite direction, or to hyperventilate by breathing deeply for 3 minutes.

In another test, the patient sits upright on an examining table. The physician tilts the patient's head back and turns it part way to one side, then gently but quickly pushes the patient backward to a lying down position. The reaction to this procedure varies according to the cause of dizziness. Patients with benign positional vertigo may experience vertigo plus *nystagmus*: rapid, uncontrollable back-and-forth movements of the eyes.

One widely used procedure, called the caloric test, involves electronic monitoring of the patient's eye movements while one ear at a time is irrigated with warm water or warm air, and then with cold water or cold air. This double stimulus causes the endolymph to move in a way similar to that produced by rotation of the head. If the labyrinth is working normally, nystagmus should result. A missing nystagmus reaction is a strong argument that the balance organs are not acting correctly.

NINCDS-supported scientists at the Johns Hopkins University in Baltimore observed that not all patients can tolerate the traditional caloric test. Some become sick when the ear is irrigated with the standard amount of water or air before physicians can measure their eye movements. So the scientists are designing a method of conducting the test more gradually by slowly adjusting the amount of water or air reaching the inner ear. Their goal is to reduce patient discomfort while allowing the test to proceed.

Some patients who cannot tolerate the caloric test are given a rotatory test. In this procedure, the patient sits in a rotating chair head tilted slightly forward. The chair spins rapidly in one direction, then stops abruptly. Depending on the cause of dizziness, the patient may experience vertigo after this rotation.

In one variation of this test, the chair is placed in a tent of striped cloth. As the chair rotates, electrodes record movements of the patient's eyes in response to the stripes. The physician evaluates these eye movements, a form of nystagmus, to determine if the patient has a disorder of the balance system.

Because disorders of balance are often accompanied by hearing loss, the physician may order a hearing test.

Hearing loss and associated dizziness could also be due to damaged nerve cells in the brain stem, where the hearing and balance nerve relays signals to the brain. To detect a malfunction, the physician may order a kind of computerized brain-wave study called a brain stem auditory evoked response test. In this procedure, electrodes are attached to several places on the surface of the patient's scalp and a sound is transmitted to the patient's ear. The electrodes measure the time it takes nerve signals generated by the sound to travel from the ear to the brain stem.

If there is reason to suspect that the dizziness could stem from a tumor or cyst, the patient may undergo a computed tomographic (CT) scan. In a CT scan, x-ray pictures are taken of the brain from several different angles. These images are then combined by a computer to give a detailed view that may reveal the damaging growth.

Sometimes, anxiety and emotional upset cause a person to feel dizzy. Certain patients may be asked to take a psychological test, to try to find out whether the dizziness is caused or intensified by emotional stress.

The many tests administered by a physician will usually point to a cause for the patient's dizziness. Disorders responsible for dizziness can be categorized as:

- peripheral vestibular or those involving a disturbance in the labyrinth.
- central vestibular or those resulting from a problem in the brain or its connecting nerves.
- systemic, or those originating in nerves or organs outside the head.

Confused signals

When someone has vertigo but does not experience faintness or difficulty in walking, the cause is probably a peripheral vestibular disorder. In these conditions, nerve cells in the inner ear send confusing information about body movement to the brain.

Ménières disease. A well-known cause of vertigo is the peripheral vestibular disorder known as Ménière's disease. First identified in

1861 by Prosper Ménière, a French physician, the disease is thought to be caused by too much endolymph in the semicircular canals and vestibule. Some scientists think that the excess endolymph may affect the hair cells so that they do not work correctly. This explanation, however, is still under study.

The vertigo of Ménière's disease comes and goes without an apparent cause; it may be made worse by a change in position and reduced by being still.

In addition to vertigo, patients have hearing loss and tinnitus. Hearing loss is usually restricted at first to one ear and is often severe. Patients sometimes feel "fullness" or discomfort in the ear and diagnostic testing may show unusual sensitivity to increasingly loud sounds. In 10 to 20 percent of patients, hearing loss and tinnitus eventually occur in the second ear.

Ménière's disease patients may undergo electronystagmography, an electrical recording of the caloric test, to determine if their labyrinth is working normally.

Attacks of Ménière's disease may occur several times a month or year and can last from a few minutes to many hours. Some patients experience a spontaneous disappearance of symptoms while others may have attacks for years.

Treatment of Ménière's disease includes such drugs as meclizine hydrochloride and the tranquilizer diazepam to reduce the feeling of intense motion during vertigo. To control the buildup of endolymph, the patient may also take a diuretic, a drug that reduces fluid production. A low-salt diet — which reduces water retention — is claimed to be an effective treatment of Ménière's disease.

When these measures fail to help, surgery may be considered. In shunt surgery, part of the inner ear is drained to reestablish normal inner ear fluid or endolymph pressure. In another operation, called vestibular nerve section, surgeons expose and cut the vestibular part of the eighth nerve. Both vestibular nerve section and shunt surgery commonly relieve the dizziness of Ménière's disease without affecting hearing.

A more drastic operation, labyrinthectomy, involves total destruction of the inner ear. This procedure is usually successful in eliminating dizziness but causes total loss of hearing in the operated ear — an important consideration since the second ear may one day be affected.

Positional vertigo. People with benign positional vertigo experience vertigo after a position change. Barbara noticed the first sign of this disorder one morning when she got up out of bed. She felt the room spinning. Frightened, she quickly returned to bed and lay down. After about 30 seconds the vertigo passed. Fearing a stroke, Barbara went to the emergency room of a hospital for a medical evaluation, which failed to show a problem. She had no symptoms for several days, then the problem returned. At this point, Barbara was referred to an otoneurologist, a physician who specializes in the ear and related parts of the nervous system.

Like Barbara, most patients with benign positional vertigo are extremely worried about their symptoms. But the patients usually feel less threatened once the disorder is diagnosed.

The cause of benign positional vertigo is not known, although some patients may recall an incident of head injury. The condition can strike at any adult age, with attacks occurring periodically throughout a person's life.

In one type of treatment, the patient practices the position that provokes dizziness until the balance system eventually adapts. Rarely, a physician will prescribe medication to prevent attacks.

Vestibular neuronitis. In this common vestibular disorder, the patient has severe vertigo. Jack experienced his first attack of this problem at 2 a.m. when he rolled over in bed and suddenly felt the room spinning violently. He started vomiting but couldn't stand up; finally, he managed to crawl to the bathroom. When he returned to bed, he lay very still — the only way to stop the vertigo. Three days later he was able to walk without experiencing vertigo, but he still felt unsteady. Gradually, over the next several weeks, Jack's balance improved, but it was a year before he was entirely without symptoms.

Unlike Ménière's disease, vestibular neuronitis is not associated with hearing loss. Patients with vestibular neuronitis first experience an acute attack of severe vertigo lasting for hours or days, just as Jack did, with loss of balance sometimes lasting for weeks or months. About half of those who have a single attack have further episodes over a period of months to years.

The cause of vestibular neuronitis is uncertain. Since the first attack often occurs after a viral illness, some scientists believe the disorder is caused by a viral infection of the nerve.

Other labyrinth problems. Inner ear problems with resulting dizziness can also be caused by certain antibiotics used to fight life-threatening bacterial infections. Probably the best-known agent of this group is streptomycin. Problems usually arise when high doses of these drugs are taken for a long time, but some patients experience symptoms after short treatment with low doses, especially if they have impaired kidneys.

The first symptoms of damage to the inner ear caused by medication are usually hearing loss, tinnitus, or unsteadiness while walking. Stopping the drug can usually halt further damage to the balance mechanism, but this is not always possible: the medicine may have to be continued to treat a life-threatening infection. Patients sometimes adapt to the inner ear damage that may occur after prolonged use of these antibiotics and recover their balance.

Balance can also be affected by a cholesteatoma, a clump of cells from the eardrum that grow into the middle ear and accumulate there. These growths are thought to result from repeated infections such as recurrent otitis media. If unchecked, a cholesteatoma can enlarge and threaten the inner ear. But if the growth is detected early, it can be surgically removed.

Brain and nerve damage

The vestibular nerve carries signals from the inner ear to the brain stem. If either the nerve or the brain stem is damaged, information about position and movement may be blocked or incorrectly processed, leading to dizziness. Conditions in which dizziness results from damage to the brain stem or its associated nerves are called central causes of dizziness.

Acoustic neuroma. One central cause of dizziness is a tumor called an acoustic neuroma. Although the most common sign of this growth is hearing loss followed by tinnitus, some patients also experience dizziness.

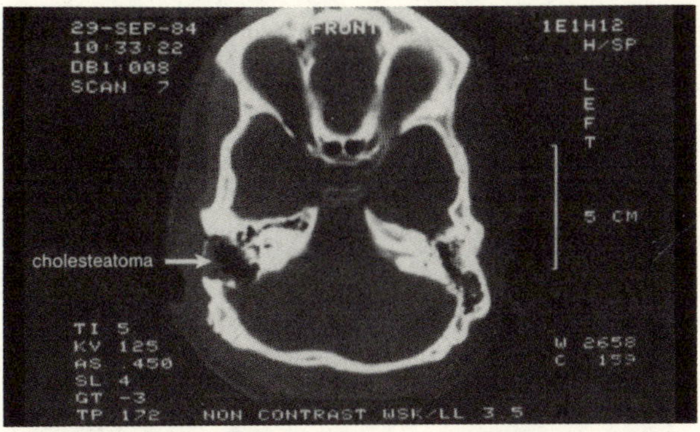

This CT scan shows a massive cholesteatoma (arrow), a tumorlike clump of cells that has grown in the middle ear, and is a likely cause of this patient's dizziness.

An acoustic neuroma usually occurs in the internal auditory canal, the bony channel through which the vestibular nerve passes as it leaves the inner ear. The growing tumor presses on the nerve, sending false messages about position and movement to the brain.

The hearing nerve running alongside the vestibular nerve can also be compressed by the acoustic neuroma, with resulting tinnitus and hearing loss. Or the tumor may press on other nearby nerves, producing numbness or weakness of the face. If the neuroma is allowed to grow, it will eventually reach the brain and may affect the function of other cranial nerves.

Computed tomography has revolutionized the detection of acoustic neuromas. If an early diagnosis is made, a surgeon can remove the tumor. The patient usually regains balance.

Stroke. Dizziness may be a sign of a "small stroke" or transient ischemic attack (TIA) in the brain stem. TIAs, which result from a temporary lack of blood supply to the brain, may also cause transient numbness, tingling, or weakness in a limb or on one side of the face. Other signs include temporary blindness and difficulty with speech. These symptoms are warning signs: one should see a physician immediately for treatment. If a TIA is ignored, a major stroke may follow.

Systemic diseases: underlying illness

Dizziness can be a symptom of diseases affecting body parts other than the brain and central nervous system. Systemic conditions like anemia or high blood pressure decrease oxygen supplies to the brain; a physician eliminates the resulting dizziness by treating the underlying systemic illness.

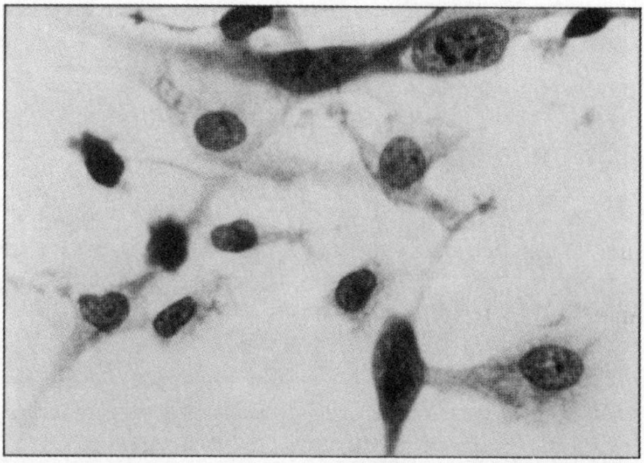

These benign cells from an acoustic neuroma were grown in tissue culture. If diagnosed early, acoustic neuromas can be removed completely with no neurological damage.

Damaged sensory nerves. We maintain balance by adjusting to information transmitted along sensory nerves from sensors in the eyes, muscles, and joints to the spinal cord or brain. When these sensory nerves are damaged by systemic disease, dizziness may result.

Multiple sensory deficits, a systemic disease, is believed by some physicians to be the chief cause of vaguely described dizziness in the aged population. In this disorder several senses or sensory nerves are damaged. The result: faulty balance.

People with diabetes, which can damage nerves affecting vision and touch, may develop multiple sensory deficits. So can patients with arthritis or cataracts, both of which distort how sensory information reaches the brain. The first step in treating multiple sensory deficits is to eliminate symptoms of specific disorders. Permanent contact lenses can improve vision in cataract patients, for example, and medication or surgery may ease pain and stiffness related to arthritis.

Symptoms of damaged sensory nerves may be relieved by a collar to eliminate extreme head motion, balancing exercises to help compensate for sensory losses, or a cane to aid balance. Some patients are helped by the drug methylphenidate, which can increase awareness of remaining sensations.

Systemic neurological disorders such as multiple sclerosis, Alzheimer's disease, Parkinson's disease, or Creutzfeldt-Jakob disease may also cause dizziness, primarily during walking. However dizziness is rarely the sole symptom of these nervous system diseases.

Low blood pressure. One common systemic disease causing dizziness is postural or orthostatic hypotension. In this disease, the heart does not move the blood with enough force to supply the brain adequately. Symptoms include sudden feelings of faintness, light-headedness, or dizziness when standing up quickly.

Because the muscles in aging blood vessels are weak and the arteries inadequate in helping convey blood to the head, older people are particularly susceptible to this condition. Older persons who do not sit or lie down at the first sensation of dizziness may actually lose consciousness.

People who have undetected anemia, or those who are taking diuretics to eliminate excess water from their body and reduce high blood pressure, are also at risk of developing postural hypotension.

A physician can easily diagnose postural hypotension: the patient's blood pressure is measured before standing abruptly and immediately afterward. Treatment is designed to eliminate dizziness by reducing the patient's blood volume.

A secondary symptom. Dizziness may also be a secondary symptom in many other diseases. Faintness accompanied by occasional loss of consciousness can be due to low blood sugar, especially when the faint feeling persists after the patient lies down.

A common cause of mild dizziness — the kind described as light-headedness — is medicine. A number of major prescription drugs may produce light-headedness as a side effect. Two types of drugs that can cause this problem are sedatives, which are taken to induce sleep, and tranquilizers, which are used to calm anxiety.

When anxiety strikes

Tranquilizers may cause a type of dizziness referred to as light-headedness — but so may anxiety. Cynthia is a young woman who becomes light-headed under a variety of stressful circumstances. The light-headedness sometimes is accompanied by heart palpitations and panic. She can produce these symptoms at will by breathing rapidly and deeply for a few minutes.

Cynthia's light-headedness is due to hyperventilation: rapid, prolonged deep breathing or occasional deep sighing that upsets the oxygen and carbon dioxide balance in the blood. The episodes are typically brief and often associated with tingling and numbness in the fingers and around the mouth. Hyperventilation is triggered by anxiety or depression in about 60 percent of dizziness patients.

Once made aware of the source of the symptoms, a patient can avoid hyperventilation or abort attacks by breath-holding or breathing into a paper bag to restore a correct balance of oxygen and carbon dioxide. If hyperventilation is due to anxiety, psychological counseling may be recommended.

Some patients who report dizziness may be suffering from a psychiatric disorder. Generally, these persons will say that they experience light-headedness or difficulty concentrating; they may also describe panic states when in crowded places. Tests of such patients reveal that the inner ear is working correctly. Treatment may include counseling.

Demystifying dizziness through research

Scientists are working to understand dizziness and its sources among the complex interactions of the labyrinth, the other sense organs, and the brain. The research is offering new insights into the basis of balance, as well as improvements in diagnosis, treatment, and prevention of dizziness.

Innovative surgery. Delicate surgical instruments and operating microscopes have made possible new methods to help patients with dizziness. The symptoms of benign positional vertigo, for example, may be relieved by a microsurgical ear operation called a singular neurectomy, in which a tiny portion of the vestibular nerve is divided and cut.

Patients with Ménière's disease may benefit from a microsurgical operation called the cochleosacculotomy. In this procedure, a small curette or wire loop is used to reach into the vestibule of the inner ear and remove the fluid-filled saccule. An investigator at the Massachusetts Eye and Ear Institute in Boston has found that this operation relieves symptoms of vertigo in about 80 percent of patients.

Space biology. Research also promises to help astronauts who suffer from dizziness or space sickness. In one study, a scientist aboard a space shuttle conducted experiments to find out why half the astronauts who have space sickness at the start of a flight overcome this problem before the end of the mission. The investigator from the Massachusetts Institute of Technology found that the space traveler's brain no longer relies on the gravity-sensitive inner ear structures for information about position and motion. Instead, the astronaut's brain realizes that the inner ear is sending false information and starts to depend more on the eyes to find out about the body's movements. This finding may enable space biologists to train astronauts before launch to avoid space sickness.

During that same space mission, a German scientist performed experiments that raised questions about the theory behind the caloric test. According to that theory, alternate heating and cooling of the endolymph causes the fluid to form wave-like swirling patterns called convection currents. These currents make the brain think the head is moving. The result is nystagmus.

In space, however, lack of gravity should prevent convection currents from forming, so the eyes were expected to remain still. Instead, they moved just as though the test were being done on Earth in normal gravity. These experiments indicate there is more than one explanation for why the caloric test works: when the endolymph is warmed, the fluid expands and moves the cupula, the top of the cochlear duct. The movement of the cupula cues the brain that the head is moving, and the eyes respond.

This research helps scientists interpret methods used to test vestibular function. It also promises to increase our understanding of the balance system.

Currently, scientists at the Johnson Space Center in Houston and at the Good Samaritan Hospital in Portland are preparing to study space sickness and vestibular function in a microgravity (near zero gravity) laboratory. The astronauts' vestibular function will be analyzed in a series of experiments, including studies to test whether visual input becomes more important in maintaining balance as weightlessness increases. The scientists anticipate that this research will help all sufferers of motion sickness, not just astronauts.

Improved diagnosis. Back on Earth, improvements are being made in measuring precisely the eye movements of patients undergoing diagnostic tests for dizziness. Investigators at the NINCDS-funded research center at the University of California at Los Angeles have developed a computer-controlled chair in which a patient is shifted into a variety of body positions to stimulate the labyrinth. Eye responses are measured with newly designed computerized instruments. To further stimulate eye movements, a set of computer-generated visual patterns can be moved with the chair or independently of it.

These instruments will extract much information about a patient's ability to integrate information from the eyes and the inner ear, and will help distinguish patients with different disorders of the balance system.

Signaling the brain. To understand dizziness, scientists must find out how stimuli to the labyrinth are translated into information that the brain can use to maintain balance. How, for example, is information from the inner ear sent to the brain and interpreted? Among the scientists studying this question is an NINCDS grantee at the University of Chicago who is looking at the different ways hair cells react to the movement of inner ear fluid. He has identified a characteristic pattern of electrical response in hair cells. The next step is to discover how these messages are interpreted by the nerve cells carrying information to the brain.

Another NINCDS grantee, at the University of Minnesota, is studying the activity of the brain when it sends balance-preserving signals from the sense organs to the muscles. In one experiment, healthy persons are rotated in the dark at a constant rate. After a few minutes they no longer think they are moving. This is because the inner ear only senses changes in the rate of movement. If the lights are turned on and both the inner ear and the room rotate at the same constant speed, again the person doesn't sense movement. Both the ear and the eyes are fooled into thinking there is no motion.

But the investigator found that if the chair and the room are accelerated, the patient develops what is described as sensory conflict. The acceleration of the chair tells the inner ear that there is movement. But the eyes tell the brain that the body is stationary. How patients react in these conflict situations reveals how the brain puts together various types of sensory information to maintain balance. The results of this and related experiments will help scientists build a mathematical model of the balance system.

Hope for the future

For those who are healthy, equilibrium is a sense often taken for granted. People can't see their labyrinth, even though it is as much a sense organ as the ears or the eyes. But when it is injured, an ability vital to everyday living is lost.

Scientists already understand a great deal about the labyrinth's function and the way the brain maintains balance. Further research into this complex system should help those who are incapacitated by dizziness when the balance system goes awry.

Voluntary health organizations

The following organizations provide information on dizziness or on inner ear diseases that cause dizziness:

Acoustic Neuroma Association
P.O. Box 398
Carlisle, PA 17013
(717) 249-4783

American Academy of Otolaryngology-Head and Neck Surgery
Suite 302
1101 Vermont Avenue,
NW. Washington, DC 20005
(202) 289-4607

Better Hearing Institute
P.O. Box 1840
Washington, DC 20013
(703) 642-0580
(800) 424-8576 (Toll free)

National Hearing Association
721 Enterprise
Oak Brook, IL 60521
(312) 323-7200

Human tissue banks

The study of ear tissue from patients with dizziness and deafness is invaluable in research. Temporal bones willed by people with balance or hearing problems and by people with normal hearing can be used to help research scientists and physicians training to be otolaryngologists. Physicians in training study the basic anatomy of the temporal bone and develop their surgical skills. Scientists use the bones for research on the inner ear and on congenital disorders that cause deafness. Middle ear bones (ossicles) and the eardrum are also used as grafts to surgically correct sound transmission problems of the middle ear.

NINCDS supports four temporal bone banks that supply scientists in every state with tissue from patients who have dizziness or deafness. The donated temporal bone includes the eardrum, the entire middle and inner ear, and the nerve tissues which combine into the brain stem. For information about tissue donation and collection, write to:

National Temporal Bone Bank
Eastern Center
Massachusetts Eye and Ear Infirmary
243 Charles Street
Boston, MA 02114
(617) 523-7900, ext. 2711

National Temporal Bone Bank
Midwestern Center
University of Minnesota
Box 396-Mayo
Minneapolis, MN 55455
(612) 624-5466

National Temporal Bone Bank
Southern Center
Baylor College of Medicine
Neurosensory Center — Room A523
Houston, TX 77030
(713) 790-5470

National Temporal Bone Bank Center
Western Center
UCLA School of Medicine
31-24 Rehabilitation Center
Los Angeles, CA 90024
(213) 825-4710

Glossary

acoustic neuroma: tumor of the vestibular nerve that may press on the hearing nerve, causing dizziness and hearing loss.

balance system: complex biological system that enables us to know where our body is in space and to keep the position we want. Proper balance depends on information from the labyrinth in the inner ear, from other senses such as sight and touch, and from muscle movement.

benign positional vertigo: condition in which moving the head to one side or to a certain position brings on vertigo.

brain stem auditory evoked response (BAER): diagnostic test in which electrodes are attached to the surface of the scalp to determine the time it takes inner ear electrical responses to sound to travel from the ear to the brain. The test helps locate the cause of some types of dizziness.

caloric test: diagnostic test in which warm or cold water or air is put into the ear. If a person experiences certain eye movements (nystagmus) after this procedure, the labyrinth is working correctly.

cholesteatoma: a tumor-like accumulation of dead cells in the middle ear. This growth is thought to result from repeated middle ear infections.

computed tomography (CT) scan: radiological examination useful for examining the inside of the ear and head.

diuretic: drug that promotes water loss from the body through the urine. Used to treat hypertension, diuretics may bring on dizziness due to postural hypotension.

dizziness: feeling of physical instability with regard to the outside world.

endolymph: fluid filling part of the labyrinth.

hair cells: specialized nerves found in the semicircular canals and vestibule. Fibers (hairs) sticking out of one end of the hair cells move when the head moves and send information to the brain that is used to maintain balance.

Hyperventilation: repetitive deep breathing that reduces the carbon dioxide content of the blood and brings on dizziness. Anxiety may cause hyperventilation and dizziness.

inner ear: contains the organs of hearing and balance.

labyrinth: organ of balance, which is located in the inner ear. The labyrinth consists of the three semicircular canals and the vestibule.

Ménière's disease: condition that causes vertigo. The disease is believed to be caused by too much endolymph in the labyrinth. Persons with this illness also experience hearing problems and tinnitus.

middle ear: the space immediately behind the eardrum. This part of the ear contains the three bones of hearing: the hammer (malleus), anvil (incus), and stirrup (stapes).

multiple sensory deficits: condition associated with dizziness in which damage to nerves of the eye and arms or legs reduces information about balance to the brain.

neurologist: physician who specializes in disorders of the nervous system.

nystagmus: rapid back-and-forth movements of the eyes. These reflex movements may occur during the caloric tests and are used in the diagnosis of balance problems.

orthostatic hypotension: see *postural hypotension*.

otologist: physician who specializes in diseases of the ear.

peripheral vestibulopathy: vestibular disorder in which the vestibular nerve appears inflamed and paralyzed. Patients may have one or several attacks of vertigo.

postural hypotension (also called *orthostatic hypotension*): sudden dramatic drop in blood pressure when a person rises from a sitting, kneeling, or lying position. The prime symptom of postural hypotension, which is sometimes due to low blood volume, is dizziness or faintness. The condition can be dangerous in older persons, who may faint and injure themselves.

semicircular canals: three curved hollow tubes in the inner ear that are part of the balance organ, the labyrinth. The canals are joined at their wide ends and are filled with endolymph.

stroke: death of nerve cells due to a loss of blood flow in the brain. A stroke often results in permanent loss of some sensation or muscle activity.

TIA: see *transient ischemic attack.*

tinnitus: noises or ringing in the ear.

transient ischemic attack (TIA): temporary interruption of blood flow to a part of the brain. Because a TIA may signal the possibility of a stroke, it requires immediate medical attention. During a TIA, a person may feel dizzy, have double vision, or feel tingling in the hands.

vertigo: severe form of dizziness in which one's surroundings appear to be spinning uncontrollably. Extreme cases of vertigo may be accompanied by nausea.

vestibular disorders: diseases of the inner ear that cause dizziness.

vestibular nerve: nerve that carries messages about balance from the labyrinth in the inner ear to the brain.

vestibular neuronitis: another name for peripheral vestibulopathy.

vestibule: part of the labyrinth, located at the base of the semicircular canals. This structure contains the endolymph and patches of hair cells.

Chapter 11

Epilepsy

Epilepsy

Convulsion, seizure, fit, falling sickness . . . the English language is rich in words that capture the stark drama of a severe epileptic attack. The victim cries out, falls to the floor unconscious, the limbs twitch, saliva bubbles at the mouth. Bladder control may be lost. Within minutes the attack is over. The victim comes to, exhausted, dazed, embarrassed. That is the picture most people have in mind when they hear the word epilepsy. But that type of seizure — the *grand mal* attack — is only one form of epilepsy. There are many other epilepsies, each with characteristic signs and symptoms.

Take Lisa, for example. She is an intelligent 15-year-old high school student with long dark hair and lashes to match. Lisa has suffered from *absence seizures* (sometimes called *petit mal* epilepsy) for some time. In an absence seizure there is a momentary lapse in consciousness. Lisa is briefly "out of it." But there is no dramatic fall. Sometimes there may be purposeless movements — an arm jerk, for example — but in Lisa's case there is no noticeable symptom, not even the blink of an eye. Immediately following the seizure Lisa can resume whatever she was doing. But her attacks happen so often — several hundred times a day — that she cannot concentrate in school and is in danger of failing her sophomore year. Moreover, she is so frightened and ashamed of the attacks that she won't tell her friends what is wrong.

In still a third form of the disorder, commonly called *psychomotor* epilepsy, the patient may laugh, talk strangely, walk around in circles, or make other automatic movements like lip-smacking or chewing. On rare occasions, the victim may strike out at walls or furniture as though angry or afraid. These attacks are also brief. Upon recovery, the individual will be confused and have no memory of what happened.

The strange symptoms and sometimes bizarre behavior of patients with epilepsy have contributed to age-old superstitions and prejudice. As long ago as 400 B.C., Hippocrates repeated the popular folklore that epilepsy was a visitation of the gods — a "sacred disease." He had the wisdom to question folklore, however. Hippocrates suspected that epilepsy was a disorder of the brain. And he was right.

Supercharged cells

Nowadays, scientists know that epilepsy is not a disease with a single cause. Rather, it is a set of symptoms associated with abnormal nerve cell activity in the brain. Normally, each nerve cell (neuron) generates small bursts of electrical impulses. The impulses, moving from neuron to neuron, and communicating with the body's muscles, sense organs, and glands, underlie all human behavior — our thoughts, feelings, actions. The pattern of activity has been likened to tiny flashes of light flicking on and off in the brain, weaving a constantly changing pattern on an "enchanted loom."

In epilepsy, the pattern of nerve cell activity is disturbed. Instead of small bursts of electrical impulses, a group of nerve cells fires a storm of strong bursts like a platoon of soldiers all firing at once. Moreover, the firing comes with machine-gun rapidity. Whereas normal nerve cells generate electrical impulses up to 80 times a second, an epileptic neuron can fire at rates of 500 times a second, disturbing the normal activity of the brain.

If the abnormal activity is confined to only a part of the brain, the seizure is described as partial, and the area of the brain involved is called the epileptic focus. Partial seizures sometimes affect the temporal lobes at the sides of the brain near the ears. Nerve centers there are associated with speech and hearing, with emotions and memory, and so disturbances in this part of the brain can account for the odd movements (automatisms) and behavior of psychomotor seizures.

In contrast, generalized seizures affect the whole brain, resulting in the unconsciousness, convulsions, and subsequent amnesia of a grand mal seizure. Similarly, seizures in absence epilepsy are generalized, with lapses of consciousness and occasional automatisms, but without convulsions. Sometimes, what begins as a partial seizure can develop into a generalized seizure if the abnormal cell behavior spreads throughout the brain.

The epilepsies are classified into subtypes within the broad categories of partial and generalized seizures. (See Table on page 184.) These divisions, and the more accurate descriptive terms neurologists prefer — generalized tonic-clonic seizure instead of grand mal; absence instead of petit mal; complex partial seizure instead of psychomotor seizure — mark important advances in understanding and controlling epilepsy. The more precise classifications of seizures enable physicians to devise better treatments. The good news is that seizures can be successfully controlled in over half the patients with epilepsy through daily medication with antiepileptic drugs.

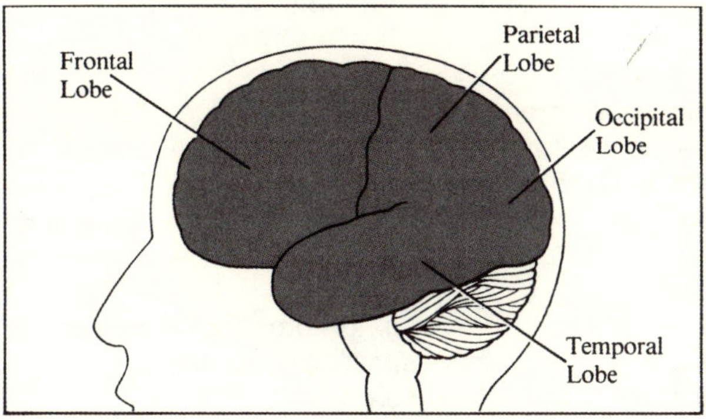

The principal lobes of the human cerebral cortex.

The story of the ongoing conquest of epilepsy is closely bound up with the history of neurology. Epilepsy is the second most prevalent neurological disorder in the United States (following stroke). Over 2 million Americans at present have epilepsy: one out of 100 persons. A century ago conditions were far worse. Not only were there few treatments, but epileptic patients were regarded as undesirables whose condition might be contagious. Many patients were placed in hospitals or institutions "for epileptics only." Faced with the challenge of so many suffering souls, pioneering neurologists of the 19th century turned their attention to the disorder and began the search for causes and cures that continues in the present.

Taking the lead in epilepsy research in America today is the National Institute of Neurological and Communicative Disorders and Stroke (NINCDS), one of the 11 Institutes of the National Institutes of Health in Bethesda, Md. Through the Epilepsy Branch of its Neurological Disorders Program, the Institute supports basic and clinical research on epilepsy throughout the country and conducts a vigorous drug screening and development program. The Institute's own clinical research activities include intensive study of epilepsy patients in its intramural program at the Clinical Center, the research hospital of the National Institutes of Health, and the support of several Comprehensive Epilepsy Programs located in the major geographic regions of the country. Individuals screened at these facilities may participate as outpatients or as inpatients in clinical research studies. The Comprehensive Epilepsy Programs also provide training for health professionals in all phases of research, care, and treatment for epilepsy.

International Classification of Epileptic Seizures

Generalized Seizures
- Tonic-clonic (grand mal)
- Absence (petit mal)
- Infantile spasms
- Other (myoclonic seizures, akinetic seizures, undetermined, etc.)

Partial Seizures
- Simple partial seizures (e.g., disturbances in movement only)
- Complex partial seizures (psychomotor, other)
- Secondarily generalized seizures

The table is a condensed form of the new internationally accepted descriptive terms and classifications of epileptic seizures.

Is it epilepsy?

Two steps are vital in screening and treating patients with suspected epilepsy. One, obvious but nontrivial, is a confirmation of the diagnosis. The second is a precise description of the pattern of seizures: their type or types, frequency, and duration.

Sometimes a child has a convulsion during the course of illness with high fever. Sometimes an adult has a seizure in reaction to anesthesia or a strong drug. Neither individual can be said to have epilepsy unless seizures recur in the absence of the original triggering event.

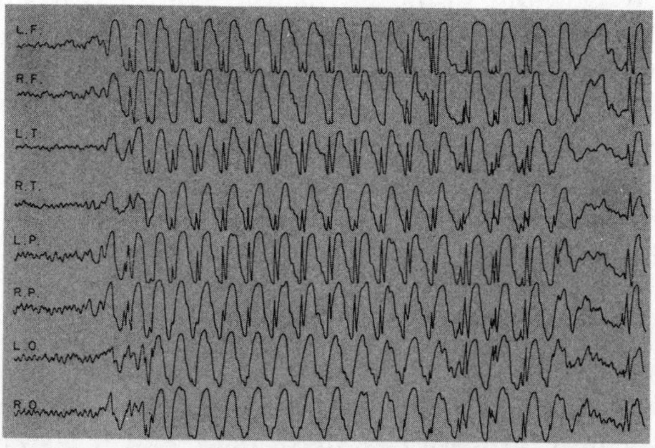

At far left are normal brain wave patterns recorded from eight sites in the brain. They are followed by the steep "spike and wave" EEG pattern associated with absence seizures.

Sometimes patients with certain forms of mental illness show behavior that mimics a complex partial seizure. Other individuals with psychological problems may suffer seizures, even what appear to be generalized tonic-clonic attacks, but their brain cells show no abnormal activity. These "psychogenic" seizures indicate that the patient has serious problems such as the need for attention, dependency, or the avoidance of stress, but the condition is not epilepsy.

In making a diagnosis of epilepsy, physicians are guided by some general rules-of-thumb. Three-fourths of all patients with epilepsy have their first attacks before the age of 18. Usually a parent will bring a child to the family doctor and describe the symptoms, helpfully noting when seizures occur and how long they last. While this information is enormously useful, the most secure confirmation of the diagnosis can only come from observation of a seizure together with electrical recordings that show the abnormal brain cell activity. These recordings are the familiar wavy line tracings of the electroencephalogram (EEG) obtained from electrodes placed on the surface of the patient's head.

Many cases of epilepsy develop for no known reason. Sometimes the disorder runs in families, as in absence epilepsy, which always has its onset in children or young people. On the whole, however, genetic factors are considered to play a secondary role, as contributing or predisposing factors to epilepsy rather than a primary cause. Epilepsy can occur as a complication of infection, head injury, or other

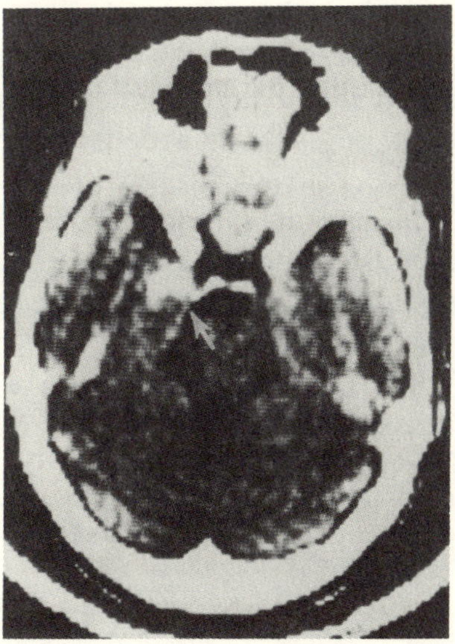

The arrow points to a lesion in the left temporal lobe that showed up in this CT scan of an epilepsy patient.

conditions affecting the brain. Epilepsy may also be associated with cerebral palsy, mental retardation, or rarer neurological conditions such as tuberous sclerosis. For these reasons, the examining physician will always make an exhaustive search for underlying causes.

A CT scan — a computerized X-ray image of the brain — may show up a tumor or cyst, for example, or reveal excess fluid in the brain — hydrocephalus. If these conditions can be treated successfully, the seizures may stop. A lumbar puncture, in which cerebrospinal fluid is withdrawn from the spinal cord, may reveal the presence of infection or other abnormalities. In any case, a thorough medical history of the patient, including details of birth and the health of other family members will be taken, and a battery of physical, mental, and neurological tests will be conducted.

The unique pattern

Every epileptic patient is unique in the symptoms, frequency, duration, and type (or types) of seizures he or she experiences. It is essential to describe the seizure pattern in detail because it is on that basis that the physician will determine treatment. Drugs used to treat epilepsy are selected according to the type of seizure the patient experiences. Other forms of treatment, such as surgery, may be appropriate for carefully selected patients with particular forms of epilepsy.

Some patients, particularly ones with complex partial seizures, experience a distinctive warning sign before a seizure, called an aura. The aura is itself a form of partial seizure, but one in which the patient retains awareness. Sometimes the warning sign may be a peculiar odor, a feeling in the pit of the stomach, or a sound. One neurologist describes a patient who was an ardent racetrack gambler. The man invariably heard the roar of the crowd followed by the name of the favorite in the race just before falling unconscious. Another patient heard rock music. Because patients retain consciousness during the aura, they occasionally may be able to learn methods of warding off the more severe attack.

Drugs are the answer for the majority of patients whose seizures can be controlled, however, and the sizable gains that have been made in recent years can be chalked up to the availability of more and better drugs administered in doses suited to the individual patient.

Taking the seizure's measure

In 1966, NINCDS began a research program of intensive long-term EEG monitoring of epilepsy patients. Electrodes placed on the patient's head transmit brain-wave data to nearby recording equipment. At the same time a television camera provides both full length and head views of the patient as he or she sits, lies, eats, or sleeps over the course of the day. The video image is displayed on a screen along with the brain wave recordings so that observers can simultaneously compare the EEG tracings with the patient's behavior. The recording sessions are 6 hours long and continue daily over a period of months.

Intensive monitoring has led to an extensive library of invaluable data on epilepsy and has paid off for many a patient whose seizures had been intractable — impossible to control. Often such patients experience seizures that are difficult to classify — a complex partial seizure that looks like an absence spell, for example, or vice versa. Interestingly, in some patients intensive monitoring shows up occasional abnormalities in the EEG between seizures. The technique also reveals that many epileptic patients experience psychogenic seizures some of the time. Sometimes, too, the EEG shows an epileptiform pattern but the patient shows no outward signs of a seizure.

Refinements in technology have made it possible to free the patient from the hospital setting and still conduct long-term EEG monitoring. The brain wave signals are detected by electrodes fitted into headgear that the patient wears. The signals are then amplified and converted to electronic signals stored on a tape recorder cassette that the patient also wears while moving about at home, school or work. Automated analysis of EEG data is also an improvement in technology, allowing reliable data to be derived from the recordings without an observer having to study the tapes hour after hour.

The treatment program

Knowledge of the types of seizures a patient suffers paves the way for effective treatment. There are now 16 antiepileptic drugs on the market. Some work on several different types of seizure. Others, especially some of the new drugs, are suited to specific types of epilepsy.

The history of drugs in the treatment of epilepsy is a spotty one. The first effective antiepileptic drugs were bromides, introduced by an astute English physician, Sir Charles Locock, in 1857. He noted that the bromides had a sedative effect and seemed to reduce seizures in some patients. Over 50 years later came phenobarbital, introduced as a sedative in 1912. Phenobarbital and related compounds quickly proved superior to the bromides in controlling seizures, and side effects were less severe. Surprisingly, these early drugs were useful in treating the most severe form of epilepsy — grand mal — as well as partial seizures. They had no effect on absence epilepsy.

The next advances waited until the thirties and forties, when the pharmaceutical industry began to grow rapidly and scientists developed ways of testing the anticonvulsant properties of drugs in experimental animals. Phenytoin (Dilantin®) was introduced in 1938 and remains a drug of major importance in treating grand mal and partial seizures. Other drugs were introduced in the fifties and sixties but, by the late sixties and seventies, there was a marked decline in new drug research. Amendments to the food and drug laws in 1962 required that new drugs had to be proven to be effective as well as safe. The new rules, plus the opinion that the market for new antiepileptic drugs was too small to warrant the investment in time or money, discouraged antiepileptic drug research as a commercial enterprise.

To remedy that situation, NINCDS supported the clinical testing of several promising compounds in the late sixties and early seventies, and thus facilitated the introduction of carbamazepine (Tegretol®) in 1974 and clonazepam (Clonopin®) in 1975 to the general public. That experience led to the establishment of an Antiepileptic Drug Development Program that includes an Anticonvulsant Screening Project within the Epilepsy Branch of NINCDS. Institute scientists have now screened over 4,000 compounds submitted by research chemists in universities or private industry. When a compound appears promising, NINCDS will cooperate with developers in conducting the next steps in drug development: toxicity studies in animals; analysis of how the drug works and how it affects behavior; and, eventually, clinical testing in normal volunteers and in patients.

Reports in the mid-seventies that valproic acid was a highly effective drug in treating absence seizures and was already available in Europe led NINCDS to press for licensing of the drug in the United States. NINCDS-supported clinical trials were among the data presented to the Food and Drug Administration that helped expedite approval of the drug in 1978.

Tailoring the dosage

Even when the neurologist is armed with an accurate picture of a patient's seizures, the drugs prescribed may not work. The seizures may be too varied and too frequent, the drugs may simply not help particular individuals, or side effects may be too toxic. Sometimes the problem is one of dosage, however, or of finding the right combination of drugs administered in the right proportion at the right time of day. For these reasons, patients with intractable seizures who undergo long-term EEG monitoring also have frequent blood samples taken to measure the amount of drug circulating in the bloodstream. At the beginning of the study, a patient may be weaned off all medication. Then drugs may be introduced gradually, increasing the amounts or changing the medication to arrive at the ideal treatment: dosages sufficient to control seizures with a minimum of side effects. Similar studies to devise the best medication program are highly recommended for all epilepsy patients.

Surgery to remove an epileptic focus in the brain is sometimes successful in preventing seizures in patients whose epilepsy cannot be controlled by drugs. In deciding which patients may benefit, surgeons will consider the location of the brain area involved and its importance in everyday behavior. Neurosurgeons will avoid operating in areas of the brain that will interfere with speech, language, hearing or other major faculties.

Occasionally, surgery is performed to sever the connections between the two halves of the brains, the cerebral hemispheres. Such surgery can prevent the spread of abnormal discharges from one side of the brain to the other. Usually, such drastic surgery has little effect on behavior. Patients go about their normal activities as usual. It was only when research scientists began to set up experiments that deliberately studied what each half of the brain contributed to behavior that they discovered that the hemispheres were not like Siamese twins, identical in every way. While there is considerable similarity in structure, each hemisphere has special abilities and makes its own contribution to how a person sees, feels, or acts in the world. This is another instance of how concern for epilepsy has opened the door to new and fascinating discoveries about the nervous system.

In addition to drugs and surgery, treatment for epilepsy has also included special diets and new psychological approaches. Some years ago, it was discovered that a diet rich in fats and low in carbohydrates led to a condition in the body called ketosis that benefits some epilepsy patients. Unfortunately most people hate the diet. It makes them feel sick and they lose weight.

One psychological approach to treating epilepsy involves training patients in methods that might allow them to control their brain waves. In the experimental technique called biofeedback, patients learn to correlate brain cell activity with visual images or sounds that are provided. They try to modify the sights or sounds and in this way alter the electrical activity in the brain. Biofeedback appears to help some patients, but how and why it does so remain tantalizing questions.

The patient as a person

Sometimes people with epilepsy achieve complete control of seizures in the hospital only to have frequent seizures when they return home. The problem may be failure to take medication. Such "noncompliance" is not uncommon, especially in young people who may rebel against the idea that anything is wrong with them. Antiepileptic drugs are strong and can have unwanted side effects such as drowsiness, nausea, or other unpleasantness. One antiepileptic drug has a tendency to increase appetite. Many patients gain weight when taking it — enough to discourage use of the drug.

When a patient is at home there are other factors that may increase the chances of having seizures. The normal pressures of everyday living may create stresses that can trigger seizures. On the other hand, the child who cannot participate fully in school activities, or the adult who cannot drive a car or suffers occasional seizures at work, may feel rejected, depressed, angry or frustrated — often a combination of emotional states that can lower the threshold for seizures.

Recent findings about patients monitored at home point up the relations between mental states and seizure activity. In one study it was noted that children with absence seizures tended to have more seizures at times when they were bored or idle, not when they were fully occupied or interested in some activity. Seizure activity also tended to increase during family discussions of their problem, or even when donning the headgear and cassette and thus being reminded of their condition.

Doctors and others who work closely with patients know that the problems the individual with epilepsy faces do not end with medication. The psychological, social, vocational and emotional needs of patients — and those close to them — are equally important.

The Comprehensive Epilepsy Programs established by NINCDS were designed to evaluate the multiple needs of epileptic patients and families, to encourage clinical research, and to demonstrate to health professionals how to improve the quality of care. Patients are seen by a multidisciplinary team of specialists: neurologists, psychologists, social workers, educators, rehabilitation experts — who pool their observations and devise an individualized program of total physical and psychological rehabilitation. The goal for patients who are accepted for long-term inpatient care is high: When the patient leaves the hospital, his or her seizures should be in good control and the patient able to participate more effectively in society — go to school, find employment, or work at home with a newfound ability to live more fully and independently.

The concept of comprehensive centers arose from the memory of the old hospitals labeled "for epileptics only" a century ago. Leading investigators thought, instead of maintaining permanent holding areas for epileptic patients, why not create way stations where individuals would be welcomed, provided with a full array of services, and discharged to a better life?

Most patients accepted in Comprehensive Epilepsy Programs in the United States are teenagers or young adults with intractable seizures. Those of school age spend part of their days in a classroom working with specially trained teachers. The atmosphere is relaxed and informal. Patients also work with physical and occupational therapists, psychologists, and other staff members to gain self-confidence and learn new skills. Lisa, the frightened 15-year-old, is now a patient in a Comprehensive Epilepsy Program conducted by the University of Virginia in Charlottesville.

An important part of the program is training the patient in the use of medication. Step by step, the patients learn what medications they must use and how to select their daily intake of drugs from the medication cart and set up their own "pill box." Eventually they assume complete responsibility for maintaining their medication and taking their drugs.

The rehabilitation of patients also entails education and counseling for family members. Like the patient, family members must learn to live with epilepsy and neither pamper nor blame the patient — nor anyone else — for the disorder.

The educational process cannot stop with patients and families alone. Even enlightened societies seem mired in the Dark Ages at times, with ignorance and attitudes of fear and rejection of patients with epilepsy. The excellent work of health voluntary organizations such as the Epilepsy Foundation of America has done much to combat ignorance and prejudice through publications, films, radio and television spots, and other activities aimed at public and professionals alike. These efforts gained impetus with the establishment of the congressionally mandated Commission for the Control of Epilepsy and Its Consequences in 1976. The commission, composed of a cross section of lay and professional people from the continental United States and Puerto Rico, submitted its report to the president and to Congress with recommendations for research, care, and treatment of epilepsy patients, as well as programs of education and prevention aimed at society at large.

As a result, the stigma attached to epilepsy has slowly begun to abate and there has been a renewed research effort to solve the riddle of epilepsy. NINCDS can now report that many of the commission's recommendations applicable to the institute have been carried out, and research directed at all phases of understanding and treating epilepsy has been measurably increased.

The research view

Fundamental research on epilepsy focuses on why neurons in the brain become epileptic, how such neurons are able to recruit neighboring cells in spreading the abnormal discharge, and what can be done about it. The research has benefitted from a battery of new tools and techniques that have emerged in the past decade or so. For example, investigators have been able to create new animal models of epilepsy. Exposure of certain species of animals to repeated electrical stimulation of their brains appears to sensitize certain cells. This "kindling" of cells later leads to the spontaneous generation of seizures. Injections of certain chemicals into the brain can also induce spontaneous seizures.

To understand the microscopic events that make a normal nerve cell epileptic, neuroscientists have isolated individual cells and grown them in tissue culture. They can then expose the cells to a variety of drugs and chemicals and observe what happens. Scientists have also dissected and studied cell parts. For example, the nerve cell membrane is crucial both in generating electrical impulses inside a nerve cell and in conducting impulses between cells. Not surprisingly, then, much research in epilepsy — indeed in all neuroscience today — focuses on details of membrane structure, on how molecules move in and out of membranes, and on how the cell body nourishes and repairs the membrane.

The ability of electrical impulses to move from cell to cell also depends on a series of chemical events occurring in the nerve cell. The nerve impulse generated inside a neuron starts its journey to the next cell along a long thin fiber that extends from the cell body. That fiber, the axon, ends a short distance away from the neighboring cell. To aid the electrical impulse to cross that little gap, called the synapse, scientists now know that the parent cell secretes tiny packets of chemicals called neurotransmitters from the axon tip. These molecules excite the second cell in such a way that it can generate an electrical impulse. Not all neurotransmitters are "exciters," however. Sometimes the chemicals inhibit the neighboring cell so that it cannot fire off an electrical impulse.

Some authorities now believe that epilepsy may occur sometimes because there is not enough of an important inhibitory transmitter in the brain. Without a means to curb their behavior, the nerve cells may go haywire, creating an electrical storm. The finding that the new drug valproic acid enhances the effects of a major inhibitory transmitter in the brain called GABA, short for gamma-aminobutyric acid, lends support to the idea.

Much of the basic research on the mechanisms of epilepsy involves drug studies. Scientists do not yet understand how anti-epileptic drugs work. Therefore many chemical experiments with epileptic and normal neurons make use of phenobarbital, phenytoin, or other anticonvulsants in order to get a better understanding of what these drugs do in the brain.

Other lively areas of research on epilepsy concern brain cell metabolism: What nutrients do nerve cells need? How do they store and use energy? Ultimately, the source of energy for nerve cells is

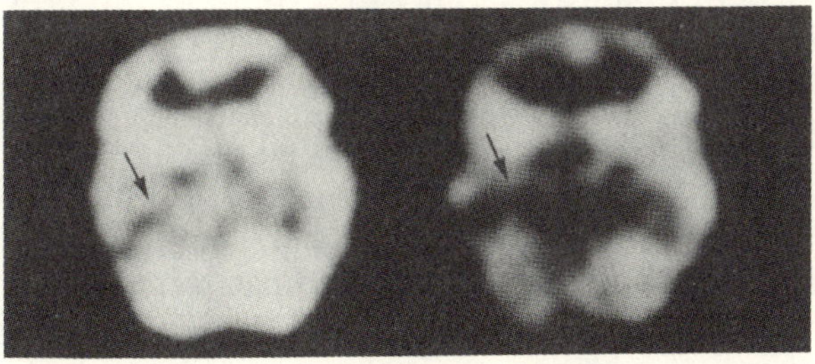

PET scans compare the same brain section during a seizure (left arrow) and between seizures (right arrow). Highly active epileptic neurons take up radioactive glucose which emits gamma rays, producing the light-colored area at central left in the left scan. That same area shows less nerve cell activity (darker image) in the scan at the right.

the blood supply to the brain, so investigators are studying cerebral blood flow in normal individuals and epileptic patients. Some neurologists believe that the depletion of energy reserves in the brain following a major seizure may lead to further damage to nerve cells. Such depletions may be especially critical in children or young adults whose brains are still actively growing.

Among the exciting new techniques for studying metabolic changes in the living brain is a new form of brain imaging called positron emission tomography (PET). The technique is based on the fact that active brain cells are high energy users, burning fuel. The animal or human subject is injected with a nutrient substance like glucose, a form of sugar used by the brain. The sugar molecules are labelled with a harmless radioactive element. The brain cells that are most active will take up more of the labelled sugar and then broadcast their location in the brain by virtue of their radioactivity: Detectors placed outside the head pick up the high-energy gamma rays emitted by the cells. A computer analyzes the data and produces a color-coded image of the brain so that the active areas show up as "hot" spots, bright in color compared to surrounding tissue. Investigators hope that PET studies will reveal any short- or long-term changes in the brain associated with seizure activity. Potentially, positron emission tomography should play an important role in evaluating new therapies and in other research studies in animals and human patients.

Is epilepsy inevitable?

While the search goes on to find out how and why brain cells become epileptic and to devise better means of treatment, concerned individuals and groups have argued forcefully for programs of prevention. Many cases of epilepsy need never happen.

Prevention of epilepsy applies first of all to the pregnant woman. Good prenatal care, adequate diet, avoidance of cigarettes, alcohol, and other drugs, quality care at the time of labor and delivery — all are ways of improving the chances that a newborn arrives in the world healthy and at full term. The developing nervous system is especially vulnerable to shortages of oxygen. Some specialists believe that some cases of epilepsy that show up later in life may be due to oxygen deficiencies in the brain at critical times in early development.

Prevention also means pressing the fight against infection, especially against those organisms that show a predilection for the nervous system. Bacterial meningitis is still a serious problem in infancy, all too often leaving the lifelong complication of epilepsy in its wake. Infections and parasites are a major problem in the many parts of the world where medical treatment is scanty and immunization programs rare. Conditions like tuberculosis and malaria still flourish in many countries, and malaria alone gives rise to thousands of cases of epilepsy worldwide every year.

While Western nations may have less to worry about in terms of infectious and parasitic causes of epilepsy, they must and can do more to prevent accidental head injury. The Epilepsy Foundation of America calculates that 8,000 new cases of epilepsy occur every year as a result of head trauma. Half of those cases result from motor vehicle accidents. Improved safety devices, lowering the speed limit, and the mandatory use of helmets for motorcyclists are demonstrated ways of lowering the toll of head injuries on the nation's roads. The use of protective headgear in competitive sports is equally important in preventing head injury.

Prevention also applies to the individual who has a first seizure. It is vital to seek early diagnosis and treatment. Not only can early examination determine if the patient has epilepsy, it can also establish a course of treatment. Medication may forestall future seizures and may also prevent any secondary damage to the brain from uncontrolled seizures.

The child who has a seizure during a bout of illness with high fever — the so-called "febrile seizure" — is a special case. In the past, some physicians routinely prescribed prophylactic treatment — daily medication with phenobarbital or other antiepileptic drugs — as a preventive measure. Other physicians thought that seizures accompanying fever were not necessarily signs of future epilepsy, but complications of the infection that would leave no lasting effects. Further, they thought that the long-term use of powerful antiepileptic drugs in children might in itself prove damaging to the developing brain, in addition to having annoying side effects. In 1980, experts met at the National Institutes of Health to discuss the issue. The consensus of the meeting was that prophylactic treatment was generally not necessary in children with fever-related seizures unless certain other conditions were present: a history of epilepsy in other members of the family; signs of nervous system impairment; or a more complicated pattern of seizure that suggested future problems.

Preventive treatment with antiepileptlc drugs also has been tried in a clinical research study of patients with head injuries. One group of patients was given antiepileptic medication while a matched control group was not. Patients in the drug group did experience fewer seizures, but the total number of patients treated was small, and further studies are indicated.

If you have epilepsy

Anyone personally concerned with epilepsy should first of all seek medical treatment. The existence of the Comprehensive Epilepsy Programs and of comparable centers throughout the country means that highly sophisticated care, especially for the most difficult or intractable cases, is within reach.

You, as a patient with epilepsy, and your close friends and relatives also owe it to yourselves to be informed about the disorder. The battle against superstition and prejudice begins at home. The NINCDS and voluntary agencies such as the Epilepsy Foundation of America, are your strong allies in providing information and advice on all phases of living with the disorder. Included in that advice is the simple information of what to do — and what not to do — in case of a seizure. Federal law is also your strong ally. New legislation prohibits discrimination against the handicapped in employment by any firm receiving any amount of federal funds. Similar antidiscrimination laws require that all buildings, programs, or facilities funded in part by the federal government must provide access for the handicapped. This means that individuals with epilepsy cannot be denied access to educational, recreational, or other activities on the grounds of a history of seizures.

Thus, slowly but surely, society is freeing many of its valuable members from the bonds of ignorance and prejudice that have kept them out of the mainstream. As knowledge advances and better treatments appear, more and more people with epilepsy will cease to think of themselves as patients and will participate fully in the art of living.

Health voluntary organizations

The major health voluntary organization devoted to epilepsy research, care, treatment, and education is the Epilepsy Foundation of America. The national office and local chapters provide information, publications, and advice to all concerned with seizure disorders.

Epilepsy Foundation of America
4351 Garden City Drive
Landover, Md. 20785
(301)459-3700

The National Easter Seal Society, Inc., provides information and services through its member clinics. Epilepsy is frequently a complication of cerebral palsy and other handicapping disorders and the society's clinics offer rehabilitative and other services.

National Easter Seal Society, Inc.
2023 West Ogden Avenue
Chicago, Ill. 60602
(312)243-8400

The National Head Injury Foundation, Inc. is a new organization developing programs of education and prevention of head injury as well as of support and rehabilitation of patients and families.

The National Head Injury Foundation, Inc.
280 Singletary Lane
Framingham, Mass. 01701
(617) 879-7473

Human tissue banks

The study of brain and other tissue from persons with neurological disorders is invaluable in research, especially in conditions like epilepsy, where the cause is obscure. NINCDS supports two national specimen banks, one in Los Angeles and one near Boston. For information about tissue donation and collection write:

Dr. Wallace Tourtellotte, Director
Human Neurospecimen Bank
VA Wadsworth Hospital Center
Los Angeles, Calif. 90073

Dr. Edward D. Bird, Director
Brain Tissue Bank
Mailman Research Center
McLean Hospital
115 Mill Street
Belmont, Mass. 02178

NINCDS information

For additional information concerning epilepsy research conducted through the Epilepsy Branch of NINCDS, direct inquiries to:

Office of Scientific and Health Reports
National Institute of Neurological and
Communicative Disorders and Stroke
National Institutes of Health
Building 31, Room 8A-06
Bethesda, Md. 20205
(301) 496-5751

Chapter 12

Friedreich's Ataxia

Friedreich's Ataxia

What is Friedreich's ataxia?

Friedreich's ataxia is an inherited disease of the central nervous system, first identified in the early 1860s by Nikolaus Friedreich of Heidelberg, Germany. Symptoms usually begin in childhood or youth as the result of deterioration in areas of the brain controlling muscle coordination, the spinal cord, and nerves. People with Friedreich's ataxia usually suffer from reduced muscle coordination and an irregular gait. Both arms and legs may become weak, and tasks requiring good coordination, like writing, may become difficult. There may be impaired speech. The spine may begin to curve to one side and the feet may become rigid or deformed. There may be numbness and loss of sensation in all parts of the body, and some patients experience vision and hearing problems. A few patients suffer mental impairment. Diabetes is present in many Friedreich's ataxia patients and, in some patients, the heart muscles may be weakened.

How often does the disease occur?

Friedreich's ataxia is not common. According to a recent survey, there are about 8,600 patients in the United States with the disorder.

What causes Friedreich's ataxia?

Friedreich's ataxia is caused by an abnormality in one of the genes — the biological "building blocks" that are passed from parents to their children and that determine a person's physical characteristics, from the color of the hair and eyes to the organization of the nervous system. The disorder develops only when a person inherits the defective gene from both parents. This is called a recessive inheritance pattern. If only one parent contributes a defective gene, the child becomes a "carrier" of Friedreich's ataxia but never develops the disorder. Carriers appear neurologically normal, and sometimes may not know they are carriers until an afflicted child is born to them.

The precise chemical abnormality in the gene responsible for Friedreich's ataxia has not yet been discovered. Nor is there yet any test to identify carriers or to detect Friedreich's ataxia in a child before birth.

Can patients expect to recover from the disease?

Occasionally Friedreich's ataxia appears to have become arrested, and these remissions may last 5 to 10 years or longer. However, in most cases the disease is slowly but steadily progressive. Most patients are seriously incapacitated within 20 years of the beginning of symptoms. The average age of death used to be 36 years, but modern hygiene and heart care have lengthened the average life span. Nearly three-quarters of deaths are from heart failure.

Can Friedreich's ataxia be treated?

As with many degenerative diseases of the nervous system, there is no specific treatment. Exercise may be beneficial, especially for people whose illness begins later in life and develops more slowly. In the exceptional case, braces can be useful for foot drop, and surgical fixation of a joint by fusion of the joint surfaces (arthrodesis) may be of value. A good, normal diet should be followed. Some of the complications of Friedreich's ataxia, such as diabetes and a weak heart, are treatable.

What research is being done?

The National Institute of Neurological and Communicative Disorders and Stroke (NINCDS), a unit of the National Institutes of Health and the agency within the federal government with primary responsibility for brain research, sponsors research on various forms of ataxia. NINCDS-supported studies encompass enzyme metabolism, genetic investigations, and efforts to find animals in which the ataxias can be induced experimentally and studied in the laboratory. The ultimate goal of NINCDS research is to prevent Friedreich's ataxia through greater understanding of how the normal nervous system works, and discovery of the specific malfunction that gives rise to this disorder.

Several nongovernment organizations also support research, along with their patient service and educational programs.

Is help available?

Yes. Three private voluntary health agencies are active in the field of Friedreich's ataxia. They are:

> Friedreich's Ataxia Group in America, Inc.
> P.O. Box 11116
> Oakland, California 94611
> (415) 658-7014

National Ataxia Foundation
6681 Country Club Drive
Minneapolis, Minnesota 55427
(612) 546-6220

Muscular Dystrophy Association, Inc.
810 Seventh Avenue
New York, New York 10019
(212) 586-0808

You may wish to contact them for any additional information they can provide.

Chapter 13

Headache

Headache

For 2 years, Jim suffered the excruciating pain of cluster headaches. Night after night he paced the floor, the pain driving him to constant motion. He was only 48 years old when the clusters forced him to quit his job as a systems analyst. One year later, his headaches are controlled. The credit for Jim's recovery belongs to the medical staff of a headache clinic. Physicians there applied the latest research findings on headache, and prescribed for Jim a combination of new drugs.

• Joan was a victim of frequent migraine. Her headaches lasted 2 days. Nauseated and weak, she stayed in the dark until each attack was over. Today, although migraine still interferes with her life, she has fewer attacks and less severe headaches than before. A specialist prescribed an antimigraine program for Joan that included improved drug therapy, a new diet and relaxation training.

• An avid reader, Peggy couldn't put down the new mystery thriller. After 4 hours of reading slumped in bed, she knew she had overdone it. Her tensed head and neck muscles felt as if they were being squeezed between two giant hands. But for Peggy, the muscle-contraction headache and neck pain were soon relieved by a hot shower and aspirin.

An estimated 40 million Americans experience chronic headaches. For at least half of these people, the problem is severe and sometimes disabling. It can also be costly: headache sufferers make over 8 million visits a year to doctor's offices. Migraine victims alone lose over 64 million workdays because of headache pain.

Understanding why headaches occur and improving headache treatment are among the research goals of the National Institute of Neurological and Communicative Disorders and Stroke (NINCDS). As the focal point for brain research in the federal government, the NINCDS also supports and conducts studies to improve the diagnosis of headaches and to find ways to prevent them.

Why does it hurt?

What hurts when you have a headache? Several areas of the head can hurt, including a network of nerves which extends over the scalp, and certain nerves in the face, mouth, and throat. Also sensitive to pain, because they contain delicate nerve fibers, are the muscles of the head and blood vessels found along the surface and at the base of the brain.

The bones of the skull and tissues of the brain itself, however, never hurt, because they lack pain-sensitive nerve fibers.

The ends of these pain-sensitive nerves, called ociceptors, can be stimulated by stress, muscular tension, dilated blood vessels, and other triggers of headache. Once stimulated, a nociceptor sends a message up the length of the nerve fiber to the nerve cells in the brain, signaling that a part of the body hurts. The message is determined by the location of the nociceptor. A person who suddenly realizes "My toe hurts," is responding to nociceptors in the foot that have been stimulated by the stubbing of a toe.

A number of chemicals help transmit pain-related information to the brain. Some of these chemicals are natural painkilling proteins called endorphins, Greek for "the morphine within." One theory suggests that people who suffer from severe headache and other types of chronic pain have lower levels of endorphins than people who are generally pain free.

When you should see a physician

Not all headaches require medical attention. Some result from missed meals or occasional muscle tension and are easily remedied. But some types of headache are signals of more serious disorders, such as head injury, and call for prompt medical care. These include

- Sudden, severe headache
- Headache associated with convulsions
- Headache accompanied by confusion or loss of consciousness
- Headache following a blow on the head
- Headache associated with pain in the eye or ear
- Persistent headache in a person who was previously headache free
- Recurring headache in children
- Headache associated with fever
- Headache which interferes with normal life

A headache sufferer usually seeks help from a family practitioner. If the problem is not relieved by standard treatments, the patient may then be referred to a specialist — perhaps an internist or neurologist. Additional referrals may be made to psychologists.

Diagnosis: What the physician looks for

Diagnosing a headache is like playing "Twenty Questions". Experts agree that a detailed question-and-answer session with a patient can often produce enough information for a diagnosis. Many types of headaches have clear-cut symptoms which fall into an easily recognizable pattern.

Patients may be asked: How often do you have head-aches? Where is the pain? How long do the headaches last? When did you first develop headaches?

The patient's sleep habits and family and work situations may also be probed.

Most physicians will also obtain a full medical history from the patient, inquiring about past head trauma or surgery and about the use of medications. A blood test may be ordered to screen for thyroid disease, anemia, or infections which might cause a headache. X rays may be taken to rule out the possibility of a brain tumor or blood clot.

A test called an electroencephalogram (EEG) may be given to measure brain activity. EEGs can indicate a malfunction in the brain, but they cannot usually pinpoint a problem that might be causing a headache.

A physician may suggest that a patient with unusual headaches undergo a computed tomographic (CT) scan. The CT scan produces images of the brain that show variations in the density of different types of tissue. The scan enables the physician to distinguish, for example, between a bleeding blood vessel in the brain and a brain tumor. The CT scan is an important diagnostic tool in cases of headache associated with brain lesions or other serious disease. Experts generally agree, however, that this sophisticated and expensive technology is not required to diagnose simple or periodic headache.

An eye exam is usually performed to check for weakness in the eye muscle or unequal pupil size. Both of these symptoms are evidence of an aneurysm — an abnormal ballooning of a blood vessel. A physician who suspects that a headache patient has an aneurysm may also order an angiogram. In this test, a fluid which can be seen on an X ray is injected into the patient and carried in the bloodstream to the brain to reveal any abnormalities in the blood vessels there.

Thermography, an experimental technique for diagnosing headache, promises to become a useful clinical tool. In thermography, an infrared camera converts skin temperature into a color picture, or thermogram, with different degrees of heat appearing as different colors. Skin temperature is affected primarily by blood flow. Research scientists have found that thermograms of headache patients show strikingly different heat patterns from those of people who never or rarely get headaches.

A physician analyzes the results of all these diagnostic tests along with a patient's medical history in order to arrive at a diagnosis.

Headaches are diagnosed as

- Vascular
- Muscle contraction
- Traction
- Inflammatory

Vascular headaches — a group that includes the well-known migraine — are so named because they are thought to involve abnormal function of the brain's blood vessels or vascular system. Muscle contraction headaches appear to involve the tightening or tensing of facial and neck muscles. Traction and inflammatory headaches are symptoms of other disorders, ranging from stroke to sinus infection. Some people have more than one type of headache.

Migraine headaches: A painful malady

The most common type of vascular headache is migraine. Migraine headaches are usually characterized by severe pain on one or both sides of the head, an upset stomach and, at times, disturbed vision.

Basketball star Kareem Abdul-Jabbar remembers experiencing his first migraine at age 14. The pain was unlike the discomfort of his previous mild headaches.

"When I got this one I thought, 'This is a headache'," he says. "The pain was intense and I felt nausea and a great sensitivity to light. All I could think about was when it would stop. I sat in a dark room for an hour and it passed."

Symptoms of migraine. Abdul-Jabbar's sensitivity to light is a standard symptom of the two most prevalent types of migraine-caused headache: classic and common.

The major difference between the two types is the appearance of neurological symptoms 10 to 30 minutes before a classic migraine attack. These symptoms are called an aura. The person may see flashing lights or zigzag lines, or may temporarily lose vision. Other classic symptoms include speech difficulty, weakness of an arm or leg, tingling of the face or hands, and confusion.

The pain of a classic migraine headache is described as intense, throbbing, or pounding and is felt in the forehead, temple, ear, jaw, or around the eye. Classic migraine starts on one side of the head but may eventually spread to the other side. An attack lasts 1 to 2 pain racked days.

The common migraine — a term that reflects the disorder's greater occurrence in the general population — is not preceded by an aura. But some people experience a variety of vague symptoms beforehand, including mental fuzziness, mood changes, fatigue, and unusual retention of fluids. During the headache phase of a common migraine, a person may have diarrhea and increased urination, as well as nausea and vomiting. Common migraine pain can last 3 or 4 days.

Both classic and common migraine can strike as often as several times a week, or as rarely as once every few years. Both types can occur at any time. Some people, however, experience migraines at predictable times — near the days of menstruation or every Saturday morning after a stressful week of work.

The migraine process. Research scientists are unclear about the precise cause of migraine headaches. There seems to be general agreement, however, that a key element is blood flow changes in the brain. People who get migraine headaches appear to have blood vessels that overreact to various triggers.

Scientists have devised one theory of migraine which explains these blood flow changes and also certain biochemical changes that may be involved in the headache process. According to this theory, the nervous system responds to a trigger such as stress by creating a spasm in the nerve-rich arteries at the base of the brain. The spasm closes down or constricts several arteries supplying blood to the brain, including the scalp artery and the carotid or neck arteries.

As these arteries constrict, the flow of blood to the brain is reduced. At the same time, blood-clotting particles called platelets clump together — a process which is believed to release a chemical called serotonin. Serotonin acts as a powerful constrictor of arteries, further reducing the blood supply to the brain.

Reduced blood flow decreases the brain's supply of oxygen. Symptoms signaling a headache, such as distorted vision or speech, may then result, similar to symptoms of stroke.

Reacting to the reduced oxygen supply, certain arteries within the brain open wider to meet the brain's energy needs. This widening or dilation spreads, finally affecting the neck and scalp arteries. The dilation of these arteries triggers the release of pain-producing substances called prostaglandins from various tissues and blood cells. Chemicals which cause inflammation and swelling, and substances which increase sensitivity to pain are also released. The circulation of these chemicals and the dilation of the scalp arteries stimulate the pain-sensitive nociceptors. The result, according to this theory: a throbbing pain in the head.

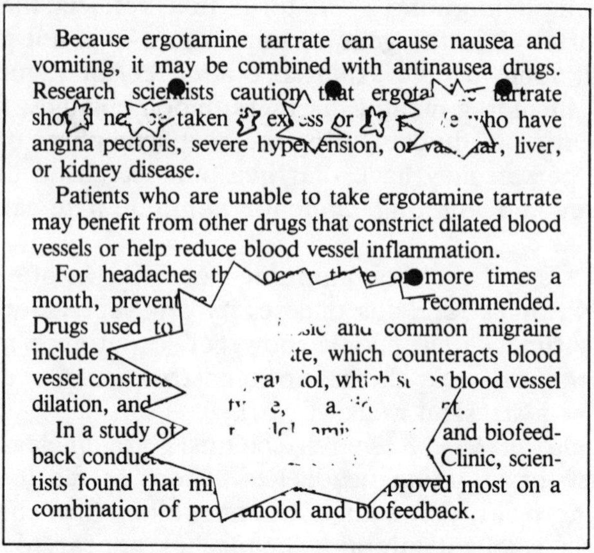

Because ergotamine tartrate can cause nausea and vomiting, it may be combined with antinausea drugs.
angina pectoris, severe hypertension, or vascular, liver, or kidney disease.
Patients who are unable to take ergotamine tartrate may benefit from other drugs that constrict dilated blood vessels or help reduce blood vessel inflammation.
month,
recommended.
include
vessel
dilation,
In a study of
and biofeedback
Clinic, scientists found that
most on a combination of
biofeedback.

If you were about to experience a classic migraine headache, you might find it difficult to read this pamphlet. You could lose part of your vision temporarily and see zigzag lines and black dots. Such visual problems—and other neurological symptoms—often precede classic migraine.

Women and migraine. Although boys and girls seem to be equally affected by migraine, the condition is more common in adult women than in men. Both sexes may develop migraine in infancy, but most often the disorder begins between the ages of 5 and 35.

The relationship between female hormones and migraine is still unclear. Women may have "menstrual migraine" — headaches around the time of their menstrual period — which may disappear during pregnancy. Other women develop migraine for the first time when they are pregnant. Some are first affected after menopause.

The effect of oral contraceptives on headaches is perplexing. Scientists report that some migrainous women who take birth control pills experience more frequent and severe attacks. However, a small percentage of women have fewer and less severe migraine headaches when they take birth control pills. And normal women who do not suffer from headaches may develop migraines as a side effect when they use oral contraceptives. Investigators around the world are studying hormonal changes in migrainous women in the hope of identifying the specific ways these naturally occurring chemicals cause headaches.

Triggers of headache. The existence of a migraine personality is a controversial theory which suggests that migraine patients are compulsive, rigid, and perfectionistic. Most scientists believe, however, that not all migraine patients have these traits and that not all individuals with these personality characteristics have migraine.

Rather than focusing on character traits, says one headache specialist, it would be better to view people who get migraines as having an inherited abnormality in the regulation of blood vessels.

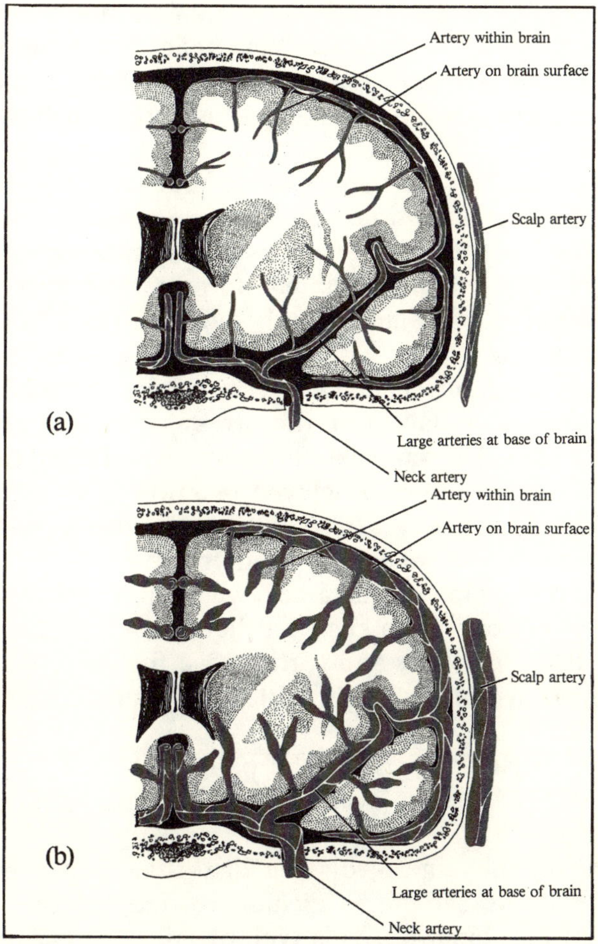

One theory of the migraine process: (a) a patient's nervous system responds to a trigger such as stress by creating a spasm in the arteries at the base of the brain. The spasm and the release of serotonin reduce blood flow to the brain. Blood-borne oxygen is decreased, causing the "aura" of neurological symptoms; (b) arteries in and around brain tissue then dilate or widen to meet the brain's energy and oxygen needs. Pain-producing chemicals are released and nerve endings on the scalp are stimulated. The patient then feels a throbbing pain in the head.

Many sufferers have a family history of migraine, but the exact hereditary nature of this condition is still unknown.

"It's like a cocked gun with a hair trigger," explains the specialist. "A person is born with a potential for migraine and the headache is triggered by things that are really not so terrible."

These triggers include stress and other normal emotions, as well as biological and environmental conditions. Fatigue, glaring or flickering lights, the weather, and even certain foods can set off migraine. It may seem hard to believe that eating such seemingly harmless foods as yogurt, nuts, and lima beans can result in a painful migraine headache. However, some scientists believe that these foods and several others contain chemical substances, such as tyramine, which constrict arteries — the first step of the migraine process. Other scientists believe that foods cause headaches by setting off an allergic reaction in susceptible people.

While a food-triggered migraine usually occurs soon after eating, other triggers may not cause immediate pain. Scientists report that people can develop migraine not only during a period of stress, but also afterwards when their vascular systems are still reacting. The "preacher monday-morning headache" is named for those clergymen who get migraines a day after the stress of delivering a Sunday sermon. Migraines that wake people up in the middle of the night are also believed to result from a delayed reaction to stress.

Other forms of migraine. In addition to classic and common, migraine headache can take several other forms:

Patients with hemiplegic migraine have temporary paralysis on one side of the body, a condition known as hemiplegia. Some people may experience vision problems and vertigo — a feeling that the world is spinning. These symptoms begin 10 to 90 minutes before the onset of headache pain.

In ophthalmoplegic migraine, the pain is around the eye and is associated with a droopy eyelid, double vision, and other sight problems.

Basilar artery migraine involves a disturbance of a major brain artery. Preheadache symptoms include vertigo, double vision, and poor muscular coordination. This type of migraine occurs primarily in adolescent and young adult women and is often associated with the menstrual cycle.

Benign exertional headache is brought on by running, lifting, coughing, sneezing, or bending. The headache begins at the onset of activity, and pain rarely lasts more than several minutes.

Status migrainosus is a rare and severe type of migraine that can last 72 hours or longer. The pain and nausea are so intense that people who have this type of headache must be hospitalized. The use of certain drugs can trigger status migrainosus. Neurologists report that many of their status migrainosus patients were depressed and anxious before they experienced headache attacks.

Headache-free migraine is characterized by such migraine symptoms as visual problems, nausea, vomiting, constipation, or diarrhea. Patients, however, do not experience head pain. Headache specialists have suggested that unexplained pain in a particular part of the body, fever, and dizziness could also be possible types of headache-free migraine.

Treating migraine headache

During the Stone Age, pieces of a headache sufferer's skull were cut away with flint instruments to relieve pain. Another unpleasant remedy used in the British Isles around the ninth century involved drinking "the juice of elderseed, cow's brain, and goat's dung dissolved in vinegar." Fortunately, today's headache patients are spared such drastic measures.

Drug therapy, biofeedback training, stress reduction, and elimination of certain foods from the diet are the most common methods of preventing and controlling migraine and other vascular headaches. Joan, the migraine sufferer, was helped by treatment with a combination of an antimigraine drug and diet control.

Regular exercise, such as swimming or vigorous walking, can also reduce the frequency and severity of migraine headaches. Joan found that yoga and whirlpool baths helped her relax.

During a migraine headache, temporary relief can sometimes be obtained by using cold packs or by pressing on the bulging artery found in front of the ear on the painful side of the head.

Drug therapy. There are two ways to approach the treatment of migraine headache with drugs: prevent the attacks, or relieve symptoms after the headache occurs.

For infrequent migraine, drugs can be taken at the first sign of a headache in order to stop it, or to at least ease the pain. People who get occasional mild migraine may benefit by taking aspirin or acetaminophen at the start of an attack. Aspirin raises a person's tolerance to pain and also discourages clumping of blood platelets. Small amounts of caffeine may be useful if taken in the early stages of migraine. But for most migraine sufferers who get moderate to severe headaches, and for all cluster patients, stronger drugs may be necessary to control the pain.

One of the most commonly used drugs for the relief of classic and common migraine symptoms is ergotamine tartrate, a vasoconstrictor which helps counteract the painful dilation stage of the headache. For optimal benefit, the drug is taken during the early stages of an attack. If a migraine has been in progress for about an hour and has passed into the final throbbing stage, ergotamine tartrate will probably not help.

Because ergotamine tartrate can cause nausea and vomiting, it may be combined with antinausea drugs. Research scientists caution that ergotamine tartrate should not be taken in excess, or by people who have angina pectoris, severe hypertension, or vascular, liver, or kidney disease.

Patients who are unable to take ergotamine tartrate may benefit from other drugs that constrict dilated blood vessels or help reduce blood vessel inflammation.

For headaches that occur three or more times a month, preventive treatment is usually recommended. Drugs used to prevent classic and common migraine include methysergide maleate, which counteracts blood vessel constriction, propranolol, which stops blood vessel dilation, and amitriptyline, an antidepressant.

In a study of propranolol, amitriptyline, and biofeedback conducted by the Houston Headache Clinic, scientists found that migraine patients improved most on a combination of propranolol and biofeedback. Patients who had mixed migraine and muscle-contraction headaches received the greatest benefit from a combination of propranolol, amitriptyline, and biofeedback.

Another recent study showed that propranolol may continue to prevent migraine headaches even after patients have stopped taking the drug. The scientists who conducted the study speculate that long-term therapy with propranolol may have a lasting effect on blood vessels, training them to react less than usual to the triggers of migraine.

Antidepressants called MAO inhibitors also prevent migraine. These drugs block an enzyme called mono-amine oxidase which normally helps nerve cells absorb the artery-constricting chemical, serotonin.

MAO inhibitors can have potentially serious side effects — particularly if taken while ingesting foods or beverages that contain tyramine, a substance that closes down arteries.

Several new drugs for the prevention of migraine have been developed in recent years, including papaverine hydrochloride, which produces blood vessel dilation, and cyproheptadine, which counteracts serotonin.

All these antimigraine drugs can have adverse side effects. But they are relatively safe when used carefully. To avoid long-term side effects of preventive medications, headache specialists advise patients to reduce the dosage of these drugs and then to stop taking them as soon as possible.

Biofeedback and relaxation training. Drug therapy for migraine is often combined with biofeedback and relaxation training. Biofeedback is a space-age word for a technique that can give people better control over such body function indicators as blood pressure, heart rate, temperature, muscle tension, and brain waves. Thermal biofeedback allows a patient to consciously raise hand temperature. Some patients who are able to increase hand temperature can reduce the number and intensity of migraines. The mechanism of this handing-warming effect is being studied by research scientists.

"To succeed in biofeedback," says a headache specialist, "you must be able to concentrate and you must be motivated to get well."

A patient learning thermal biofeedback wears a device which transmits the temperature of an index finger or hand to a monitor. While the patient tries to warm his hands, the monitor provides feedback either on a gauge that shows the temperature reading or by emitting a sound or beep that increases in intensity as the temperature increases. The patient is not told how to raise hand temperature, but is given suggestions such as "Imagine that your hands feel very warm and heavy."

"I have a good imagination," says one headache sufferer who traded in her medication for thermal biofeedback. The technique decreased the number and severity of headaches she experienced.

In another type of biofeedback called electromyographic or EMG training, the patient learns to control muscle tension in the face, neck, and shoulders.

Either kind of biofeedback may be combined with relaxation training, during which patients learn to relax the mind and body.

Biofeedback can be practiced at home with a portable monitor. But the ultimate goal is to wean the patient from the machine. The patient can then use biofeedback anywhere at the first sign of a headache.

The antimigraine diet. Scientists estimate that a small percentage of migraine sufferers will benefit from a treatment program focused solely on eliminating headache-provoking foods and beverages.

Other migraine patients may be helped by a diet to prevent low blood sugar. Low blood sugar, or hypoglycemia, can cause dilation of the blood vessels in the head. This condition can occur after a period without food: overnight, for example, or when a meal is skipped.

People who wake up in the morning with a headache may be reacting to the low blood sugar caused by the lack of food overnight.

Treatment for headaches caused by low blood sugar consists of scheduling smaller, more frequent meals for the patient. A special diet designed to stabilize the body's sugar-regulating system is sometimes recommended.

For the same reason, many specialists also recommend that migraine patients avoid oversleeping on weekends. Sleeping late can change the body's normal blood sugar level and lead to a headache.

Beyond migraine: Other vascular headaches

After migraine, the most common type of vascular headache is the toxic headache produced by fever. Pneumonia, measles, mumps, and tonsillitis are among the diseases that can cause severe toxic vascular headaches. Toxic headaches can also result from the presence of foreign chemicals in the body. Other kinds of vascular headaches include "clusters," which cause repeated episodes of intense pain, and headaches resulting from a rise in blood pressure.

Chemical culprits. Repeated exposure to nitrite compounds can result in a dull, pounding headache that may be accompanied by a flushed face. Nitrite, which dilates blood vessels, is found in such products as heart medicine and dynamite. Hot dogs and other meats containing sodium nitrite can also cause headaches.

"Chinese restaurant headache" can occur when a susceptible individual eats foods prepared with mono-sodium glutamate (MSG) — a staple in many Oriental kitchens. Soy sauce, meat tenderizer, and a variety of packaged foods contain this chemical, which is touted as a flavor enhancer.

Vascular headache can also result from exposure to poisons, even common household varieties like insecticides, carbon tetrachloride, and lead. Children who eat flakes of lead paint may develop headaches. So may anyone who has contact with lead batteries or lead-glazed pottery.

Painters, printmakers, and other artists may experience headaches after exposure to art materials that contain chemicals called solvents. Solvents, like benzene, are found in turpentine, spray adhesives, rubber cement, and inks.

Drugs such as amphetamines can cause headaches as a side effect. Another type of drug-related headache occurs during withdrawal from long-term therapy with the antimigraine drug ergotamine tartrate.

Jokes are often made about alcohol hangovers, but the headache associated with "the morning after" is no laughing matter. Fortunately, there are several suggested remedies for the pain, including ergotamine tartrate. The hangover headache may also be reduced by taking honey, which speeds alcohol metabolism, or caffeine, a constrictor of dilated arteries. Caffeine, however, can cause headaches as well as cure them. Heavy coffee drinkers often get headaches when they try to break the caffeine habit.

Cluster headaches. Cluster headaches, named for their repeated occurrence in groups or clusters, begin as a minor pain around one eye, eventually spreading to that side of the face. The pain quickly intensifies, compelling the victim to pace the floor or rock in a chair. "You can't lie down, you're fidgety," explains a cluster patient. "The pain is unbearable." Other symptoms include a stuffed and runny nose and a droopy eyelid over a red and tearing eye.

Cluster headaches last between 30 and 45 minutes. But the relief people feel at the end of an attack is usually mixed with dread as they await a recurrence. Clusters can strike several times a day or night for several weeks or months. Then, mysteriously, they may disappear for months or years. Many people have cluster bouts during the spring and fall. At their worst, chronic cluster headaches can last continuously for years.

Cluster attacks can strike at any age, but usually start between the ages of 20 and 40. Unlike migraine, cluster headaches are more common in men and do not run in families. Research scientists have observed certain physical similarities among people who experience cluster headache. The typical cluster patient is a tall, muscular man with a rugged facial appearance and a square, jutting or dimpled chin. The texture of his coarse skin resembles an orange peel. Women who get clusters may also have this type of skin.

Studies of cluster patients show that they are likely to have hazel eyes and that they tend to be heavy smokers and drinkers. Paradoxically, both nicotine, which constricts arteries, and alcohol, which dilates them, trigger cluster headaches. The exact connection between these substances and cluster attacks is not known.

Despite a cluster headache's distinguishing characteristics, its relative infrequency, and similarity to such disorders as sinusitis can lead to misdiagnosis. Some cluster patients have had tooth extractions, sinus surgery, or psychiatric treatment in a futile effort to cure their pain.

Research studies have turned up several clues as to the cause of cluster headache, but no answers. One clue is found in the thermograms of untreated cluster patients, which show a "cold spot" of reduced blood flow above the eye.

The sudden start and brief duration of cluster headaches can make them difficult to treat. By the time medicine is absorbed into the body, the attack is often over. However, research scientists have identified several effective drugs for these headaches. The anti-migraine drug ergotamine tartrate can subdue a cluster, if taken at the first sign of an attack. Injections of dihydroergotamine, a form of ergotamine tartrate, are sometimes used to treat clusters.

Some cluster patients can prevent attacks by taking propranolol or methysergide. Investigators have also discovered that mild solutions of cocaine hydrochloride applied inside the nose can quickly stop cluster headaches in most patients. This treatment may work because it both blocks pain impulses and it constricts blood vessels.

Another option that works for some cluster patients is rapid inhalation of pure oxygen through a mask for 5 to 15 minutes. The oxygen seems to ease the pain of cluster headache by reducing blood flow to the brain.

In chronic cases of cluster headache, certain facial nerves may be surgically cut or destroyed to provide relief. These procedures have had limited success. Some cluster patients have had facial nerves cut only to have them regenerate years later.

Painful pressure. Chronic high blood pressure can cause headache, as can rapid rises in blood pressure like those experienced during anger, vigorous exercise, or sexual excitement.

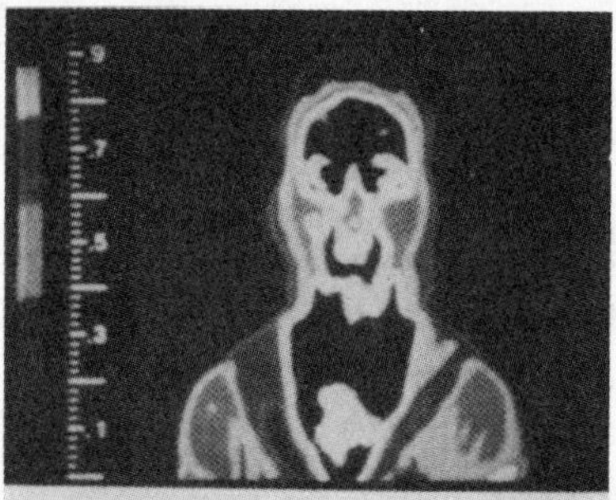

A thermogram of a normal person shows a symmetrical heat pattern on the individual's forehead.

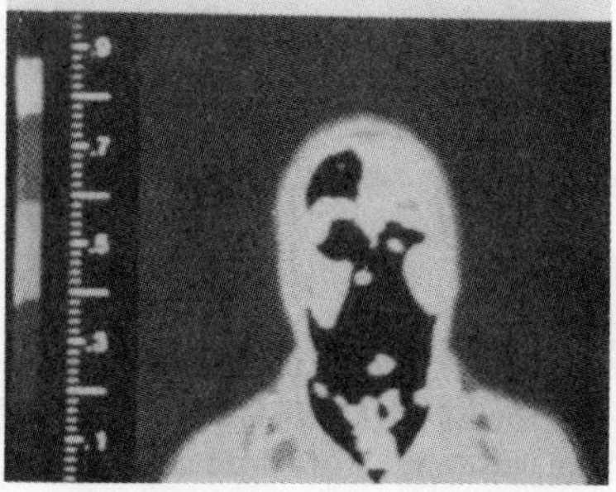

A cluster headache patient's thermogram shows a cold area (appears white) of reduced blood flow on the left side of the forehead.

The severe "orgasmic headache" occurs right before orgasm and is believed to be a vascular type. Since sudden rupture of a cerebral blood vessel can also occur during orgasm, this type of headache should be promptly evaluated by a doctor.

Muscle-contraction headaches: The everyday menace

It's 5:00 p.m. and your boss has just asked you to prepare a 20-page briefing paper. Due date: tomorrow. You're angry and tired and the more you think about the assignment, the tenser you become. Your teeth clinch, your brow wrinkles, and soon you have a splitting tension headache.

Tension headache is named not only for the role of stress in triggering the pain, but also for the contraction of neck, face, and scalp muscles brought on by stressful events. Tension headache is a severe but temporary form of muscle-contraction headache. The pain is mild to moderate and feels like pressure being applied to the head or neck. The headache usually disappears after the period of stress is over.

By contrast, chronic muscle-contraction headaches can last for weeks, months, and sometimes years. The pain of these headaches is often described as a tight band around the head or a feeling that the head and neck are in a cast. "It feels like somebody tightening a giant vise around my head," says one patient. The pain is steady, and is usually felt on both sides of the head. Chronic muscle-contraction headaches can cause sore scalps — even combing one's hair can be painful.

Many scientists believe that the primary cause of the pain of muscle-contraction headache is sustained muscle tension. Other studies suggest that restricted blood flow may cause or contribute to the pain.

Occasionally, muscle-contraction headaches will be accompanied by nausea, vomiting, and blurred vision, but there is no preheadache syndrome, as with migraine. Muscle-contraction headaches have not been linked to hormones or foods, as has migraine, nor is there a strong hereditary connection.

Research has shown that for many people, chronic muscle-contraction headaches are caused by depression and anxiety. These people tend to get their headaches in the early morning or evening when conflicts in the office or home are anticipated.

Emotional factors are not the only triggers of muscle-contraction headaches. Certain physical postures, such as holding one's chin down while reading, can lead to head and neck pain. Tensing head and neck muscles during sexual excitement can also cause headache. So can prolonged writing under poor light, or holding a phone between the shoulder and ear, or even gum-chewing.

More serious problems that can cause muscle-contraction headaches include degenerative arthritis of the neck and temporomandibular joint dysfunction, or TMJ. TMJ is a disorder of the joint between the temporal bone (above the ear) and the mandible or lower jaw bone. The disorder results from poor bite and jaw clenching.

Treatment for muscle-contraction headache varies. The first consideration is to treat any specific disorder or disease that may be causing the headache. For example, arthritis of the neck is treated with anti-inflammatory medication, and temporomandibular joint dysfunction may be helped by corrective devices for the mouth and jaw.

Acute tension headaches not associated with a disease are treated with muscle relaxants and analgesics like aspirin and acetaminophen. Stronger analgesics, such as propoxyphene and codeine, are sometimes prescribed. As prolonged use of these drugs can lead to dependence, patients taking them should have periodic medical checkups and follow their physicians' instructions carefully.

Nondrug therapy for chronic muscle-contraction headaches includes biofeedback, relaxation training, and counseling. A technique called cognitive restructuring teaches people to change their attitudes and responses to stress. Patients might be encouraged, for example, to imagine that they are coping successfully with a stressful situation. In progressive relaxation therapy, patients are taught to first tense and then relax individual muscle groups. Finally, the patient tries to relax his or her whole body. Many people imagine a peaceful scene — such as lying on the beach or by a beautiful lake. Passive relaxation does not involve tensing of muscles. Instead, patients are encouraged to focus on different muscles, suggesting that they relax. Some people might think to themselves, Relax or My muscles feel warm.

People with chronic muscle-contraction headaches may also be helped by taking antidepressants or MAO inhibitors. Mixed muscle-contraction and migraine headaches are sometimes treated with barbiturate compounds, which slow down nerve function in the brain and spinal cord.

People who suffer infrequent headaches may benefit from a hot shower or moist heat applied to the back of the neck. Cervical collars are sometimes recommended as an aid to good posture. Physical therapy, massage, and gentle exercise of the neck may also be helpful.

When headache is a warning

Like other types of pain, headaches can serve as warning signals of more serious disorders. This is particularly true for headaches caused by traction or inflammation.

Traction headaches can occur if the pain-sensitive parts of the head are pulled, stretched, or displaced, as, for example, when eye muscles are tensed to compensate for eyestrain. Headaches caused by inflammation include those related to meningitis, as well as those resulting from diseases of the sinuses, spine, neck, ears, and teeth. Ear and tooth infections and glaucoma can cause headaches. In oral and dental disorders, headache is experienced as pain in the entire head, including the face.

Traction and inflammatory headaches are treated by curing the underlying problem. This may involve surgery, antibiotics, or other drugs.

Characteristics of the various types of traction and inflammatory headaches vary by disorder:

- ***Brain tumor.*** Brain tumors are diagnosed in about 11,000 people every year. As they grow, these tumors sometimes cause headache by pushing on the outer layer of nerve tissue that covers the brain or by pressing against pain-sensitive blood vessel walls. Headache resulting from a brain tumor may be periodic or continuous. Typically, it feels like a strong pressure being applied to the head. The pain is relieved when the tumor is destroyed by surgery, radiation, or chemotherapy.
- ***Stroke.*** Headache may accompany several conditions that can lead to stroke, including hypertension or high blood pressure, arteriosclerosis, and heart disease. Headaches are also associated with completed stroke; the latter occurs when brain cells die from lack of sufficient oxygen.

Many stroke-related headaches can be prevented by careful management of the patient's condition through diet, exercise, and medication.

Mild to moderate headaches are associated with so-called "little strokes," or transient ischemic attacks (TIAs), which result from a temporary lack of blood supply to the brain. The head pain occurs near the clot or lesion that blocks blood flow.

The similarity between migraine and symptoms of TIA can cause problems in diagnosis. The rare person under age 40 who suffers a TIA may be misdiagnosed as having migraine; similarly, TIA-prone older patients who suffer migraine may be misdiagnosed as having stroke-related headaches.

• *Spinal tap*. About one-fourth of the people who undergo a lumbar puncture or spinal tap develop a headache. Many scientists believe these headaches result from leakage of the cerebrospinal fluid that flows through pain-sensitive membranes around the brain and down to the spinal cord. The fluid, they suggest, drains through the tiny hole created by the spinal tap needle, causing the membranes to rub painfully against the bony skull. Since headache pain occurs only when the patient stands up, the "cure" is to remain lying down until the headache runs its course — anywhere from a few hours to several days.

• *Head trauma*. Headaches may develop after a blow to the head, either immediately or months later. There is little relationship between the severity of the trauma and the intensity of headache pain. One cause of trauma headache is scar formation in the scalp. Another is ruptured blood vessels which result in an accumulation of blood called a hematoma. This mass of blood can displace brain tissue and cause headaches as well as weakness, confusion, memory loss, and seizures. Hematomas can be drained to produce rapid relief of symptoms.

• *Arteritis and meningitis*. Arteritis, an inflammation of certain arteries in the head, primarily affects people over age 50. Symptoms include throbbing headache, fever, and loss of appetite. Some patients experience blurring or loss of vision. Prompt treatment with corticosteroid drugs helps to relieve symptoms.

Headaches are also caused by infections of meninges, the brain's outer covering, and phlebitis, a vein inflammation.

• *Tic douloureux*. Tic douloureux, or trigeminal neuralgia, results from a disorder of the trigeminal nerve. This nerve supplies the face, teeth, mouth, and nasal cavity with feeling and also enables the mouth muscles to chew. Symptoms are headache and intense facial pain that comes in short, excruciating jabs set off by the slightest touch to or movement of trigger points in the face or mouth. People with tic douloureux often fear brushing their teeth or chewing on the side of the mouth that is affected. Many tic douloureux patients are controlled with drugs, including carbamazepine. Patients who do not respond to drugs may be helped by surgery on the trigeminal nerve.

• *Sinus infection*. In a condition called acute sinusitis, a viral or bacterial infection of the upper respiratory tract spreads to the membrane which lines the sinus cavities. When one or all four of these cavities are filled with bacterial or viral fluid, they become inflamed, causing pain and sometimes headache. Treatment of acute sinusitis includes antibiotics, analgesics, and decongestants.

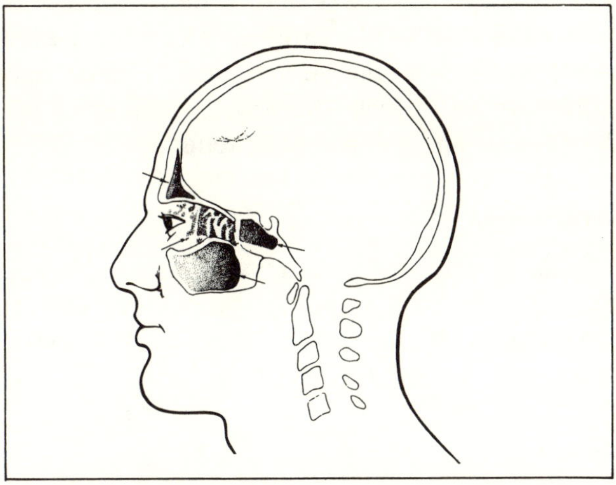

Acute sinusitis headaches can occur when one or all four of the sinus cavities fill with bacterial or viral fluid. The particular cavity affected determines the location of the sinus headache.

Chronic sinusitis may be caused by an allergy to such irritants as dust, ragweed, animal hair, and smoke. Research scientists disagree about whether chronic sinusitis triggers headache.

A childhood problem

Like adults, children experience the infections, trauma, and stresses that can lead to headaches. In fact, research shows that as young people enter adolescence and encounter the stresses of puberty and secondary school, the frequency of headache increases.

Migraine headaches often begin in childhood or adolescence. According to a recent health interview survey, over a million children age 16 and under experience migraine and other vascular headaches.

Children with migraine often have nausea and excessive vomiting. Some children have periodic vomiting, but no headache — the so-called "abdominal migraine." Research scientists have found that these children usually develop headaches when they are older.

Phenobarbital, cypropheptadine, and certain anticonvulsant drugs are used to treat migraines in children. A diet may be prescribed to protect the child from foods that trigger headache. Sometimes psychological counseling or even psychiatric treatment for the child and the parents is recommended. NINCDS-supported scientists at the State University of New York in Albany find that thermal biofeedback can help children with migraines control their headaches.

Childhood headache can be a sign of depression. Parents should alert the family pediatrician if a child develops headaches along with other symptoms, such as a change in mood or sleep habits. Antidepressant medication and psychotherapy are effective treatments for childhood depression and related headache.

Research intervenes

Modern methods of diagnosis and treatment enable physicians and psychologists today to help about 90 percent of chronic headache patients, according to the director of a major U.S. headache clinic. These methods are based on years of scientific research. New research should lead to even more advanced techniques of headache management.

Some scientists explore the role that certain foods play in causing this disorder. Others are more concerned with the function of the autonomic nervous systems of headache-prone people. The autonomic nervous system automatically controls a variety of essential body functions, including the flow of blood throughout the body and the working of the pupils of the eyes.

At the Philadelphia College of Osteopathic Medicine, scientists supported by the National Institute of Neurological and Communicative Disorders and Stroke are gauging the autonomic nervous system activity of normal controls and headache patients with a technique called "pupillometry." This technique measures the response of the iris, or eye muscle, to light and darkness. Migraine, cluster, and muscle-contraction headache patients are included in the study. Each patient sits in a chair with his or her head in a chin rest. The eye is stimulated with light and then with darkness. A television camera in front of the patient picks up the reaction of the iris and translates it into a graph which provides clues about the functioning of the patient's autonomic nervous system.

Another experiment with the pupillometer involves measuring eye muscle reaction to light and darkness after stress. In this study, stress is simulated by dipping the patient's arm in very cold water for up to 20 seconds.

Preliminary findings from these studies suggest that, under stress-free conditions, the autonomic nervous systems of both people with common migraine and of people without headaches react normally. Paradoxically, migraine patients during stress show reduced autonomic nervous system activity, a condition that should prevent the decreased blood flow thought to cause headaches.

However, NINCDS-supported scientists at Southern Illinois University in Carbondale report a different connection between blood flow and migraine headache.

Using an infrared light sensor that measures the diameter of blood vessels, the investigators have found that, after stress, blood flow returns to normal more quickly in headache-free people than in patients with migraine and muscle-contraction headache. This finding supports the theory that restricted or decreased blood flow may cause or contribute to headache.

The scientists also found that different types of headaches are characterized by different blood flow patterns. After stress, the temporal arteries in the foreheads of migraine patients expand to a greater degree than the arteries of muscle-contraction headache patients. People with the same type of headache also show differences in blood flow patterns — offering evidence that there are a variety of causes for each headache type.

Testing new treatments. Scientists are also developing new therapies and analyzing the effectiveness of current treatment methods for headache. The research team at Southern Illinois University is comparing a biofeedback method that monitors blood flow with a method that monitors muscular tension in the head. This research should lead to improved understanding of individual differences in treatment response.

Several scientists are studying the value of biofeedback and other forms of treatment carried out in the patient's home. Home-based programs may be a boon to patients in rural areas who have limited access to medical care and cannot afford frequent visits to headache specialists.

In NINCDS-supported research at the State University of New York in Albany, scientists are comparing the effectiveness of a standard office-based relaxation training program for muscle-contraction, migraine, and mixed-headache patients, with a similar program conducted by patients at home. Patients in the home-based program are seen in the office once a month, but rely heavily on manuals, cassettes, and portable biofeedback devices.

Preliminary results suggest that home-based and office-based programs are equally effective. "If these relaxation techniques are learned at home," speculates the investigator, "they may transfer more readily to the home situation — where they will be used to cope with daily stresses."

Furthermore, at the University of Washington in Seattle, an NINCDS-supported investigator is finding that home-based treatment involving only dietary changes is as effective in treating migraine patients as a home-based program of biofeedback and stress management.

Thermal biofeedback training, which involves the conscious warming of parts of the body through thought control, is believed to work because it gives people a feeling of control over their headaches. An NINCDS-supported study at Midwest Research Institute in Kansas City, Missouri, raises the possibility that this feeling of control is a more important factor in decreasing headaches than is the actual warming of the hands.

Patients who had frequent migraines were told that they would be given one of two types of biofeedback: "real temperature biofeedback," where a sound indicated their real hand temperature, or "bogus biofeedback," where a prerecorded sound emitted from the monitor would be unrelated to the patient's effort to warm the hands. Neither the patients nor the technicians training them knew whose feedback was real or bogus. Throughout the 6 weeks of training, the scientists emphasized to the patients that biofeedback should become an integral part of their lives because it was giving them control over their headaches.

Patients in the bogus biofeedback group had a success rate that rivaled the one in the real biofeedback group. More than 80 percent of patients in both groups reduced the frequency and intensity of their headaches, as well as the quantity of medication they had been taking to control pain.

"It isn't so much the physical mechanism of migraine that matters," explains the principal investigator, "but a person's ability to cope with the syndrome and to take charge of his or her body. The emphasis on self-control is what made these people improve."

Another important area of research is the study of beta-blocking drugs like propranolol, which are used to prevent migraine.

Beta-blockers stop the activities of beta receptors — cells in the brain and heart which control the dilation of blood vessels. The ability of beta-blockers to halt the dilation of blood vessels in the brain is believed to be a major reason for their antimigraine action. But, because the drugs also affect heart receptors — slowing the heart rate — they cannot be used by people who have certain heart conditions.

This problem may be resolved by NINCDS-supported research at Massachusetts General Hospital in Boston. A research team there is using biochemical techniques to find out if there is a certain type of beta receptor that exists in the blood vessels of the brain but not in the heart. The discovery of this receptor could lead to the development of beta-blocking agents that would affect brain receptors only.

Another NINCDS-funded study at the University of Kansas Medical Center is comparing the effectiveness of propranolol with that of the antidepressant amitriptyline in the prevention of migraine. Physical and psychological characteristics of migraine patients are being correlated with their responses to the two drugs.

Investigators supported by the National Institutes of Health General Clinical Research Center at the University of Colorado in Denver are studying the antimigraine properties of a class of drugs called calcium-channel blockers. Research on these drugs is also under way at the U.S. Air Force Medical Center, Wright-Patterson AFB in Ohio. Calcium-channel blockers interfere with the constriction of arteries, an effect that appears to be responsible for reducing the frequency of headaches in patients studied so far.

High technology in diagnosis. Physicians of the future may diagnose their patients' headaches with the aid of a computer. A computer might take a patient's medical history, store information on headache characteristics, and keep data on patients and their treatments. Programs might even be devised to explain to patients the way to take prescribed medications and the side effects of those drugs.

Scientists at Beth Israel Hospital in Boston are taking the first steps toward computer-assisted headache practice in a study funded by the National Library of Medicine. They are creating a working model for a headache interview program in which a computer will collect patient histories and symptoms. The scientists envision that an "automated physician's assistant" will eventually free health care providers from collecting routine medical information, allowing them to devote more time to physical examination and treatment.

A final word of hope

If you suffer from headaches and none of the standard treatments help, do not despair. Some people find that their headaches disappear once they deal with a troubled marriage, pass their law board exams, or resolve some other stressful problem. Others find that if they control their psychological reaction to stress, the headaches disappear.

"I had migraines for several years," says one woman, "and then they went away. I think it was because I lowered my personal goals in life. Today, even though I have 100 things to do at night, I don't worry about it. I learned to say no."

For those who cannot say no, or who get headaches anyway, today's headache research offers hope. The work of NINCDS-supported scientists around the world promises to improve our understanding of this complex disorder and how to treat it.

Where to get help

Finding a clinic or physician who specializes in headache is a task made easier by the National Migraine Foundation. The foundation provides a list of clinics in the U.S. as well as the names of physicians in a specific geographic area who are members of the American Association for the Study of Headache. The foundation also supports research and education in migraine headache.

National Migraine Foundation
5252 North Western Avenue
Chicago, Illinois 60625
(312) 878-7715

Inquiries about NINCDS research on headache may be directed to:

Office of Scientific and Health Reports
National Institute of Neurological and
Communicative Disorders and Stroke
Building 31, Room 8A-06
National Insitutes of Health
Bethesda, Maryland 20205
(301) 496-5751

Chapter 14

Head Injury

Head Injury

Driving home late at night from a high school graduation party, Frank lost control of his car. The car went off the road and struck a tree. Frank, only 18 years old, survived severe injuries — a fractured skull and a blood clot on the brain — but his life has never returned to normal.

Despite immediate surgery in the local hospital, Frank was comatose for 3 weeks. He then required hospital care for another 3 months. Now at home for more than 2 years, the left side of his body remains weak and he has such serious memory problems that he cannot hold a job or continue his schooling. He is quiet, but occasionally gets angry and breaks things or threatens his family. His parents are having trouble coping with the heavy emotional and financial burden that has resulted from the accident. They do not know where to get help for him nor are they aware of support systems for the family.

Frank's story is a common one. According to one estimate, each year between 400,000 and 500,000 Americans suffer head injuries severe enough to cause death or admission to a hospital. Of course, many of these people do not experience head injuries as severe as Frank's. And not all are involved in car accidents. Some people receive head injuries while playing sports; others are hurt in falls; still others are victims of crime.

But the most common cause of severe head injuries is motor vehicle accidents. The more serious the injury, the more likely it is to have been caused by a motor vehicle.

Victims of car accidents and other causes of serious head injury face years of disability and lost productivity. Like Frank, many of these patients struggle to regain memory and the ability to concentrate.

National brain research institute

Finding ways to restore Frank's capabilities, and to help the thousands of head-injured people like him, is a major goal of the National Institute of Neurological and Communicative Disorders and Stroke (NINCDS), the leading federal agency responsible for research on head trauma. The NINCDS is the focal point for brain research in the United States. As a unit of the National Institues of Health in Bethesda, Md., NINCDS supports and conducts studies to find more effective ways to repair brain damage, to improve rehabilitation techniques, and to prevent the devastating consequences of head injury.

A major health problem

Much of what we know about head injuries in this nation comes from a survey supported by the NINCDS:

- Almost 1 million people in the United States suffer from the effects of head injuries.
- More than 400,000 patients with new injuuies of the head are admitted to U.S. hospitals each year.
- About 100,000 victims of trauma, including head injury, die each year — many before reaching a hospital.

The survey found that head injuries occur most often among people aged 15 to 24 years. Young men are more than twice as likely as women to suffer a head injury.

Two other age groups are at high risk of head injury: the elderly and infants. The elderly are likely to injure themselves in falls; infants and children may be dropped from an adult's arms, tumble down stairs, or fall from high chairs or changing tables. Abused children may also suffer from head injuries.

Too often, children are injured in automobile accidents because they were not protected with safety seats or seat belts. Children struck by moving vehicles can also receive head injuries.

According to another study supported by NINCDS, children are more likely than adults to be hit by cars and thus risk head injury. That same study revealed that children are more apt than adults to survive severe head trauma. Nevertheless, there is still a substantial death rate among head-injured children.

Because the victims of head trauma are usually young people, the cost to society is high — almost $4 billion annually. This figure includes the direct expense of medical treatment, indirect costs of rehabilitation and support services, and the patient's lost income.

A middle-aged woman expresses the human side of these statistics: "My husband had a head injury 10 years ago. Now he's in a nursing home. He's only 45 years old, and he'll probably have to stay there the rest of his life. My children miss his guidance and compassion."

No two injuries are alike

The injuries that prevent head-trauma victims from participating fully in society are as varied as the functions of the brain.

Lying within the bony protection of the skull, and encased in a watery fluid, the brain works by means of signals that are passed from nerve cell to nerve cell through a network with billions of connections. Different regions of the brain are responsible for specific functions. One part of the brain controls speech; another regulates movement. The brain stem, at the base of the brain, controls heart rate, breathing, and blood pressure, and regulates temperature.

Depending upon what areas of the brain are damaged, a head injury can produce losses in movement, sensation, intellect, and memory. There is no such thing as a typical brain injury. The effect of brain damage varies according to the location and the severity of the injury.

The outcome of a head injury is equally variable. Some victims die. Other people with serious head injuries become totally unresponsive for an indefinite time — a condition known as coma. Head-injured people may also suffer physical, emotional, intellectual, or psychological handicaps.

The more fortunate return to their regular employment and resume their social life with little or no disability. It is the goal of

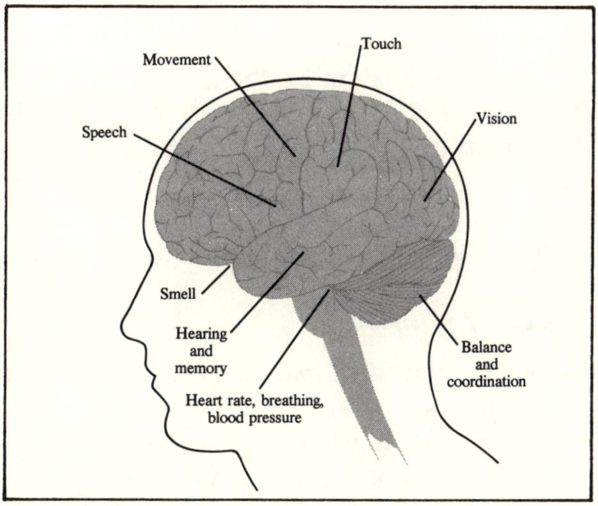

Specific parts of the brain control specific functions, like the ability to see, to smell, to remember. The effect of a head injury is partly determined by the location of the bruise or wound. Damage to the left side of the brain, for example, may result in speech problems.

NINCDS research to provide this most desirable outcome for all head-injured patients.

Preventing head injuries

"As long as we're in a motorized, highly mechanized society, we'll always have traumatic brain damage," says one head-injury expert. "We're never going to eliminate it, but we can prevent some of it."

Many of the head injuries that occur in this country each year can be prevented. Use of seat belts for every trip in an automobile — no matter how short — can lower the chance of serious head injury in accidents. Cars can be designed so that the heads of the drivers and passengers are unlikely to hit projections or hard surfaces.

Decreased alcohol consumption by drivers and pedestrians can also reduce the number of accidents causing severe head injuries.

"Both my husband and daughter are living with the effects of head injuries caused by a 20-year-old drunk driver," says one woman. "This guy drove down the street drunk after a football game and hit my family and six other people."

Motorcyclists can protect themselves from head injuries by wearing safety helmets. Studies show that riders without helmets are two to four times more likely to incur a head injury than are helmet wearers. Unhelmeted riders are three to nine times more likely to suffer fatal head injuries.

Helmets are a wise protective measure for many other activities that can lead to head injuries — construction work, for example, and such sports as bicycling, boxing, football, and rock climbing.

Parents can protect children from head injury by using approved infant and child restraint seats in automobiles. Infants and young children should be kept away from open, unguarded windows. Toddlers should not be left unattended in high chairs, buggies, or strollers, nor should they be allowed to climb out of their cribs.

Two major types of injuries

Head injuries can be placed in two categories: penetrating injuries and closed head injuries.

Penetrating injuries occur when a penetrating object — a bullet, for example, or fragments of exploding shells — lacerates the scalp, fractures the skull, enters the brain, and rips the soft tissue in its path. The resulting stretching and tearing of nerve fibers, which kills many nerve cells in the damaged area, are the primary sources of harm in many penetrating head injuries. The severity of the injury depends on the type of object, its force, and its path through the brain.

Much of what we know about how penetrating injuries damage the brain and how the damage is best treated comes from studying the many thousands of soldiers who received head injuries during World War II, Korea, and Vietnam. Almost 1,000 men who were head injured during World War II participated in a Veterans Administration study designed to determine the long-term effects of head injuries. The study found that few men considered themselves "perfectly normal" years after the injury even though the results of their neurological examinations showed that they were normal. About 80 percent of these men still had injury-related headaches 7 years after the trauma. In a similar collaborative study by the NINCDS, the Veterans Administration, and the Department of Defense, scientists are now evaluating the condition of head-injured Vietnam veterans 10 years after injury.

Penetrating injuries, however, are not limited to war. In any major hospital, surgeons are called upon to treat penetrating head injuries caused by objects such as a steak knife or an ice pick.

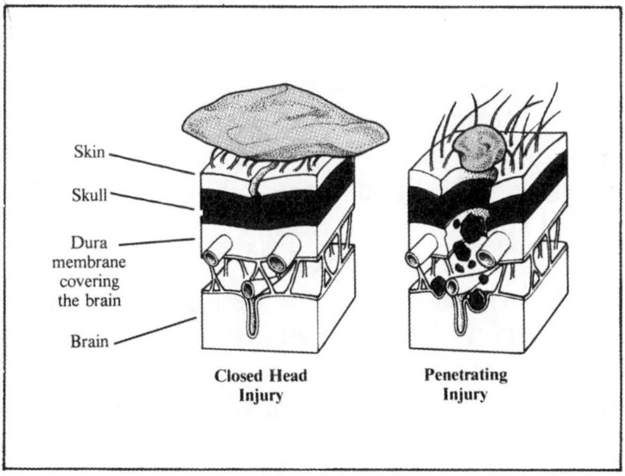

In this closed head injury (left), a large stone fractures the skull. But the skull helps absorb the blow, preventing the rock or bone fragments from entering the brain. In the penetrating injury (right), however, a small pellet fractures the skull, sending bone fragments ripping into the brain.

Even do-it-yourself home repair may cause penetrating injuries. Great care must be taken when using stud guns and power staplers. The force of the gun can easily drive a nail or screw through a thin wall or board, and the object may then become a dangerous flying missile that could pierce the head and cause a serious head injury.

Closed head injury is the most common type of head injury outside a war zone. In a closed head injury, damage is caused by the collision of the head with another surface such as a large stone. Although no object penetrates the brain, it may still be severely damaged.

A person's head hitting a car windshield is an example of closed head injury. When a person without a seat belt is thrown forward in a car that stops suddenly, the brain can be hurled against the inside of the skull. The soft brain collides with bone that is not only hard but has rough protrusions. This same kind of force can also squeeze and twist the brain in ways that are damaging.

In closed head injury, the blow may also injure the scalp and fracture the skull.

Where is the damage?

Regardless of the source of the head injury, the area of the brain damaged partly determines the resulting symptoms.

- ***Focal lesions.*** Focal lesions, injuries that affect single, specific part of the brain, are of two types: *contusion*, which is like a bruise of a portion of the brain, and *hematoma*, which is a mass of blood resulting from bleeding in a confined space.

A contusion is a frequent result of severe head injury, occurring in almost 90 percent of cases. A contusion can occur at the point where an object strikes the head, or a distant point where the jostled brain hits the hard surface of the skull.

The symptoms of a brain contusion vary according the severity and location of the bruise. Some patients may be confused, restless, delirious, or even unconscious; others may develop severe headache paralysis, or seizures which may lead to epilepsy.

A hematoma, which is generally considered a severe symptom of head injury, may accompany a contusion. Hematomas occur when a blood vessel is torn at the time of impact and blood leaks into the brain or its covering membrane (the dura). Intracerebral hematomas are formed within the brain tissue. Extracerebral hematomas occur between the brain and the skull — either below or above the dura. A hematoma may be as small as a letter on this page or it may involve a large part of the brain.

Hematomas can result in increased pressure on the brain, causing further brain injury.

• ***Diffuse lesions.*** Focal lesions are confined to one brain site, but *diffuse lesions* are spread out and involve several areas of the brain. Billions of brain cells in these areas are distorted by the twisting, stretching, and compressing forces unleashed during the injury. This distortion can be temporary or can damage the nerve cells so severely that they die.

A physician describing the type of diffuse lesion suffered by a patient may use such terms as *mild concussion*, *concussion*, or *disuse axonal injury*.

The least harmful form of diffuse lesion is the mild concussion, which occurs, for example, when a tall person bumps his or her head on the top of a low staircase and "sees stars." This sort of injury is reversible and probably leaves no ill effects.

In the mild concussion, a person experiences temporary neurological problems but does not lose consciousness. Mild concussions frequently occur in sports-related injuries. A blow to the head in a football game may cause confusion for a few seconds, and 5 to 10 minutes later the player may not remember the injury or events just before it. With more powerful blows, the player has longer periods of confusion and forgets events just after as well as just before the injury.

A person who has a full concussion loses consciousness for a period of time and also the memory of events just before and after the impact. Many people have no lasting ill effects from a concussion; however, some may show permanent subtle changes in personality or more prolonged memory loss.

In both the mild and severe concussions, the regions in the base of the brain involved in breathing and heart rate — called the brain stem — are temporarily disturbed. The parts of the brain that control memory are also affected.

Diffuse axonal injuries, the third type of diffuse lesion, involve a damaged brain stem as well as torn brain axons, the fiber-like projections from nerve cells that help transmit chemical "messages" from the brain to the body.

Diffuse axonal injuries range from mild to severe. All forms involve coma, a loss of consciousness triggered by brain stem damage. Recovery of consciousness is followed by confusion and memory lapses. Some patients recover to resume all normal activities, but others suffer intellectual, memory, and personality losses.

A severe diffuse axonal injury involves the tearing of many nerve fibers throughout the brain and brain stem. Patients with this type of injury remain deeply unconscious for a long time. They often have extensive loss of intellect, sensation, and movement. Some of them will die.

Coma

Brain damage caused by a head injury may cause a patient to lose consciousness for a prolonged period of time. Such a person is considered to be in a state of coma. Someone in a coma does not respond normally to stimulation. A comatose patient's eyes are closed, and he or she does not speak or move voluntarily. As one young man wrote about his brother who was in a coma after a car accident: "His body is whole, his brain is physically all there, but his mind, at least for now, is gone."

Coma can last from 6 to 24 hours or longer, depending on the severity of brain damage. Occasionally, a person remains unconscious for months or even years.

While in a coma, a patient must be given special care to survive. In an extended coma without intensive care, muscles will shrink and the body will become vulnerable to infection.

When patients first come out of a coma, they may follow people around the room with their eyes or blink in response to simple questions.

"My daughter was in a coma for 3 weeks," says one woman. "She woke up slowly. Physically, she was in good shape, but most of her mental processes were impaired. She didn't recognize us, and I don't think she knew who she was."

People often emerge from a coma with a combination of physical, intellectual, and psychological difficulties that need specialized attention. Recovery usually occurs gradually, with patients acquiring more and more ability to respond. Some patients never progress beyond very basic responses, but many recover full awareness.

Bill, for example, was in a coma for 4 months. He was left with few physical problems but many intellectual and emotional difficulties that prevent him, 8 years later, from taking care of himself. Susan, who was 8 years old when she received a head injury, was in a coma for 2 weeks. The only remaining effect of her injury is occasional headaches.

A threat to survival

In addition to causing direct damage to the brain, a head injury may be complicated by pressure on the brain resulting from brain swelling or edema. These consequences of head injury can be life threatening.

Although poorly understood, brain swelling is thought to be partly the result of dangerously increased blood flow to the brain. The head injury disrupts the normal action of the brain's blood vessels, causing them to expand with blood and take up more space within the skull. Because the skull is a rigid container, this swelling may cause increased pressure on the brain. The brain is compressed and receives insufficient oxygen.

Swelling may occur immediately after injury, or be delayed by minutes or hours. The most common visible sign of brain swelling is a decrease in the patient's alertness. Some patients may lapse into unconsciousness. If the swelling can be controlled, it may not cause permanent damage. Uncontrolled, it may lead to the patient's death.

Treatment for severe prolonged brain swelling is difficult, so the symptom is best taken care of at the earliest stages. The increased pressure in the brain caused by swelling may be monitored by any of several measuring devices developed through biomedical research. One such device is placed in the brain during a minor surgical procedure called ventriculostomy. This device is attached to fluid-filled spaces of the brain called ventricles and then hooked up to a wall monitor.

Because currently used pressure-monitoring instruments require opening the skull, infection is a potential problem. Scientists and engineers at Case Western Reserve University are developing a totally implantable miniature electronic sensor (not physically connected to a monitor) that could record pressure on the brain for long periods of time without the risk of infection. The development of this device is supported by the Division of Research Resources of the National Institutes of Health.

Brain edema, the excessive accumulation of water and other fluids within the brain, also causes increased pressure within the skull. Edema often occurs where the brain has been bruised — around a contusion, for example.

The same devices used to monitor brain swelling are also used to check for edema.

Immediate care saves lives

Two decades ago, 90 percent of patients with severe head injury died. Scientific research has lowered this percentage. As a result of modern emergency-room, surgical, and intensive-care treatment, at least 50 percent now survive.

Emergency treatment before the patient reaches the hospital is a critical aspect of head-injury care. Proper immediate care may prevent additional damage to brain tissue from inadequate blood flow or insufficient oxygen supply.

The rescue team that cares for a head-injured victim at the scene of an accident usually consists of a paramedic and an emergency medical technician. They will first determine the location and severity of the victim's injuries. The team will then test the injured person's neurological condition — level of consciousness and the eye's pupil response, for example — and such vital signs as heart rate and blood pressure. They will also examine the patient for broken bones — particularly a broken neck. A head-injured patient will probably be splinted onto a rigid support to keep the neck immobile and prevent spinal cord injury.

The medical team will quickly transport the patient to a hospital with a staff qualified to care for head injuries, or to a special facility called a shock trauma center. While in transit, the patient will be given needed care and the rescue team will establish radio communication with a physician in the hospital or trauma center.

If the patient is deeply unconscious, the emergency medical team may insert a mouth tube to help breathing. This procedure is sometimes performed in the hospital emergency room.

When the patient arrives at the hospital, accurate and immediate evaluation and treatment of the injury is essential for survival. One patient who benefitted from speedy treatment in the hospital and the latest research in emergency-room and surgical care was James Brady. The 40-year-old presidential press secretary was shot in the head during the attempted assassination of President Reagan on March 31, 1981. Thanks to fast action by the Secret Service, Brady was taken immediately to a nearby hospital that had a skilled neurosurgical team.

A bullet had tunneled through Brady's brain, leaving a trail of bone fragments, metal, and air. The bullet, which had entered Brady's forehead above the left eye, was surgically removed from his head near the right ear.

Brady was in the hospital for 8 months. He underwent several operations in addition to the 6½-hour emergency surgery the first day. Intensive physical therapy has helped him regain a degree of coordination and balance, although he is still partially paralyzed. He also has some speech impairment. Throughout the long ordeal, Brady maintained his sense of humor and interest in his work. His progress in rehabilitation is attributed to personal courage, to the outstanding care he received, and to the advances made possible in recent years through medical research.

Scans, surgery, and drugs

Once initial care has been provided and the patient is not in immediate danger of death, the physician will turn to an array of tests and procedures to determine the extent of damage and restore function. Because the skull completely surrounds the brain, it is difficult to tell whether the brain has been injured and, if so, the type and extent of damage.

A technique called computerized tomography (CT) scanning has helped improve diagnosis and treatment of head-injury patients. The technique, perfected after years of research, creates a series of computerized X-ray images of the brain. After special X rays are taken of the patient's head, a computer is used to reconstruct a cross-sectional view of the brain. With the CT scan, a neurosurgeon — a physician who specializes in surgery of the brain — can detect skull fractures and damage to the brain.

Surgical repair of injuries and bleeding is a common form of treatment for severe head injuries. Most hematomas require prompt surgical removal. In a study funded by NINCDS, patients with hematomas who were operated on up to 2 hours after injury had a death rate less than 30 percent, compared to 95 percent in patients operated on more than 6 hours after injury.

Head-injury patients are monitored to ensure that they have no problems breathing and that brain swelling is under control. Some patients may need a breathing tube inserted into the nose or mouth. This tube is attached to a respirator.

Drugs can also help to control brain swelling and edema. Diuretics, which help the body eliminate water, and steroids, which decrease water in the brain, are drugs commonly used for this purpose. Barbiturates, a class of drugs that reduces the activity of nerves in the brain and spinal cord, are also administered on occasion. Treatment of increased intracranial pressure with barbiturates was the result of NINCDS-sponsored research. Although scientists are not certain how barbiturates control brain swelling, they suspect that the drugs' ability to slow body functions may also reduce blood flow to the brain. Treatment for brain swelling is begun before the pressure within the skull becomes too high to respond to therapy.

Rehabilitation: A long-term goal

After receiving treatment in the hospital, the head-injury patient may be allowed to go home to complete the recovery process. Outpatient therapy may be provided at a rehabilitation center or in a hospital with a rehabilitation program.

People with more severe injuries, however, will live at a rehabilitation center for some time in order to participate in a more intensive program of physical and psychological therapy. These patients may make periodic visits home.

"I remember when Jack came home from the rehabilitation center," says a young woman. "He was visiting us for the weekend on a trial basis. On the first night, he stayed upstairs a very long time — so I went to see if he was okay. I found him crying there. 'What's the matter?' I asked. He said, 'I'm so afraid the children won't love me because I'm different now.' "

Like Jack, many people who have had a head injury are sad or depressed. Helping the patient cope with these and other effects of head injury is one goal of long-term therapy.

A number of specialists may be called upon to help rehabilitate the head-injury patient. Psychologists can help patients like Jack to understand the consequences of their injury, cope with marital and sexual difficulties, and ask for assistance when they need it.

Other experts involved in the rehabilitation process include psychiatrists and speech, physical, and occupational therapists. Services offered to the patient include instruction in basic living skills such as bathing, dressing, cooking, and reading.

Some patients benefit from memory retraining therapy, which helps them remember words by forming visual images. For example, they might picture Uncle Sam to remember "United States."

Another type of rehabilitation, called cognitive therapy, "opens the doors to understanding thinking processes" says a head-injury expert. Cognitive therapy may help people whose mental processes no longer interact in the normal, effective way. The training teaches patients to respond appropriately in a wide variety of situations, and improves attention span, self-awareness, and flexibility of thought. Techniques may include computer games, videotapes, and group role-playing sessions.

Rehabilitation may play a role even after mild head injuries, which can reduce a person's ability to process information. A patient who returns to work too soon after such an injury may not be able to succeed at ordinary tasks, especially at jobs requiring attention to several factors at once. A lawyer may not be able to follow court arguments; an insurance agent may find it hard to perform necessary calculations. Such difficulties can lead to tension, fatigue, irritability, anxiety, and depression — conditions that can only aggravate the cognitive or thought process.

Experimental occupational therapy tries to increase tolerance to fatigue and noise, thus improving work efficiency and ability to concentrate. The therapy program gives the patient increasingly abstract and complex activities to deal with — activities that are selected according to the patient's progress. The therapist also provides the patient with emotional support, while periodic tests measure patient improvement.

Occupational training and most other types of therapy are begun as soon as possible after the injury. Research has shown that this is the most effective way to approach the rehabilitation process. Exercise therapy, for example, is sometimes begun while the patient is still unconscious.

Physical troubles interfere

The patient's physical troubles often complicate the early stages of rehabilitation. The more severe the injury, the more lasting and serious will be the resulting physical problems.

Loss of muscle control and muscle weakness on one side of the body, interfering with leg and arm movement, can occur after head injury. Recurrent epileptic seizures may also be a problem. In fact, head injury is a leading cause of epilepsy. Fortunately, most seizures can be controlled with medicines.

Hematomas and skull fractures that press on the brain can cause facial paralysis, deafness, disorders in muscles controlling eye movement, and loss of the sense of smell.

Therapy for physical problems may restore old skills to damaged parts of the brain and teach new skills to brain areas that were spared by the injury.

Some physical problems, however, may be difficult to control, including relatively minor ones. "It's very embarrassing to be talking to someone, especially someone you don't know, when a rush of saliva spills from your lower lip," says one patient. "This can be controlled — but only if your every thought is to swallow. Just tell me one person whose every thought is to swallow."

Coping with personality changes

Just as important as the consequences of physical disabilities are the psychological and mental problems that are the most common result of head injury. Psychological difficulties include depression, anger, and behavior inappropriate to the situation.

Immediately following severe injury, most patients have impaired mental functions that can last for a long time. Some impairment may be permanent. Patients may have problems with abstract thinking, being unable consider an idea in general terms without having a specific example in real life.

Patients may also have difficulty concentrating and they may find it hard to remember or to learn. Scientists have found that even a mild head injury such as a concussion impairs the brain's ability to handle new information for varying periods of time.

"It takes him 10 minutes to read a sentence," says a woman about her head-injured husband, "and a few minutes later he may not remember what he read. My husband has no long-term memory and he can't follow directions. You tell him to turn off the light, he'll shut the door."

Children, like adults, may have persistent memory problems after head injuries. The ability to learn new things may be impaired, interfering with school progress. In NINCDS-funded research at the University of Texas Medical Branch in Galveston, investigators found similar patterns of memory problems in head-injured children, adolescents, and young adults. Among head-injured children, they found that nearly half later had trouble with the storage and retrieval functions of long-term memory. Those with the most severe head injuries suffered the greatest memory impairment.

Changes in personality, although harder to measure, seem to be more frequent than mental changes in head-injured patients, and are at least as disabling. One common personality change involves apathy — a reduced interest in life's activities and challenges.

An example is Cheryl, who at age 21 was knocked off her bicycle by a car, causing her to hit her forehead. Her family was overjoyed when she seemed to recover. However, when Cheryl was discharged from the hospital months later, she had a tendency to sit idly. Cheryl had no interest in doing anything, her parents complained. Doctors examined Cheryl 14 years later. Although her thinking was slow, her intellectual functions appeared normal and she'd held a job requiring above-average intelligence. But she said that she was uninterested in doing anything except mundane household chores, and that she felt surprisingly little affection for her husband and children.

Other patients may become overly optimistic — believing that things are better than they are. Or they may underestimate their disabilities.

A third common personality change is loss of social restraint and judgment. A person becomes tactless, talkative, and hurtful, and may have outbursts of rage in response to trivial frustrations. These rages occasionally become so violent that the patient may require hospitalization.

The embarrassment that some head-injury patients unintentionally cause their relatives can be a problem. "One night we took Phillip to the movies," says his wife. "He had to go to the bathroom. Normally, I would take him, but I was really involved in the film. So he went by himself. But when he came back, he couldn't find us. He started yelling, 'Janet, where are you?' It was so embarrassing. I didn't want to claim him. But of course I went and got him."

Patients may also react with psychiatric symptoms to the stress of mental disabilities and life-style readjustment. A law student might become depressed at having to change to a community college or a former accountant at having to take a menial job.

Regaining the quality of life

"Up until now," says one expert "we've attended to the acute needs of the patient. But it is becoming apparent, as more and more head-injury patients are surviving, that we need to look at the quality of their lives. Many survive at least 40 years."

Generally, the greatest recovery occurs in most patients in the first year. Some people continue to improve for years. Therapists believe that patients who receive concentrated therapy soon after their injuries will continue to improve for a longer time. Long-term therapy can lead to a patient's continued improvement over a lifetime.

One patient who had been a photographer devised her own form of therapy — creating photographic collages — which helped to express the sense of loss and change experienced after a head injury. The patient illustrated her post-injury verbal problems by photographing documents written in the unfamiliar language of Arabic. "Though I recognized alphabet, words, sentences on the page, for a period of time not a scrap of sense could I make of them," she says.

The progress made by a brain-damaged patient may be described according to one of four categories which make up the Glasgow Outcome Scale. These categories range from good recovery to the vegetative state where there is no evidence of a functioning brain.

In an NINCDS-sponsored study of survivors of severe head injury, 50 percent showed good recovery after 3 months or more, 35 percent had moderate disability, 10 percent remained severely disabled, and 5 percent were in the vegetative state.

The extent of an injury affects a person's ability to return to work — although not always to the degree expected. A recent study sponsored by NINCDS at the University of Virginia Medical Center showed that a surprising number of patients with very minor head injuries found themselves unable to work for several months. Certain jobs can be handled by someone with a serious disability, while other jobs cannot be performed with even minimal disability. In some patients, thought-process or memory problems are not apparent until they attempt to return to their occupations. For this reason, it is important for even the minimally injured patient to be tested.

The length of a person's life, as well as its quality, may be affected by a nonfatal head injury. NINCDS scientists have shown that World War I veterans whose head injuries led to later epileptic seizures had a decreased life span.

The impact on the family

When 16-year-old Lily found out that her younger sister, Fran, had been in a car accident and suffered a head injury, she felt "as if I had just been thrown into a make-believe world, one that I would just as soon not have known. I remember the endless trips to the hospital. I hated each and every one of them. My mother was there every day — all day. There was nothing else on her mind. I hated that too. In fact, I hated everything then. Fran was not the little sister I grew up with. She was a lifeless body — a part of machines and wires."

Whether it is a sister, brother, mother, or father who has been injured, the effect on the family can be dramatic. Relatives undergo tremendous emotional turmoil — from worrying whether the injured victim will survive to dealing with a mentally or physically handicapped person.

When a family member is injured, relatives need information about the condition of the patient and about the prospects for recovery. Later, they need to be taught to participate in rehabilitation and to plan for the patient's long-term care.

It is particularly difficult for a family to deal with a member who has trouble thinking, withdraws emotionally, and lacks initiative. Families need to be forewarned of ways in which the head-injury patient is likely to seem different, to experience difficulty, and to pose extra burdens. It is also important for the family to understand the reason for a patient's behavior. A person who recently awoke from a coma, for example, will probably experience confusion.

"My daughter was so confused, she couldn't find her own room," says one mother. "Things didn't look right because her visual perception was off. She'd go into the bathroom and sit 6 feet away from the toilet — all the while thinking she was on the toilet."

If a patient is disoriented and has visual, perceptual, and verbal problems, he or she can experience an overwhelming feeling of confusion and frustration. Not only does everything "look wrong," but the patient may be unable to talk about the unsettling after-effects of the injury. For that matter, the patient may have difficulty talking about anything if the part of the brain that controls speech and language is impaired. The patient's confusion and frustration can lead to a temporary state of agitation where he or she becomes verbally and physically abusive.

"I remember when Judy was in the hospital," says her mother, "and she asked for milk. I got a glass of milk for her and then had to leave her room. When I came back, she was screaming and throwing the milk at the nurse. Everyone was very upset with her. Later, I realized she wanted a milk shake but was unable to say what she wanted."

Although some patients remain combative, most people progress to a condition of greater control. Whatever the patient's disability, any denial of the problem by the family can subject the patient to more frustration and put pressure on the person to reassume responsibilities prematurely.

Even when a patient recovers, the rehabilitation process can be terrifying to relatives. Distressing effects of personality change and impaired intellectual function — no matter how temporary — can be overwhelming. One research study in Scotland found that an injured person's mental handicap tends to break up a family far more than does a physical handicap.

But many families learn to cope. "It's been 6 years since Fran's accident," writes her sister, Lily. "The waiting was worth it. Fran continues to improve; but mentally and physically she will never be the same. My sister is becoming a new person, a strong young woman whom I am growing to respect. It does no good to look for the Fran of yesterday — she is no more. There is only the Fran of today. I've learned to understand that the brain-damaged victims of head injury are new people with their own unique needs and desires. It is our responsibility to understand and accept."

Dos and don'ts of patient care

Rehabilitation experts consider family support an important factor in patient recovery. As family members struggle to assist an injured person, they may be helped by the following guidelines advocated by a rehabilitation expert with the Maryland Head Injury Foundation:

- Try to maintain a balance between pushing a patient beyond the ability to function and not encouraging the person enough.
- Consider the rate, the amount, and the complexity of materials presented to the patient. Remember that the patient usually cannot process information quickly and has a short-term memory loss. Complex materials — a 200-piece jigsaw puzzle, for example — should not be given to a patient with visual and perceptual problems.
- Try to establish a daily routine, as patients do not deal well with the unexpected.
- Use visuals — pictures, photographs, films — to augment spoken language.
- Help prevent confusion in the patient's environment. "When I brought my daughter home," says one woman, "I had put patterned paper in the drawers where her clothes were. Well, she couldn't distinguish between the clothes and the patterned paper. I had to remove the paper and keep the clothes separated by type of garment — in very organized piles."

Research fights back

The increased success of rehabilitation techniques in improving quality of life and survival rates for head-injured patients is largely due to better knowledge of the brain itself. Brain research, much of which is supported by NINCDS, continues to provide more answers. But the neuroscientist's task is made difficult by the nature of the brain: it is the most complex organ in the body. Much remains to be learned about how the brain functions normally and after injury.

NINCDS-supported scientists pursue a variety of approaches to the study of head injuries. Some research teams look at what happens to brain cells when they are injured, and explore ways to stimulate recovery and regrowth. Other investigators follow the history of head-injury patients to make better predictions of survival and extent of recovery.

Scientists will be better able to predict the outcome of head injuries as a result of information obtained through the NINCDS-sponsored Traumatic Coma Data Bank. At four U.S. medical centers, physicians feed into a national computer network information about the types of head-injured patients they see and the treatment they provide. These data will help research determine which factors influence the survival of head-injury victims, and what kind of life survivors can expect.

Scientists will also be able to compare the results of treatments used at different neurosurgical centers, and to evaluate the effectiveness of various therapies.

Consequences of head injury

An NINCDS-funded study at the Medical College of Virginia addressed the important question of what happens to patients who survive a severe head injury. Medical advances have decreased the number of deaths, but have they increased the number of severely disabled survivors? The study concluded that aggressive surgical and medical therapy enables some patients who would have died to make a good recovery without increasing the proportion of severely disabled patients. Other studies looking at patients with minor head injuries, such as concussions, indicate that subtle consequences may be more frequent and more lasting than previously believed.

Scientists hope to identify the structural and functional changes in the brain produced by a head injury. These changes could then be related to the condition of the patient after the injury and possible methods of treatment.

Looking at the brain

The development of computerized tomography (CT) has enabled neurologists to detect and identify different types of head injuries. Scientists continue to investigate new ways to use the CT scan. One study sponsored by NINCDS at the Medical College of Virginia, Richmond, is evaluating the CT scan as a tool for deciding when brain-pressure monitoring devices should be used.

Other measures of brain changes should provide valuable information for the care and treatment of the head injured. At the University of Texas, Houston, the Medical College of Virginia, and the University of California, San Diego, scientists are examining electrical activity in the brain which results from stimulating the senses of touch, hearing, and sight.

A new brain-imaging technique called positron emission tomography (PET) is helping scientists learn more about changes in brain function after injury. This research technique, whose development has been funded by NINCDS, is already used to identify areas of specific brain function in normal subjects, to locate the origins of epileptic seizures, and to evaluate brain tumors.

Unlike conventional X rays which show how the brain looks, PET shows how the brain works by depicting its chemical activity or metabolism.

Chemical activity in the brain is fueled by glucose — a form of sugar. In order to "see" the brain at work, scientists attach a harmless radioactive tag to glucose which is then given to the patient. The PET scanner "reads" the tag, showing where the glucose goes in the brain. The more active the brain cells, the greater the use of glucose.

To explore this new research technique fully, NINCDS established a national PET research program involving medical centers around the country and the NIH research facility in Bethesda, Maryland. One study at the University of Pennsylvania is using PET and CT scans to determine the cause of edema and brain swelling after head injury.

A technique similar to PET, called 2-deoxyglucose autoradiography, was used to conduct the first study of how specific brain regions function after head injury. Investigators carrying out animal experiments at the Medical College of Virginia found decreased brain activity in most areas. But a surprising finding was increased activity in one small region. This area of increased activity may somehow trigger coma-like states in animals; similar increase in activity in a certain part of the human brain may also be connected to human coma. Perhaps certain areas in animal and human brains can suppress activity in other parts of the brain — resulting in coma.

Scientists are using another imaging technique, nuclear magnetic resonance (NMR), to study the brain. NMR scanners use the magnetic properties of atoms in living tissue to produce computer-reconstructed images of the brain or other organs. These images can detect changes in cells and the structures surrounding cells. NMR scans have shown hematomas and small brain lesions not visible on a CT scan.

A new experimental technique, called the 133 xenon Cerebral Blood Flow System, does not produce an image of the brain, but allows scientists to create a map or chart of the brain's blood flow. The patient inhales a small amount of radioactive xenon gas. The amount of xenon circulating in the blood is then measured by detectors attached to the patient's head. By determining the concentration of xenon carried through blood vessels to brain tissue, scientists can produce a map of blood flow within the brain. NINCDS-supported scientists using this method at the University of Pennsylvania, the Medical College of Virginia, and the University of Texas, Galveston, found that there are marked changes in brain blood flow during the early phase of head injury. Certain areas of the brain have normal blood flow while other areas show reduced flow.

These changes in blood flow can help predict a patient's recovery, according to one of the investigators.

Drugs help reduce damage

Drug therapy can also be useful in treating head injury. Research studies suggest that barbiturates may reduce the damage caused by insufficient oxygen in the injured brain. Several groups of investigators have reported that these drugs lower the brain's energy requirements.

Other scientists are examining the role of diuretics — drugs that increase the body's excretion of fluid — in decreasing brain swelling.

In laboratory studies at the Medical College of Virginia, NINCDS-supported scientists found that apnea, a temporary breathing halt that can occur during a concussion, is caused by the release of certain body chemicals. Experimental drugs designed to block the effects of these chemicals appear to control apnea.

Other research supported by NINCDS at Albany Medical College showed that one type of serious brain swelling involves a type of support cells called astrocytes. The investigators then discovered that diuretic drugs inhibiting astrocyte swelling also reduced the death rate among head-injured animals. This work led to the synthesis of new chemicals that may have advantages in treating human head injuries.

Some scientists are examining the biochemical events that lead to brain cell death and are looking for drugs to intervene in the process. There is hope that a combination of drugs may someday control these events that inhibit the healing process.

Reestablishing connections

Skin and muscle nerves grow back and regain function after they are cut or crushed. Traditionally, however, scientists believed that damaged nerve cells in the brain and spinal cord — the central nervous system — were incapable of regeneration. But recent work shows that, under special laboratory conditions, these damaged nerve cells may be able to function again.

In NINCDS-supported experiments, nerve cells from the mammalian central nervous system sprout new branches when they are in contact with the supporting (glial) cells associated with skin and muscle nerves. This research shows that adult brain cells have the capacity for growth. But whether this property can be used to repair the injured brain — with its billions of nerve cell connections — remains to be seen.

Other studies of implanted cells offer hope for people with head injuries. Recent animal studies have shown that, in some cases, implanted embryonic nerve cells appear to connect with other nerve cells and restore disrupted functions.

The brain has also shown a remarkable ability to compensate for loss on its on. When the left half of a child's brain is damaged, for example, the language processing function normally carried out there shifts to the right half. Behavior that is suddenly controlled by a different area of the brain, however, may be somewhat altered.

Examining rehabilitation

Rehabilitation is crucial if the ever-growing numbers of severely head-injured patients are to attain a satisfactory lifestyle. Efforts expended on intensive care immediately after the injury may be wasted if subsequent therapy is inadequate. Recently, methods of therapy have been specifically designed for patients with head injuries.

In rehabilitation studies, a patient's family stability, higher intelligence, and occupational status before an injury were associated with better recovery and a more likely return to work. Lengthy periods of coma, persistent motor impairment, and seizures reduced the chances of good recovery. In addition, realistic self-appraisal, high motivation, and family support appeared important for successful rehabilitation.

Hope for the future

Rehabilitation helps many head-injured patients return to the community, even if they are different in some ways. And more patients are reaching the rehabilitation stage. Scientific research has produced improvements in emergency-room practicc, diagnosis, and surgery which allow more head-injured patients to survive. With continued research, there is hope that these head-injury victims will be able to resume their former jobs and lifestyles.

Where to get help and information

The National Head Injury Foundation was recently formed by families of head-injured patients and health professionals. The organization provides information, including a newsletter, and brings together families for mutual support.

National Head Injury Foundation
333 Turnpike Road
Southbury, MA 01701
1-800-444-NHIF
(508) 445-8106

Some local chapters of the National Easter Seal Society also have programs for the head injured.

The National Easter Seal Society, Inc.
2023 West Ogden Avenue
Chicago, Ill. 60612
(312) 243-8400

The American Speech-Language-Hearing Association can help head-injury patients locate clinical services.

American Speech-Language-Hearing Association
10801 Rockville Pike
Rockville, Md. 20852
(301) 897-5700

The National Institute of Handicapped Research (NIHR) supports research on aspects of head injury, particularly rehabilitation services. NIHR's Clearinghouse on the Handicapped provides disability-related information to handicapped individuals.

National Institute of Handicapped Research
U.S. Department of Education
Mail Stop 2305
Washington, D.C. 20202

Clearinghouse on the Handicapped
U.S. Department of Education
400 Maryland Ave., S.W.
Room 3119, Switzer Building
Washington, D.C. 20202

The Family Survival Project provides support and information to families of head-injury patients in California.

Family Survival Project
425 Bush Street
Suite 500
San Francisco, CA 94108
1-800-445-8106

The American Paralysis Association supports research on paralysis resulting from brain and spinal cord injury. The organization also publishes a free quarterly newsletter, "Progress in Research."

American Paralysis Association
P.O. Box 187
Short Hills, NJ 07078
1-800-346-2742

Human tissue banks

The study of brain and other tissue from persons with neurological disorders is invaluable in research. NINCDS supports two national human specimen banks which supply scientists around the world with tissue from patients with neurological diseases. Both banks also need tissue from patients with head injuries for use in a variety of studies. For information about tissue donation and collection, write to:

Dr. Wallace Tourtellotte, Director
Human Neurospecimen Bank
VA Wadsworth Hospital Center
Los Angeles, CA 90073

Dr. Edward D. Bird, Director
Brain Tissue Bank
Mailman Research Center
McLean Hospital
115 Mill Street
Belmont, MA 02178

NINCDS information

For additional information concerning NINCDS research on head injuries, contact:

Office of Scientific and Health Reports
National Institute of Neurological and
Communicative Disorders and Stroke
Building 31, Room 8A06
National Institutes of Health
Bethesda, MD 20205
(301) 496-5751

Chapter 15

Hearing Loss

Hearing Loss

Some years ago pollsters asked a sample of adults, "If you had to choose between becoming blind or becoming deaf, which would you choose?" A surprisingly large number chose blindness. As terrifying as a world of darkness may have seemed, a world of silence seemed even worse.

When you think about it, the reasons are not hard to fathom. Human beings are talkers, social creatures who seek out their fellow beings for conversation and contact. From birth on we cry and coo, look and listen, in our first attempts to communicate. But for over 200,000 newborns and young infants who are born deaf or suffer severe hearing loss in the first years of life, that vital communications link never gets forged. Not only are deaf children denied the wealth of experience that comes from listening to the sounds of nature, of music, and of the human voice, but they must also struggle hard to master speech and language.

For those who become profoundly hard of hearing later in life, the impact is hardly less tragic. At present, nearly 2 million Americans are either totally deaf or suffer such significant hearing loss in both ears that they cannot hear conversation, a phone ringing, traffic noises, or a fire alarm. Another 14 to 15 million are moderately to severely impaired.

All these people know the loneliness, isolation, and frustration that comes from hearing loss. They know what it's like to sit in company and miss the joke or the gist of conversation. Worse, they soon realize that society can be cruel. People are impatient. They don't like repeating their words or raising their voices. They show by facial expression and gesture how annoyed they are when talking to someone "who doesn't understand what I'm saying." It is only a short step from that attitude to the assumption that people who are hard of hearing are soft in intelligence. Ages ago, that assumption led to the vulgar use of the word *dumb* to mean stupid. *Dumb* derives from Old English roots that mean mute, unable to speak — once the common fate of those born deaf.

Fortunately, many elements in society — including the hearing impaired themselves — have rallied to fight ignorance and prejudice. Such well-known figures as Henry Fonda, Nanette Fabray, Lou Ferrigno (TV's Incredible Hulk), and *New Yorker* cartoonist and children's book author William Steig have publicly acknowledged their hearing problems. Their example, along with that of individuals as celebrated as Beethoven, Thomas Edison, Helen Keller and Winston Churchill, has helped dispel the embarrassment that many hearing-impaired people feel, an embarrassment that often makes them deny they have a problem and avoid seeking treatment or wearing a hearing aid.

Pediatricians, family physicians, ear specialists and parents are increasingly aware of the need to diagnose hearing impairments early in life, so that remedial measures and language and speech training can begin. Many lay and professional organizations have formed to aid those with hearing impairments.

In 1975, one of the 11 research institutes of the National Institutes of Health in Bethesda, Md., added *communicative disorders* to its name to emphasize its increasing attention to research on hearing, speech, and language problems. The National Institute of Neurological and Communicative Disorders and Stroke (NINCDS) is the principal federal agency supporting research on the many causes of hearing loss, as well as on prevention, treatment, and rehabilitation. Support includes the development of better hearing aids and other ways to augment hearing: research on hearing *gains*, one might say, to counter hearing *losses*.

Through basic studies of normal hearing and studies targeted on specific impairments, the primary goal of the NINCDS research program is to develop improved methods of *prevention*. But, until this goal of prevention is achieved, research attention will continue to be directed toward better therapies for the hearing impaired.

Sound and hearing

Human hearing depends on a series of mechanical and electrical events that enable sound waves in air to be converted to electrical impulses carried by nerves to the brain.

Sound itself is a form of energy. Suppose you snap your fingers. The snap generates a force that presses against the molecules of air surrounding your fingertips. The molecules are pushed out a short distance in all directions, crowding into space occupied by other air molecules so that a densely packed shell of air molecules forms. That shell — sound experts call it a "shell of compression" — in turn presses against other air molecules nearby so that they, too, are pushed out to form a second, slightly larger shell of compression, which nudges a third layer of air, and so on.

Meanwhile, the air around your fingertips has become less dense as a result of those first molecules being pushed out. A partial

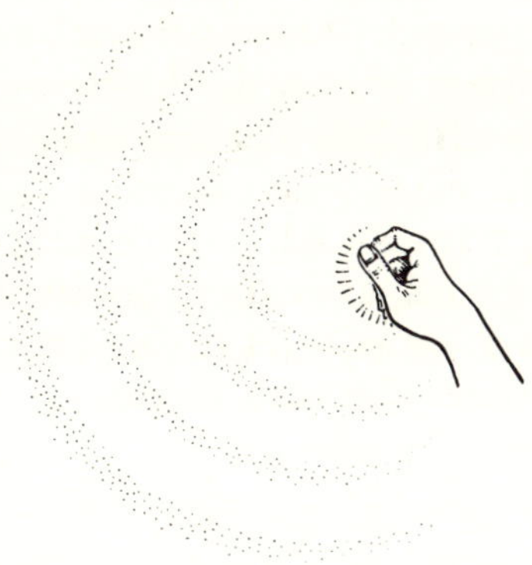

When you snap your fingers the sound energy creates shells of compression and rarefaction in air.

vacuum is created by this "rarefied" air, and the molecules that moved out now rush back to fill that vacuum. Their return creates a second partial vacuum in their wake, which the molecules of the second shell rush back and fill. And so it goes. Thus, the original sound energy generated by your fingersnap moves through the air on a "wave" which is really a succession of shells of compression and rarefaction created by molecules moving back and forth — vibrating.

The number of shells of compression that pass a given point every second determines the frequency of the sound, measured in cycles per second (cps) or Hertz (Hz). Human beings interpret frequency as pitch: the greater the frequency, the higher the pitch. How far the molecules move back and forth as they vibrate is a measure of the energy or intensity of sound. Human beings interpret sound intensity as loudness.

Our ears are sensitive to only certain ranges of frequency and intensity. Healthy young adults can hear notes as low as 20 Hz — lower than the lowest notes of a bass fiddle — as well as sounds at 20,000 Hz, beyond the upper reaches of a flute. The intensity range to which our ears respond is enormous. When sound is just audible — the threshold level of hearing — the force of sound waves acting on the ear is about 140 million times smaller than the force needed to lift a 1-ounce weight. At the other extreme, human ears can respond — painfully — to sonic booms, explosions, or the noise of jack-hammers breaking up city streets.

Because the ear can respond to such enormous ranges of sound energy, intensity is measured in ratios. That is the basis of the decibel (dB) scale. A sound 10 times more intense than another at the same frequency differs from it by 10 dB; a sound 100 times more intense differs by 20 dB. The decibel scale is usually set at an arbitrary zero level (0 dB), which does not mean the absence of sound, but the average threshold level of hearing of healthy young adults. On that basis, a whisper is about 20 dB, and normal conversation about 60 dB. The noise of a jet taking off is on the order of 160 dB — 10 quadrillion times the zero level!

Tuning in

Understanding these fundamentals of sound explains a lot of what goes on — and what can go wrong — with the hearing process. Initially, the job of the ears is to pick up sound waves and conduct them accurately to the inner ear. That the ears can manage this task with great skill and efficiency is due in part to the design of the outer and middle ear.

When sound waves enter the ear, they travel for an inch or so down a narrow tube, the external auditory canal, before striking the delicate, skin-covered tympanic membrane, or eardrum. The drum is shaped like a broad, flat cone about 1/2-inch across and less than 1/50-inch thick. The drum vibrates in tune with the sound waves striking it and transmits the vibrations accurately to three tiny bones in the middle ear, the ossicles. These bones — the malleus, the incus, and the stapes — amplify the vibrations so that the waves can pass on to the inner ear.

It's not hard to understand why specialists find the ear a stunning example of design as well as a challenge for study. For the ear's high-fidelity equipment is miniaturized. The ossicles are the smallest bones in the human body; they fit into a string-bean-seed sized cavity that has been carved out of the temporal bone of the human skull.

Two other features of the middle ear are important: One is that the compartment connects to the throat by a narrow canal with collapsible walls, the eustachian tube. When you swallow, the eustachian tube opens so that air pressure in the middle ear and throat is equalized. That mechanism protects your middle ear from harmful pressure differences that can occur in a fast-rising elevator, for example, or on takeoff and landing in an airplane. The second important middle ear feature is also protective. Muscles attached to the ossicles automatically contract in response to loud noises. These automatic reflexes may prevent strong sound pressures from damaging the delicate structures of the inner ear.

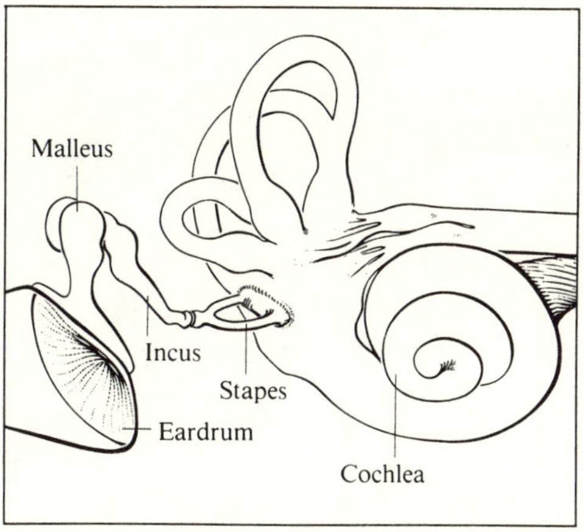

The bones of the middle ear shown in position in relation to the eardrum and inner ear.

To summarize, when the eardrum and middle ear bones are working properly, sound waves striking the drum are faithfully conducted across the middle ear and boosted in energy. The energy boost helps prepare sound waves that have been traveling in air for the more resistant watery medium of their next stop: a fluid-filled bony shell in the inner ear called the cochlea.

Conductive problems

A variety of problems can affect hearing before sound reaches the cochlea. Because these early stages in the hearing process are concerned with picking up and conducting sound signals, specialists refer to the hearing impairments involved as *conductive* problems. Among the most common problems are:

- ***External blockage***. Sometimes there is a buildup of wax in the ears. Sometimes children put things in their ears. Sometimes a bug crawls in. These are obvious plugs that partially block sound. The removal of impacted wax and foreign objects is best left to experts to avoid the possibility of damaging the eardrum.
- ***Perforated eardrum***. A hole or a tear in the eardrum can occur as a result of injury, sudden pressure change, or infection. Ear specialists can repair or completely rebuild the eardrum using the latest techniques of microsurgery.
- ***Genetic and congenital abnormalities***. Malformations of the outer and middle ear sometimes occur in connection with hereditary disease or as a result of injuries and illnesses that affect a baby before, or

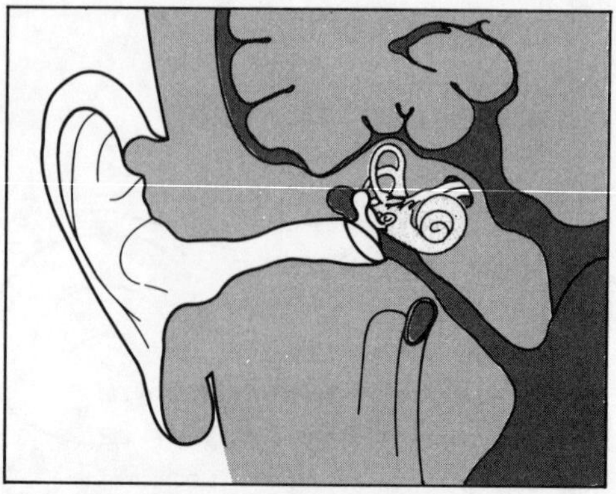

The organ of Corti, containing the auditory receptors and nerve fibers embedded in a snail-shaped bony canal, collectively called the cochlea.

around, the time of birth. Surgery can sometimes correct these problems.

• ***Otitis media***. By far the most prevalent cause of conductive impairments is a common middle ear disease, otitis media. The problem can occur at any age, but is particularly prevalent in children. An estimated two-thirds of preschoolers have at least one episode. The reason that children are so vulnerable may be that their eustachian tubes are shorter and positioned more horizontally than in adults. Infectious agents causing colds or other upper respiratory disease can easily spread to the middle ear. At the same time, mucus, pus, or other fluids accumulating in the middle ear tend not to drain off. Thus, the middle ear can become inflamed, swollen, fluid-filled and painful — the classic symptoms of otitis media that can result in temporary and sometimes permanent hearing impairment. Thanks to today's medications, most middle ear infections can be cleared up with no lasting damage.

Some children are particularly prone to middle ear disease, however, suffering five or six bouts a year. When the condition recurs that often, and is accompanied by fluid in the ear, it is called chronic otitis media with effusion (also serous otitis media). NINCDS-supported scientists at the University of Minnesota are currently studying chronic otitis media to determine if changes in the body's immune system are involved. One possibility is that the body's immune defenses successfully fight off the initial infection, but that some residue of the virus or infectious agent remains to stimulate an immune reaction, leading to the accumulation of fluid. NINCDS is also supporting a major Otitis Media Research Center in Pittsburgh, Pa., in association with Children's Hospital of the University Health Center. The center will study all aspects of otitis media in animals and in human patients.

Patients with chronic middle ear disease with effusion need careful supervision and treatment by ear specialists (otologists) or ear, nose, and throat specialists (otolaryngologists). Not only is there danger of permanent hearing impairment, but frequent bouts of temporary hearing loss may in themselves be serious. The auditory system, especially in the developing years, needs the regular stimulation of sound for healthy growth. Periodic episodes of hearing loss may starve the auditory cells in the brain and contribute to impairments in speech and language skills. Studies of such "auditory deprivation" are under way by NINCDS grantees at Louisiana State University in New Orleans.

Physicians treating otitis media with effusion can drain the fluid by making a small incision in the eardrum. The incision will heal and the problem may disappear. If fluids continue to build up, however, the physician may insert a small drainage tube in the eardrum in an operation called a tympanostomy. Tympanostomy tubes are sometimes dislodged accidentally and may be rejected by the body, but often they may stay in place for as long as a year and effectively

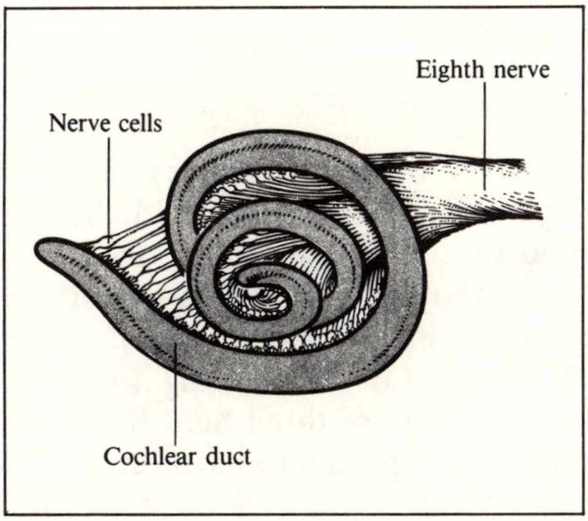

The snail-shaped cochlea has been cut away to show the center compartment, the soft cochlear duct that contains the organ of Corti. The nerve fibers stimulated by hair cells spiral around the cochlea and come together in the eighth nerve.

control the problem. Because there is a small risk that the tubes can give rise to scarring or thickening of the drum after removal, some doctors prefer not to use them, and choose instead to wait and see if the ear problem will improve in time.

• *Otosclerosis*. An example of a hereditary hearing problem that develops in adults is otosclerosis, a condition in which there is an overgrowth of bone in the middle ear. Usually the tiny stirrup-shaped stapes bone is the most affected and becomes fixed in place, impeding sound conduction. Otosclerosis can often be remedied by surgery to remove the excess bone and replace all or part of the stapes with an artificial part. Those who have undergone successful surgery describe the results as miraculous. "I was completely deaf before the operation," one woman said. "As soon as I woke up I could hear again!"

• *Presbycusis*. Specialists have coined the word *presbycusis* — literally, old hearing — to describe hearing impairments that occur in aging. While presbycusis is primarily associated with changes in the inner ear and brain (discussed later), conductive impairments may also occur. The bones of the middle ear may become stiff, for example, or the eardrum thicker and less flexible. Both those changes may reflect a less-rich blood supply to the ear as a result of heart disease, high blood pressure, or other circulatory problems in older people.

Conductive impairments can be detected in the course of an ear examination that includes a variety of diagnostic tests. Before we describe the tests, let us pick up the story of what happens to sound when it reaches the cochlea.

From ear to brain

When sound vibrates the three middle ear bones, the last in line, the stapes, presses against a membranc called the oval window. This membrane is fitted into a thin shell of bone that encloses all the inner ear structures. About an inch down from the oval window, the bone spirals to form the snail-shaped cochlea, another ministructure less than 1½-inch across at its base, rising a mere ¼-inch to its tip.

The cochlea is composed of three fluid-filled compartments. The center, and smallest, compartment is a duct of soft tissue that contains the organ of hearing, called the organ of Corti, after the Italian scientist who first described it. Like the retina of the eye, the organ of Corti contains special cells called sensory receptors that take incoming energy — light in case of the eye, sound for the ear — and transform that energy into electrical signals. The ear cells that do the transforming are called hair cells because the cell tops are fringed with fine hairs that stick up into the fluid filling the duct. The hair cells are sandwiched between two membranes: one membrane rests lightly on the hair tips; the other forms the floor, or base, of the duct, and so is called the basilar membrane.

Research had led to greater understanding of how the organ of Corti works and to a Nobel prize for the investigator who contributed significantly to that under-standing, George von Békésy. Put very simply, when the stapes kicks in the oval window, the fluid in the cochlea is stirred and sets the basilar membrane moving in a very special way: Sounds of high frequency cause the greatest movements of the membrane under hair cells at the base of the cochlea, agitating the tips of the cells' protruding hairs. Sounds of middle frequency cause maximum movements of the membrane further toward the center of the cochlea, while sounds of lowest frequencies cause peak membrane movements near the top of the cochlea.

The movements of the hairs cause changes inside the cells that lead to the production of electrical signals. These signals excite nearby nerve cells whose long fibers — some 30,000 in each ear — spiral out from the cochlea to form the eighth, or auditory, nerve which goes from the ear to the brain.

Soon after entering the brain, eighth-nerve fibers contact nerve cells in the first of many nerve centers concerned with hearing. Ultimately, the auditory signals reach the cortex, the outermost covering of the brain. The cortex contains centers associated with interpreting speech and music, with thinking, memory, learning, and other higher mental faculties.

There are a great many details and subtleties about human hearing that scientists are continuing to work out. How do we manage to block out unwanted sounds, for example, enjoying an intimate conversation in the midst of a noisy party? How do we detect subtle differences in loudness as well as pitch? What enables some of us to hear a tune for the first time and repeat it perfectly? How do we locate the source of sound and judge how near or far it is?

Much of this research requires a detailed analysis of what happens at the cochlea and at auditory centers in the brain. In recent years, NINCDS-supported scientists have been able to remove embryonic cochlear tissue and grow it in the laboratory. Small animals like guinea pigs or chinchillas are often used in these studies because their cochleas are relatively large and their brains not very complex.

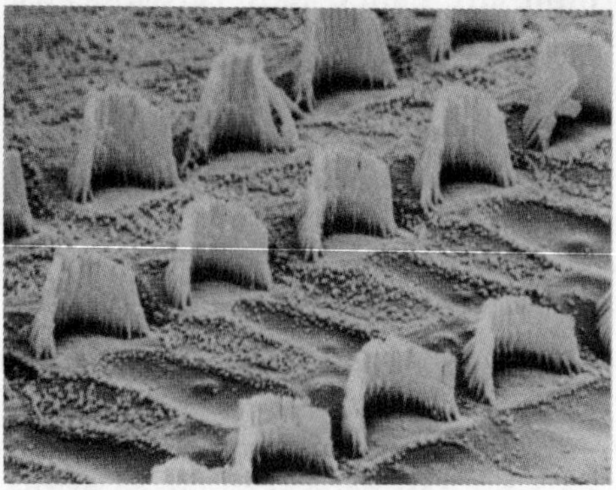

Microscopic clusters of hairs fringe the tops of auditory cells in the inner ear.

Work with human volunteers is also essential. Persons with normal hearing are often studied in experiments in which different messages are piped into each ear or where computers are used to generate garbled or synthetic speech. These studies are aimed at analyzing how people recognize speech and how they detect a meaningful message amidst noise.

Also of great interest are studies of how the two ears and the two halves of the brain work individually and together in the perception of speech, music, and other complex sounds. Experiments with hearing-impaired individuals are equally important, leading to a better understanding of the cues hearing-impaired people use to recognize speech — and how noise affects them.

Hearing problems higher up

Hearing impairments that result from damage to the sensory apparatus (the hair cells and other parts of the inner ear) or to the eighth nerve and auditory centers higher up in the brain (the neural apparatus) are often lumped together as "sensorineural" problems. These include:

Hearing loss at birth. Some 4,000 infants are born deaf every year in the United States. Close to half those cases are due to hereditary disorders.

A larger group of babies is born deaf or with major hearing impairments as a result of congenital disorders or difficult labor and delivery. Mothers who contract certain infections during pregnancy or who take certain drugs may give birth to hearing-impaired infants. Sometimes the hearing loss accompanies other prenatal or birth-related problems that result in cerebral palsy, seizures (epilepsy), or mental retardation.

Before the advent of a vaccine for German measles (rubella), this viral disease in pregnant women was a notorious cause of hearing impairment at birth. Common measles (rubeola) in pregnant women also imposed a threat to the unborn child. Fortunately, there are now vaccines for both these viral diseases so that women can (and should) be immunized well before becoming pregnant.

There are other virus infections for which no effective treatments or vaccines exist as yet. Of these, cytomegalovirus and herpes simplex type 2 virus (which causes a genital infection) can seriously affect the nervous system of infected newborns. Cytomegalovirus infection is estimated to affect 1 out of every 100 children born in the U.S. Between 5 percent and 10 percent of those children develop hearing impairments, especially for high frequencies, and have IQ scores less than 80 later on in school.

Hereditary hearing loss. It is important to realize that hereditary conditions not only can result in deafness at birth, but also account for a variety of hearing impairments occurring later. Hereditary disorders can affect the outer and middle ear, as in otosclerosis, but generally involve damage to the cochlea or higher nerve centers. Because there are so many kinds of hereditary disorders, with different risks of inheritance, couples with a history of deafness on either side of the family should consult genetic counselors for information.

- ***Trauma-induced problems.*** A severe blow to the head, an accident, stroke, brain hemorrhage, or other trauma that affects the ear or any of the auditory pathways and brain centers will obviously take its toll on hearing ability.

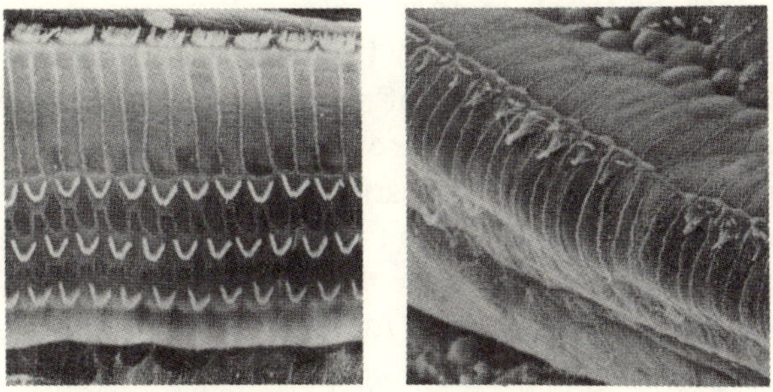

The hair cells in the left photo are normal; right photo shows that exposure to noise leads to total destruction of hair cells (lower layers) or damage (upper layer).

• *Tumors*. Patients with eighth-nerve tumors — called acoustic neuromas — may complain of hearing loss in one or both ears, headaches, dizziness, ringing in the ear (called tinnitus), or numbness over the face. Such symptoms deserve prompt attention. If an eighth-nerve tumor is detected early, surgery to remove the tumor can be completely successful, leaving no hearing or other impairment. Tumors diagnosed at later stages may have grown large enough to be life-threatening, or their surgical removal may result in hearing loss, disturbances in the sense of balance (also located in the inner ear), loss of sensation in the face, or facial paralysis.

Acoustic neuromas can occur for no known reason, but can also arise as a result of a hereditary disease called neurofibromatosis.

• *Noise damage*. Brief exposures to high intensity sound can cause a temporary, but reversible, hearing loss. But continued exposure to loud noise means trouble: Eventually the hair cells sustain permanent damage, resulting in gradual hearing loss.

During the early days of industrialization, nobody doubted that the din surrounding boilermakers, hydraulic press operators, or steel mill workers rendered their hearing less than perfect. Nowadays, specialists are concerned that the everyday sounds of our highly technological society are also wilting our hair cells. Think of the power mowers and chain saws, the disposals, stereo sets, dishwashers, and food processors we live with . . . and the sounds of airplanes, motorcycles, city and highway traffic, fire and emergency trucks. Think, too, of joggers wearing earphones or young people at rock concerts or disco clubs, and you have the reason so many hearing specialists are worried.

Concern about noise has inspired research at several major hearing laboratories supported by NINCDS. Scientists at Washington University Medical School in St. Louis, Mo., for example, are systematically changing the frequency, intensity, and duration of noise to see how each of these factors affects the structures of the inner ear. Investigators at the Central Institute for the Deaf, also in St. Louis, are analyzing the effects of noise on the inner ears of animals and also observing how such stress affects the animals' behavior. Other NINCDS-supported investigators are studying how noise damage may lead to degeneration of eighth-nerve fibers, why some people are more affected by noise than others, and why the ear, once impaired by noise, often becomes hypersensitive and more vulnerable to noise damage.

• *Drug-induced hearing loss*. Drugs as common as aspirin, the antibiotics streptomycin or neomycin, and certain of the water pills (diuretics) used to treat high blood pressure can damage the hair cells or other vital parts of the inner ear. Anyone who, while under medication, has a sudden change in hearing, or experiences dizziness or ringing in the ears (tinnitus), or has other problems with hearing or balance should report the symptoms to a physician at once. Often, changes in the prescription can eliminate the symptoms and prevent permanent damage to the ear.

Certain powerful anticancer drugs may also damage hearing. NINCDS is currently conducting research studies of patients undergoing cancer chemotherapy at the Clinical Center, the research hospital of the National Institutes of Health. Audiologists measure the patient's hearing before treatment and then at periodic intervals thereafter to determine if the drugs have affected hearing.

• *Tinnitus*. Many people have experienced one or more occasions when they felt a ringing or buzzing in the ears or inside the head. But a surprising number of people, especially in middle age or later years, complain of a constant ringing in the head for no known reason. In some cases, the symptoms may be unnoticed if a person is busy at work, talking, or otherwise distracted. For other people, however, the unpleasant sounds are present during every waking hour, interfering with all activities. In the most severe cases, tinnitus even interrupts sleep. The hapless victim is tormented by an incessant internal siren sounding off. The psychological effects on a person can be devastating.

Tinnitus is considered a sensorineural disorder, but what causes it and where in the ear or brain the trouble lies are unknown. Because excessive amounts of aspirin and related drugs produce temporary tinnitus in human beings, NINCDS-supported investigators are studying the effects of these drugs in animals. The scientists can detect whether the animal is experiencing tinnitus by first training the animal to behave in specific ways in response to typical tinnitus sounds. They then observe whether the animal behaves the same way after drug treatment. Other NINCDS grantees are studying sounds that may be generated within the cochlea itself. Still a third NINCDS-supported group at the University of Oregon is developing an ear device designed to mask the tinnitus sounds, a method of treatment that appears to help some tinnitus sufferers. A variety of tinnitus maskers can now be obtained commercially.

• *Presbycusis*. Changes associated with aging are responsible for the majority of hearing impairments in adults. Many people in their forties and fifties experience a decline in sensitivity to high frequencies. The decline is gradual and progressive so that by their sixties and seventies as many as 25 percent of the elderly are noticeably impaired. However, investigators are beginning to question whether "aging factors" *per se* are at fault. There are cultures in the world — the Mabaan people of the African Sudan, for example — where presbycusis doesn't exist. Both men and women have excellent hearing in old age. The environment of the Mabaans is exceptionally quiet by Western standards. Further, the Mabaans do not suffer from heart disease, high blood pressure, ulcers or asthma. They lead relatively stress-free lives. No conclusions can yet be drawn, except that presbycusis is clearly not an inevitable result of aging.

Many experts now think that lifelong exposure to noise, as well as the high prevalence of heart disease, high blood pressure, and other blood vessel disorders increase the odds of hearing loss in later years.

In addition, some hereditary predisposition may be involved: As one investigator puts it, "Some of us may simply be programmed to suffer a decline and fall of our hair cells or our auditory neurons starting at a particular age — as young as the twenties and thirties in some people." Further, the decline may be selective: The hair cells and inner ear structures may be healthy in some older individuals so that they can pass a hearing test for pure tones with flying colors. Yet those same people may have trouble understanding speech, especially under trying conditions. Experts suspect that the listener's confusion is associated with tissue damage or loss of nerve cells in the brain where centers for speech perception and discrimination are located.

With the realization that people are living longer, the problem of presbycusis has become an area of growing concern to the National Institute on Aging (NIA) as well as NINCDS. At present, 6 million Americans 65 or over have moderate to severe hearing losses. By the year 2000, an estimated 32 million Americans will be 65 or older. If 25 percent continue to be affected by presbycusis, that means that 8 million Americans may know only too well the limitations on activities, the lack of enjoyment, the isolation and boredom that severe hearing impairments can impose. To deal with this problem, cooperative research ventures are being initiated by the NINCDS with its sister organization, the NIA.

Currently, NINCDS-supported research on presbycusis includes programs at the University of Michigan, focusing on the causes of presbycusis and microscopic changes in the inner ear, and a program at the University of California at Los Angeles concerned with how age affects the transmission of nerve signals along the auditory pathways in the brain.

Detecting hearing loss

In the case of a simple infection or impacted wax, the diagnosis and treatment of a hearing problem may begin and end in the family doctor's office. More complicated cases call for the expertise of the otologist. He or she will conduct a thorough ear examination, note the patient's medical history, and inquire about hearing problems affecting other members of the family. Certain blood tests or other laboratory analyses may be necessary, as well as standard hearing tests. The specialist may also want X-rays of the head or the computerized X-ray images of the brain called CT scans.

Hearing tests are usually conducted by audiologists, professionals educated in the science of hearing and in the battery of tests used to assess and analyze hearing impairment. Audiologists also provide counseling and nonmedical rehabilitation for the hearing impaired, such as lipreading and hearing aid evaluation.

Persons undergoing audiological testing sit in a small soundproof room. The examination usually includes tests to determine how well the eardrum and middle ear bones conduct sound. These tests depend on inserting a snug-fitting probe with wires attached into the external canal of the ear. Then air pressure between the probe tip and the eardrum is varied at the same time that a tone is sounded through the probe tip. A machine analyzes the movements of the drum and middle ear bones, printing out the results on a graph — the "tympanogram."

The probe can also be used to check the acoustic reflex to loud noise. The tympanogram and acoustic reflex tests take only a few minutes. Since the tests depend on automatic responses of the auditory system, they can be used to test hearing in infants and others who cannot respond voluntarily.

The audiologist then measures the patient's thresholds for two-syllable words and for pure tones in a range from 250 Hz to 8000 Hz. The patient wears headphones and indicates when he or she can just barely detect sounds as the decibel level is varied. The graph that plots sound frequency against decibel level is the audiogram. The audiologist also measures the ability to discriminate speech by having the individual repeat one-syllable words. The audiologist may conduct further tests to determine the nature of the hearing loss. These tests may involve manipulations of pure tones and noises or the use of tape recordings that introduce distortions into voice or sound signals.

An EEG for hearing

In the past decade, investigators have developed ways of recording the electrical activity of brain centers associated with hearing. Electrodes are attached to the top of the head and at each side, near the ear. The individual wears earphones and sits quietly in a soundproof room listening to clicks at different intensities. A computer analyzes the nerve cell activity in response to the clicks, and displays the brain wave pattern on a video screen. Audiologists know the normal shape of the waves and the time it takes for nerve signals to move from center to center along the auditory pathways. Delays in the appearance of certain waves, or changes in their pattern, help localize the problem. Because the brain cells recorded lie in the brain stem — a core of brain tissue located below the cortex — the brain wave recording is called the auditory brain stem response. Like tympanometry, the auditory brain stem response test

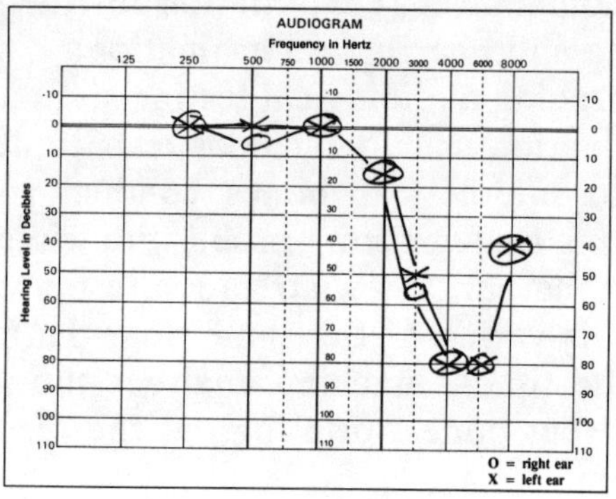

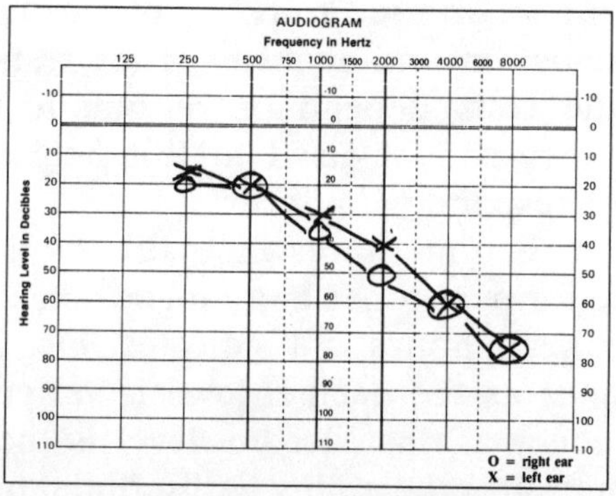

Audiograms measure how well you hear pure tones with each ear. Upper audiogram shows a typical noise-induced hearing loss—worst at around 4000 Hz. Lower audiogram shows a typical presbycusis pattern: hearing in both ears gradually worsens as frequency increases.

is automatic and so can be used to study hearing in infants. However, the test takes up to an hour and the subject must remain stationary and quiet, so testing in young children usually requires mild sedation.

Many people think that you can't measure children's hearing in the first months or years of life. Even without the newer automatic tests, however, there have always been ways of measuring infants' hearing. Parents can approach a baby from behind and sound a bell or rattle. The child who hears will be startled, and, depending on the stage of brain development, may turn toward the direction of the sound. Audiologists can also test an infant's hearing with standard pure tone tests. The infant wears earphones and sits on its mother's lap in the test room. The audiologist trains the child to associate a certain sound with the appearance of a toy or other interesting object displayed on a screen. By observing the child's behavior in response to speech or noises at various intensities, the audiologist can measure how well the child can hear.

The results of medical and audiological examinations may indicate a problem that can be helped by surgery, medication, or a hearing aid. Sometimes, preventive measures are urged: Adults with middle ear infections are cautioned to avoid flying; workers who are beginning to show noise-induced hearing losses are advised to transfer to less noisy departments or at least wear ear protection. Often, however, the hearing loss is long-standing and irreparable. In those instances, there is no instant remedy or miraculous cure. But there *are* important things that can be done.

What hearing aids do

A hearing aid amplifies sound. The aid provides the extra power to boost sound so that it can stimulate the cochlear cells. Hearing aids can benefit anyone, as long as some hearing remains. How well hearing aids work is another matter. Their effectiveness depends not only on the design of the aid (is it a quiet, high-quality, easy-to maintain instrument?), but also on how well the aid matches the individual's needs. Present-day aids are a far cry from the ear trumpets used generations ago. A modern aid is lightweight, battery-operated, and miniaturized. It can be molded to fit inside the ear, worn behind the ear, or fitted into eyeglasses.

Many individuals with hearing impairments become sensitive to amplified sound. This does not mean they cannot wear a hearing aid; it does mean that the aid must accommodate their sensitivities. Some investigators now suspect that hard-of-hearing people occasionally retain "islands of hearing" — frequency ranges where sound is still perceived at near normal levels. Such individuals might find the amplification provided by hearing aids uncomfortable. Scientists at Louisiana State University in New Orleans are currently investigating islands of hearing in hearing-impaired people to see how common the phenomenon is, and whether special aids making use of these frequencies could be designed to enable individuals to understand speech.

But no matter how well designed and appropriate to the wearer's hearing impairment, the chances of the aid benefiting the user largely depend on attitude and motivation. It is important to realize that adjustments in the aid have to be made and all wearers go through a period of learning and adaptation. In short, the recommendation and fitting of a hearing aid is not the end of an audiological examination, but the beginning of a new way of life. Follow-up in the first few weeks, proper maintenance, and periodic checkups to see how the human ear and aid are both doing are a necessary part of the process.

At the same time, a person can learn simple skills to enhance the usefulness of an aid. Speech reading (lipreading) is one. Most people already posses this skill to a remarkable degree. If you think you are no a speech reader, consider the times you have watched a TV movie where sound was not quite synchronized with lip movement.

Hearing handicaps before age 3

The problems of communication are vastly more complicated for the child who has never heard speech than for those whose hearing problems develop later.

Normally we learn to speak by imitating others and listening to the sounds we make. That instant replay — auditory feedback — allows us to correct our speech and continuously adjust the tone, rhythm, and loudness of our voices. Children who suffer a hearing loss in infancy must overcome a double hurdle: They are cut off from a major source of learning about the people, places, and things of this world. And they cannot benefit from the natural feedback system that makes speaking one's native tongue the inevitable event in development that it is for most of us.

Children who become moderately to severely impaired before age 3 (the prelingual years) can be helped by hearing aids, but as one specialist put it, "Rehabilitation begins with parent education . . . the audiologist and hearing therapist must use considerable skill in helping parents (and children) adjust to the benefits and the limitations of a hearing aid." How much progress can be made also depends on what other handicaps a child may have. Visual problems, movement disorders or mental retardation compound the basic communication and learning problems.

It is testimony to human resourcefulness and to progress in hearing research that people no longer despair of overcoming the problems of hearing loss in infancy. In times past, those afflicted often remained mute or chose not to make vocal sounds. They communicated with the speaking world through notes, gestures, and signs — not unlike the tourist struggling in a foreign land. Society tended to enforce the communications barrier by ignoring the problem or else relegating deaf people to special schools or institutions. One result has been that deaf people have tended to form a separate culture among themselves, employing their own means of communication and seeking each other's company. Even today, 95 percent of deaf people marry other deaf people. Many have the native intelligence and creativity to succeed at professional careers, but communication and social barriers continue to work against their achieving their full potential.

At the end of the 19th century, authorities urged reforms in education aimed at solving the problem of the isolation of the deaf: Enforce a strictly oral mode of speech training, they declared. Forbid children to use any form of sign language, finger spelling, or other manual communication. Instead, teach speech reading and vocal training exercises so that the deaf will have to master the sounds of speech and the principles of spoken language. This strictly oral approach has been effective in many cases, and remains the guiding philosophy of many training centers and schools for the deaf throughout the world.

In the United States, however, opposition to the oral-only tradition remained active, in part due to the efforts of such teachers as Thomas Gallaudet, for whom Gallaudet College for the Deaf in Washington, D.C., is named. Gallaudet believed that the all-important goal for the deaf individual was to be able to communicate with *anyone*. He strongly advocated sign language. Others agreed, urging that whatever means aided communication — speech reading, vocal training, gestures, or sign language — should be encouraged. Today this "total communication" approach, as it has come to be called, coexists with the oral-only school, each with strong adherents and notable successes.

Important in the development of the total communication approach has been the growing use of American Sign Language, *Ameslan*. Ameslan uses subtle combinations of hand, face, and body movements to comprise a vocabulary and grammar that are distinct from English. Ameslan "signers" now make it possible for profoundly hearing-impaired people who have learned the language to watch the television news or attend some public meetings. In the hands of the creative actors and writers of the National Theater of the Deaf, Ameslan has also developed as a vehicle for imaginative expression in poetry and drama.

Hearing horizons today . . .

The hearing-impaired individual has more learning opportunities and communications aids available now than at any other time in history. Legislation enacted in 1973 prohibits discrimination against the handicapped in employment or education by any organization receiving any amount of federal funds. This has meant new opportunities for the profoundly hard of hearing in the job market and at all levels of education.

In addition, variants on the training methods followed by either oralist or total communication practitioners have been developed. "Cued speech" is an outgrowth of the desire to make speech reading more effective. Speakers learn to augment their lip movements by finger signs to indicate particular consonantal or vowel sounds. The signs clarify whether the lips are saying "bad" or "pad," "road" or "load." (Only about a third of spoken English can be understood by interpreting lip movements alone.)

There has also been renewed interest in teaching the deaf to understand speech by having the deaf person feel the muscles of the throat and neck as the speaker pronounces words. This was the method Helen Keller's teacher used, and NINCDS-supported investigators at Massachusetts Institute of Technology (Cambridge, Mass.) are currently exploring its effectiveness.

An increasing variety of amplifying devices and signals are now available for the hearing impaired. Telephones can be equipped with lights to signal when the phone is ringing and amplifiers can be built into the receiver. Other communication equipment includes teleprinters which enable a sender to type a message that is encoded electronically for transmission over the one. A decoder at the other end reconverts the signals to a printed message.

. . . and tomorrow

Meanwhile, scientists are exploring how to use the body's other sense systems as a means of communication when hearing fails. The skin is sensitive to vibrations over a range of frequencies. By attaching a set of vibrators around the waist or chest, the wearer can learn to interpret a sequence of vibrations as words and sentences. Such "vibrotactile aids" are currently being investigated by NINCDS-supported scientists at the University of Washington in Seattle and the Callier Center for Communication, Dallas, Texas.

Perhaps the most ambitious scientific program on the sign boards today is the cochlear implant, a device to aid individuals with sensorineural deafness. The implant uses tiny electrodes to apply electrical stimulation directly to auditory nerve fibers. NINCDS currently supports implant research at Stanford University, Palo Alto, Calif., the University of California at San Francisco, and the University of Washington in Seattle. In some designs, the electrodes are implanted in the cochlea itself, positioned to stimulate selected nerve fibers as they spiral around the shell. In other designs, the electrodes are applied to nerve fibers after they have been bundled together in the eighth nerve. Either way, the trick is to stimulate fibers associated with a selection of different frequencies so that the brain can distinguish different tones. So far, the implants use only a few electrodes, too crude to enable even the rudiments of speech to be encoded and deciphered. But in the few instances where profoundly deaf individuals have volunteered to have the devices surgically implanted, the hardware seems to be well tolerated and the wearers generally report pleasure in being able to hear any sound at all.

The state of the art of cochlear implants is in its infancy. A dozen or so microelectrodes cannot be expected to replace the 30,000 nerve fibers we are born with in each ear. But advances in electronics, in computers, in audio engineering, and in hearing science have been great and continue to develop at an impressive rate. Tomorrow's cochlear implants may be even more miniaturized, allowing greater numbers of fibers to be stimulated with less risk that the implant itself may damage tissue. And if, in the end, the cochlear implant is not the ideal device, the same kind of thinking that led imaginative men and women to try it in the first place will stimulate other research directions, ultimately more successful solutions for the problems of the hearing impaired. That is the hope through research.

Voluntary health organizations

There are many organizations concerned with the problems of the hearing impaired. One of the largest groups is the American Speech-Language-Hearing-Association, which is both a professional and lay organization. Another important professional organization is the

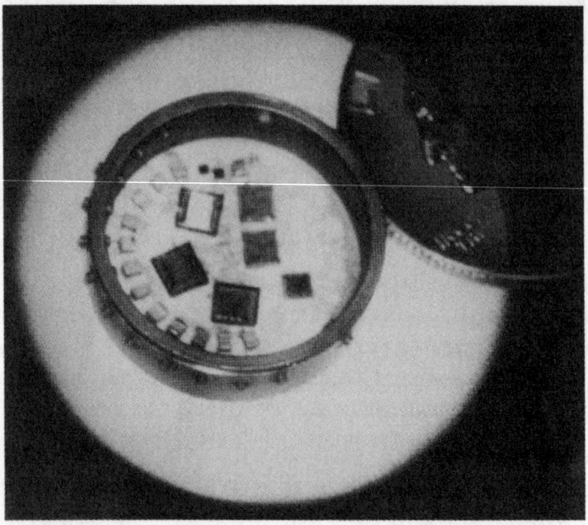

NINCDS-sponsored scientists at Stanford have developed a 12-channel radio receiver-stimulator that is smaller in diameter than the U.S. quarter in the background. The device is attached to a cochlear electrode array to form a cochlear implant.

American Academy of Otolaryngology/Head Neck Surgery, which provides information to the general public.

Some groups espouse particular philosophies in speech education and training. The Alexander Graham Bell Association for the Deaf, for example, adopts the oralist approach. All the groups listed provide literature advice, and can generally indicate schools and other resources available in local communities. Some organizations, like the National Easter Seal Society, have local chapters providing information and rehabilitation for a variety of handicapping conditions. One organization, the Better Hearing Institute, provides information on a toll-free Hearing HelpLine: (800) 424-8576. In addition, some organizations also support research. Most can supply practical information for individuals interested in donating temporal bone tissue to Temporal Bone Banks for research study. The temporal bone of the skull, collected at autopsy, contains the organs of hearing and balance and is valuable source material for scientists studying the tissue changes that occur in communicative disorders.

Organizations:

Alexander Graham Bell Association for the Deaf, Inc.
3417 Volta Place N.W.
Washington, DC 20007
(202) 337-5220

American Academy of Otolaryngology/Head and Neck Surgery
1101 Vermont Avenue, N.W., Suite 302
Washington, DC 20005
(202) 289-4607

American Speech-Language-Hearing Association
10801 Rockville Pike
Rockville, MD 20852
(301) 897-5700

American Tinnitus Association
P. O. Box #5
Portland, OR 97207
(503) 248-9985

Better Hearing Institute
1430 K St., N.W.
Washington, DC 20005
Toll-free Hearing HelpLine: (800) 424-8576

The Deafness Research Foundation
55 East 34th Street
New York, NY 10016
(212) 684-6556

National Association for Hearing and Speech Action
10801 Rockville Pike
Rockville, MD 20852
(301) 897-8682 (Call Collect)

National Association of the Deaf
Suite 301
814 Thayer Avenue
Silver Spring, MD 20910
(301) 587-1788

National Black Association for Speech, Language, and Hearing
P.O.Box 50214
Washington, DC 20004

National Easter Seal Society, Inc.
2023 West Ogden Avenue
Chicago, IL 60612
(312)243-8400

National Hearing Association
Suite 308
1010 Jorie Boulevard
Oak Brook, IL 60521
(312) 323-7200

Self-Help for Hard of Hearing People, Inc.
P.O. Box 34889
Bethesda, MD 20034
(301) 365-3548

Publications

The following publications are published for people with hearing impairment and others concerned with the problem. (Subscription prices are not given since they are subject to change.)

Silent News
193 Main Street
Lincoln Park, NJ 07035

Deaf American
(Published by the National Association of the Deaf, listed above)

NINCDS Information

Additional information concerning hearing research supported by the Communicative Disorders Program of the National Institute of Neurological and Communicative Disorders and Stroke can be obtained from:

Office of Scientific and Health Reports
National Institute of Neurological and
Communicative Disorders and Stroke
Building 31, Room 8A-06
National Institutes of Health
Bethesda, MD 20205
(301)496-5751

Chapter 16

Joseph Disease

Joseph Disease

What is Joseph disease?

Joseph disease is a fatal genetic disorder of the nervous system that cripples and paralyzes while leaving the intellect intact. The disease is characterized by weakness in the arms and legs and a general loss of motor control that eventually confines the patient to a wheelchair. Symptoms appear when a defective gene causes a breakdown and loss of cells in specific areas of the brain known as the striatum, the cerebellum, and the substantia nigra, but what sets this process in motion is still unknown. There is, as yet, no effective treatment.

Joseph disease, first documented in the 1970s, is named for Antone Joseph, a Portuguese sailor with the defective gene who came to California in 1845. The disease occurs primarily in people of Portuguese ancestry, but it has also been found in other ethnic groups, nationalities, and races.

What are its symptoms?

Some symptoms of Joseph disease resemble those of other neurological disorders such as multiple sclerosis and Parkinson's disease. A careful diagnosis is therefore important and should be made by a physician with expertise in neurology. Symptoms of Joseph disease include

- weakness in the arms and legs
- spasticity, especially in the legs
- awkward body movements
- staggering, lurching gait — easily mistaken for drunkenness
- difficulty with speech and swallowing
- involuntary eye movements
- double vision
- bulging appearance of the eyes
- frequent urination.

Symptoms most commonly begin between the ages of 15 and 35, but may appear a little earlier or much later in life. Progression may be fast or slow, and life expectancy ranges from 10 to 30 years after the disease begins.

How is Joseph disease inherited?

Joseph disease is an autosomal dominant disorder. This means that each child of an affected parent has a 50 percent chance of inheriting the defective gene. Joseph disease does not skip generations, but people at risk who escape the disease will not pass it on to their children or future generations. However, since there is no test yet to identify carriers of the defective gene, and since symptoms sometimes do not appear until later in life, people at risk must decide whether to have children without knowing for sure whether they might pass the gene on. As with any inherited disorder, Joseph disease is not contagious and cannot be "caught" by people who are not at risk.

How is the disease diagnosed?

Joseph disease is diagnosed by identifying the typical symptoms in a family in which the disease occurs. Characteristic features include progressive difficulty in walking and speech beginning in the late teen years or in the 20s through the 50s. The gait is abnormal due to spasticity, and speech is slurred because of spastic weakness in the throat muscles. The Joseph disease patient may be unable to look upward or inward, and the eyes may oscillate from side to side.

Late-onset Joseph disease, the type that begins when a patient is 70 or older, is characterized by an uncoordinated gait that may cause the patient to stumble or fall, the slurring speech, and the loss of muscle in the arms and legs.

Neurologists have classified Joseph disease into three types, depending on age at onset and characteristic symptoms. But it is uncertain whether the three types are subtypes of the same disease or three separate diseases. Because the three types have at times borne different names, the plural term *Joseph diseases* has been used.

What research is being done?

The National Institute of Neurological and Communicative Disorders and Stroke (NINCDS) conducts and supports research on all disorders of the nervous system, including Joseph disease. Much of this research is relevant to different aspects of Joseph disease, and may lead to treatment, a cure and, eventually, prevention.

NINCDS is studying normal and defective genes to understand how inherited characteristics are transmitted. With such knowledge and improved genetic engineering techniques, intervention and a cure for inherited disorders like Joseph disease might be possible.

One thrust of Joseph disease research is to find a "genetic marker" which could be used to identify carriers of the defective gene before they have children. NINCDS-supported scientists developed techniques that allowed them to find one such marker for Huntington's disease. They are now using this knowledge and looking for additional markers so that a presymptomatic test can be developed for people at risk for Huntington's. Investigators hope that the new genetic methodology used in this work can be applied to the development of a test for Joseph disease.

A number of other neurological disorders share symptoms with Joseph disease, and research conducted on these disorders should benefit Joseph disease patients. NINCDS scientists are studying the degeneration of the brain's cerebellum that occurs in the ataxias. This type of degeneration produces the kind of spasticity and tremor seen in Joseph disease. NINCDS research on motor neuron diseases, including amyotrophic lateral sclerosis and spastic paraplegia, focuses on the deterioration of certain nerve cells in the spinal cord that also degenerate in Joseph disease.

Much NINCDS-supported research on Parkinson's disease is relevant to Joseph disease. The brain's substantia nigra area is under study because it deteriorates in both disorders. The development of drugs that will increase dopamine — a brain chemical missing in Parkinson's disease — may produce an effective therapy for symptoms of Joseph disease. Investigators using a special imaging technique called positron emission tomography (PET) have already produced the first pictures of dopamine at work in the living brain. Further studies with PET may increase our understanding of dopamine's possible connection to Joseph disease.

Some scientists are studying the role of enzymes in olivopontocerebellar atrophy, a rare inherited neurological disorder similar to Joseph disease. These studies may uncover an enzyme defect that could also be responsible for Joseph disease.

Some patients with Joseph disease have high blood glucose levels and abnormal glucose tolerance test results. Research has also shown that some patients have reduced levels of homovanillic acid (a nervous system chemical) in their spinal fluid. These abnormalities are of special interest to scientists studying Joseph disease.

How can I help research?

The National Institute of Neurological and Communicative Disorders and Stroke and the National Institute of Mental Health support two national human brain specimen banks, one at the Wadsworth Veterans Administration Hospital in Los Angeles and the other at McLean Hospital near Boston. These banks supply investigators around the world with tissue from patients with neurological and psychiatric diseases. Both banks need brain tissue from Joseph disease patients to enable scientists to study this disorder more intensely. Prospective donors should write to:

Dr. Wallace W. Tourtellotte, Director
Human Neurospecimen Bank
VA Wadsworth Medical Center
Building 212, Room 31
Los Angeles, California 90073
Telephone: (213) 824-4307 (Call collect.)

Dr. Edward D. Bird, Director
Brain Tissue Bank, Mailman Research Center
McLean Hospital
115 Mill Street
Belmont, Massachusetts 02178
Telephone: (617) 855-2400 (Call collect 24 hours a day.)

Where can I get help?

The International Joseph Diseases Foundation is a voluntary, nonprofit organization of concerned people including patients, their families and friends, and health-care professionals. The foundation provides information about the disease, supports and conducts clinical research, and helps patients find medical, social, and genetic counseling services.
Contact:

International Joseph Diseases Foundation, Inc.
P.O. Box 2550
Livermore, California 94550
Telephone: (415) 455-0706

NINCDS information

For additional information concerning Joseph disease research supported by the National Institute of Neurological and Communicative Disorders and Stroke, contact:

Office of Scientific and Health Reports
National Institute of Neurological and
Communicative Disorders and Stroke
Building 31, Room 8A-06
National Institutes of Health
Bethesda, Maryland 20892
(301) 496-5751

Chapter 17

Lipid Storage Disease

Lipid Storage Disease

What are lipid storage diseases?

Lipid storage diseases are hereditary conditions in which large amounts of complex fatty materials (lipids) accumulate in tissues. This excessive and dangerous storage of fats can cause mental retardation, enlarged spleens and livers, bone degeneration, and even death.

Ten lipid storage diseases have been identified along with their major symptoms:

Gaucher's disease — enlarged spleen and liver, eroded bones, possible mental retardation or dementia

Niemann-Pick disease — enlarged spleen and liver, probable mental retardation

Krabbe's disease — mental retardation

Metachromatic leukodystrophy — mental retardation or psychological disturbances

Fabry's disease — skin rash, kidney failure, pain in the hands and feet

Tay-Sachs disease — mental retardation, blindness, muscular weakness

Tay-Sachs variant (Sandhoff's disease) — mental retardation, blindness, muscular weakness

Generalized gangliosidosis — mental retardation, enlarged liver, skeletal deformities

Fucosidosis — mental deterioration, muscle spasticity and weakness, thick skin

Farber's disease — hoarseness, joint deformities, mental retardation

What causes these diseases?

Lipids are normally found in every cell of the human body. When cells become worn out and must be replaced, these lipids are routinely broken down into simpler materials by a variety of enzymes. Each enzyme breaks down a specific portion of the lipid molecule.

However, some people are born with a genetic defect that prevents the body from producing enough of a needed enzyme — or from producing the enzyme at all. In these cases, the lipid that is normally broken down by this enzyme accumulates in certain tissues

— signifying the onset of a lipid storage disease. Gaucher's disease, for example, is caused by the absence or deficiency of the enzyme glucocerebrosidase; the fat that accumulates is called glucocerebroside.

How are lipid storage diseases classified?

Lipid storage diseases are classified as infantile, juvenile, or adult types, depending on age at onset.

How are these diseases inherited?

Lipid storage diseases are caused by an abnormality in one of the genes — the biological "message units" on chromosomes that are passed from parents to children and that determine a person's physical characteristics. All of the lipid storage disorders except Fabry's disease develop when a person inherits a defective gene from both parents. This is called a recessive inheritance pattern. Each child of affected parents has a 1-in-4 chance of inheriting a defective gene from both parents and developing the disorder. If only one parent has a defective gene, each child has a 50 percent chance of becoming a carrier. Carriers, other than some who bear a gene for Fabry's disease, do not show any of the signs or symptoms of the disorder.

Fabry's disease, primarily a disorder of males, is inherited from a carrier mother. When a carrier mother has a son, he has a 50 percent chance of getting Fabry's disease. When the mother has a daughter, the child has a 50 percent chance of being a carrier. Some female carriers of Fabry's disease may have mild to severe symptoms of the disorder.

Adult Gaucher's, Tay-Sachs, and Niemann-Pick diseases are found predominantly in Ashkenazi Jews of Eastern and Central European descent. Two-thirds of Gaucher's patients are of Ashkenazi Jewish ancestry. One in 13 Ashkenazi Jews carries the defective gene for Gaucher's disease and about 1 in 30 carries the Tay-Sachs gene.

How common are lipid storage diseases?

The most common lipid storage disorder is the adult form of Gaucher's disease, which affects an estimated 20,000 people in the United States. There are approximately 2,000 patients with Fabry's disease in the U.S., and about 600 people have Niemann-Pick disease. Screening and genetic counseling have significantly reduced the number of Tay-Sachs cases to fewer than 50 in America.

The other lipid storage disorders are extremely rare.

How are these diseases diagnosed?

Most lipid storage diseases strike in infancy. They are identified first through such physical symptoms as poorly developing motor skills, and neurological symptoms such as mental retardation. Diagnosis can be confirmed by a blood test that measures enzyme activity in the patient's white blood cells. Another way to confirm the diagnosis is through skin biopsy. A small sample of skin is taken from the patient and grown in a cell culture. The activity of a particular enzyme in the cultured skin cells is then measured. Both of these techniques are also useful for detecting carriers of lipid storage diseases.

Scientists with the National institute of Neurological and Communicative Disorders and Stroke (NINCDS) have developed diagnostic tests that predict whether a child with Gaucher's disease will eventually experience nervous system problems. These tests will help scientists plan a course of treatment and provide precise genetic counseling for such patients.

Lipid storage diseases can also be diagnosed prenatally through amniocentesis, a procedure, usually done around the 14th week of pregnancy, that involves removing a sample from the sac of fluid surrounding the fetus. Cells that have come from the skin and mucous membrane of the fetus are grown in culture. In another 3 to 4 weeks, enzyme activity can be measured from the resulting cell culture.

A new test for genetic defects in the fetus — chorionic villi sampling — gives results faster and earlier in pregnancy than amniocentesis. However, the safety of this experimental technique — for both mother and fetus — has not yet been determined. The procedure is performed around the 10th week of pregnancy. An obstetrician inserts a slender tube through the vagina into the uterus. A tissue sample is then taken from the chorion, a membrane surrounding the fetus. Genetic analysis of chorion cells can be performed within 24 hours.

Can patients expect to recover from these diseases?

Lipid storage diseases are fatal for patients who develop brain damage. Death can occur 18 months after disease onset, although some patients may live 4 to 5 years. The rate of deterioration for brain-damaged patients varies by disease and severity of symptoms.

When the brain is not involved — such as in the adult form of Gaucher's disease, Fabry's disease, and some cases of Niemann-Pick — patients may have a normal life span.

Can these diseases be treated?

A totally effective treatment for these diseases does not exist at present. However, NINCDS has a study under way of a treatment called enzyme replacement therapy.

In enzyme replacement therapy, enzymes are taken from the placentas of human newborns, purified, and injected into the bloodstream to replace the patient's missing or inactive enzymes. This treatment is similar to the therapy used by diabetics to help overcome their insulin shortage.

However, enzyme replacement has not yet been perfected. It is difficult to obtain the large quantities of highly purified enzymes needed to treat every patient with lipid storage disease. And the treatment is not totally efficient. A significant amount of the injected enzyme fails to go to the cells where the lipids are stored. Instead, sugar molecules that make up part of the enzyme and control its fate direct it to other cells that do not have high lipid concentrations. Scientists are now working on ways to increase the supply of enzymes and to improve their delivery to the lipid-laden cells that need them most.

Gaucher's patients without nervous system involvement should benefit from a recently developed technique which modifies the structure of the enzyme so that it is directed to the specific cells in which the fatty material accumulates.

Another possible way to treat lipid storage diseases is with total bone marrow replacement. Cells in the bone marrow produce the needed enzymes. However, bone marrow transplants are risky and expensive. Thus, enzyme replacement therapy seems to offer the most hope for the future as an effective treatment for lipid storage diseases.

What research is being done?

NINCDS research scientists have identified and cloned the gene for the defective enzyme in Gaucher's disease. Gene identification is expected to aid in the development of improved methods of diagnosis. Cloning of the gene, a process in which exact copies are created, should lead to large-scale production of the enzyme product needed to treat patients. Institute scientists and grantees are also trying to identify and clone the genes for several other lipid storage diseases, including Niemann-Pick and Fabry's diseases.

Other studies are testing the effectiveness of procedures that direct needed enzymes to the cells where lipids are stored. One way, for example, to help reduce deadly lipid accumulation in the brain might be to move enzymes through the cell barrier that protects the brain from foreign substances. Enzymes normally cannot pass through this "blood-brain barrier," but scientists are now trying to open the barrier temporarily by injecting concentrated sugar solutions into a neck artery. Even using this technique, however, only small amounts of enzymes have so far been able to cross the barrier into the brain.

Future prospects

Scientists may someday use genetic engineering techniques to develop strains of bacteria or yeasts capable of producing enough enzymes to treat all lipid storage disease patients. These enzymes may even be adapted to travel only to areas of high lipid concentration where they are most needed.

Experts are also hopeful that gene transplants may be available in the future to patients with lipid storage diseases. Scientists would insert a normal gene capable of producing the needed enzyme into a patient's cells. This procedure could eventually eliminate lipid storage diseases.

Is help available?

Five voluntary agencies are actively involved with the lipid storage diseases. They are:

Gaucher's Disease Research Foundation
9319 Meadow Hill Road
Ellicott City, Maryland 21043
(301) 837-3596

National Foundation for Jewish Genetic Diseases
250 Park Avenue
New York, New York 10177
(212) 682-5550

National Genetics Foundation, Inc.
Room 1240
555 West 57th Street
New York, New York 10019
(212) 586-5800

National Lipid Diseases Foundation
1201 Corbin Street
Elizabeth, New Jersey 07201
(914) 337-2992

National Tay-Sachs and Allied Diseases Association, Inc.
92 Washington Avenue
Cedarhurst, New York 11516
(516) 569-4300

The U.S. Government's National Center for Education in Maternal and Child Health responds to public queries on lipid storage diseases.

National Center for Education in Maternal and Child Health
3520 Prospect Street, N.W.
Washington. D.C. 20057
(202) 625-8400

NINCDS information

For additional information concerning lipid storage disease research supported by the National institute of Neurological and Communicative Disorders and Stroke, contact:

Office of Scientific and Health Reports
National Institute of Neurological and
Communicative Disorders and Stroke
Building 31, Room 8A-06
National institutes of Health
Bethesda, Maryland 20205
(301)496-5751

Chapter 18

Multiple Sclerosis

Multiple Sclerosis

Multiple Sclerosis

Former Notre Dame football coach Ara Parseghian summed it up: "I spend my life working with beautiful young adults, the kids who play for me, but there are hundreds of thousands of other beautiful young adults in this country who are struck down in the prime of life by multiple sclerosis. They need our help." Ara Parseghian knows: his sister and daughter have multiple sclerosis (MS).

These men and women, and others like them throughout the world, have one of the more common disorders affecting the brain and spinal cord, which together comprise the central nervous system.

Yet, considerable confusion exists about multiple sclerosis. As one young woman with MS wrote, "Most people, I now realize, don't know what multiple sclerosis is — they often confuse it with muscular dystrophy. Ignorance of the disease, I had learned, compounds the patient's problem." (The muscular dystrophies are a major group of neuromuscular disorders which are distinctly different from MS, and occur primarily in children.)

However, there is no reason for people to remain uninformed. Knowledge of MS gained during the past two decades of research has expanded at a rate greater than occurred during the entire 100 years following the initial description of the disorder by the great French neurologist, Jean-Martin Charcot. A better understanding of what we do know often can aid those with MS in learning to cope and live with it; and it can provide families and friends with important insights about ways to help and the value of their support.

But we do not stop here. Researchers throughout the world are committed to finding the cause of MS and to developing effective methods of treatment and prevention. In this country, these efforts are spearheaded by the National Institute of Neurological and Communicative Disorders and Stroke (NINCDS), and the National Multiple Sclerosis Society, which was a major force behind establishing the Institute. This research will continue until the answers are found.

The MS population

Most of the estimated 250,000 young American men and women diagnosed with MS are between the ages of 20 and 40. Usually their

The World Distribution of Multiple Sclerosis

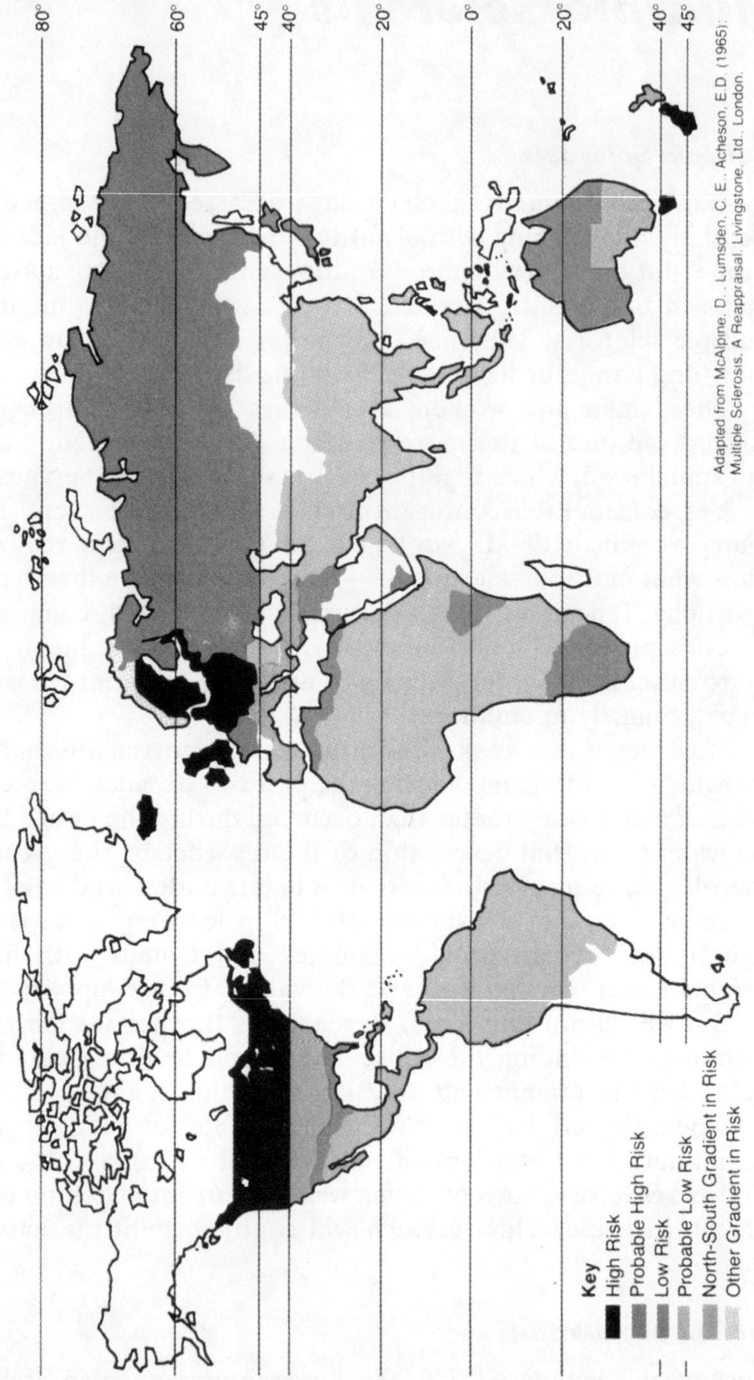

families have had little or no known familiarity with MS. Thus, they are struck at the prime of life by an unexpected disorder, and frequently have no prior knowledge or experience to guide them.

At the time of diagnosis, patients learn that since MS affects the central nervous system, both the sensory and motor (muscle) functions of the body may be impaired and that the symptoms may vary unpredictably, and last for differing amounts of time. Initially, symptoms usually will come and go (termed a "relapsing" course). Most often, patients will find that symptoms improve after an attack; only rarely will symptoms initially get progressively worse.

Most patients also learn that MS is not a killer. In fact, the majority of persons with MS can expect to live their normal life span. Recent studies have indicated that at least half of those persons with MS can still engage in a majority of the activities they performed before developing MS, as long as 15 to 20 years after onset of the disorder. These MS patients have a relapsing course and some — who have mild or infrequent symptoms — may never know they have MS. In the remaining half of MS patients, the degree of severity varies. Some persons with chronic MS have a slowly progressive course, while a small percent develop a more rapid, severely incapacitating form. This variability and unpredictability stems from the very nature of the disorder.

The nature of MS

The brain and spinal cord, where MS occurs, send out and receive signals from all parts of the body. Therefore, symptoms of MS can be experienced anywhere in the body, depending upon the specific site or sites in the brain or spinal cord which are affected.

Nerves, following orders from the brain, control functions within the human body. This mammoth task seems all the more impressive when you realize that each nerve is composed of individual cells, called "neurons." Each nerve cell communicates with its neighbor by passing along the brain's messages, called impulses. Just as a chain's strength depends on its weakest link, a nerve is only as strong as its weakest cell in controlling the body's activities.

Nerve cells in the central nervous system (CNS) — which includes the brain and spinal cord — send out long fibers called axons. For example, nerve cells in the brain which control leg movement have axons which extend to the lower part of the spine. Many are normally surrounded by a fatty covering which insulates them and speeds up the passage of messages along the nerve fibers. MS is a disease of this covering which is called "myelin." The disease process causes destruction of patches of myelin (demyelination) in an erratic and seemingly random fashion. Thus, messages which ordinarily travel at 225 miles per hour are slowed to a fraction of that figure. Although we do not yet know whether destroyed myelin actually repairs itself in the human brain and spinal cord, there is some indication that, initially, myelin may be partially restored at these "demyelinated" areas which begin to dot the central nervous system. Messages may still get through, but they are slower and weaker. The nervous system can sustain a certain amount of demyelination. But eventually, at "multiple" sites throughout the brain and spinal cord — in the process for which multiple sclerosis was named — scar or "sclerosed" tissue forms in place of myelin. At these "multiple" sites, impulses then are blocked or greatly slowed down and the message is lost. This causes the symptoms of MS.

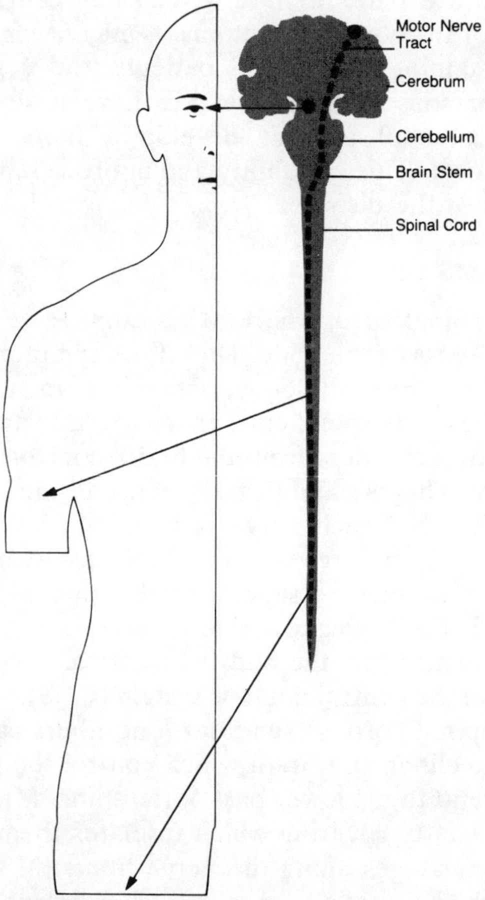

Usually MS symptoms occur and disappear (or lessen) in varying and unpredictable episodes. The pattern can take many forms. Symptoms may occur only once and not return; or they may recur sporadically. In this case, symptom severity either will stay the same or become progressively worse. Finally, a small number of persons with MS experience symptoms which can become progressively more severe. Exacerbations (the occurrence and sometimes worsening of symptoms) are considered by many doctors to be a sign of demyelination, while remissions (periods of cessation or lessening of symptoms) are thought by some doctors to signify myelin repair, although this remains to be proved. Symptom type and severity are determined by the extent and location of myelin damage; by the type of function ordinarily performed by the nerve; and by whether that function is specific or general.

During periods of remission, symptoms will either lessen or disappear completely. Although scientists do not yet know what determines the extent of symptom improvement during remission, some have suggested that — if myelin repair indeed does occur — the extent of repair might influence the degree of symptom improvement. Because the course of MS is so dependent upon the course of demyelination — which varies with every person with MS — no two persons will have the identical experience. In fact, experiences can, and often do, differ completely.

MS symptoms

One of the most common initial manifestations of MS is optic neuritis, a fleeting disorder of the optic nerve which is involved in vision. Optic neuritis often produces "blind spots" in the center of vision and can cause blurriness or transient blindness. It also can affect color vision of one eye. These disturbances usually do not last for long periods of time, but they may recur in the same eye or affect the other eye. Very rarely are they permanent. The course of optic neuritis usually is benign, and vision returns to normal, although some disturbances in color vision may remain. About half of the persons with optic neuritis never develop MS. But since the other half do eventually develop other MS symptoms, optic neuritis is strongly suspected to be related to — or actually a partial form of — MS. Occasionally after optic neuritis, blurred vision may occur following exercise or hot baths. Other visual disturbances such as double vision or the sensation of objects moving or shaking may occur.

Because nerves can be damaged anywhere in the body, any of a number of MS symptoms may occur. However, *rarely* will any patient experience all or a majority of these. Moreover, many of these symptoms can be minimized by supportive treatment. In addition to the visual disturbances mentioned above, other possible sensory symptoms include dizziness and, *rarely*, deafness. Occasionally, sensory symptoms may be manifested as pain. Muscle symptoms may include impaired coordination, weakness, intention tremor (mild shaking when performing a muscular task), and spasticity (muscle rigidity), especially at night. Numbness or feelings of "pins and needles" may occur, but this rarely creates discomfort. Other symptoms may include: bladder problems (frequency or urgency of urination or incontinence), bowel difficulty (constipation), and sexual impotence (of either physical or psychological origin).

Depression also may be encountered in MS. Initially, a period of depression may set in after diagnosis, but this usually gives way to acceptance of the condition. In fact, some patients actually live with a degree of disease-produced euphoria. Nonetheless, some patients may experience depression while adjusting to the disease, or may actually consider it part of the disease process.

On the positive side, patients are spared any mental disability, except in rare instances. They remain as bright, alert and capable as they were before onset of MS. Patients sometimes worry that their memory is worsening, but this usually is a reflection of the normal aging process or a symptom of depression rather than loss of any mental ability. These symptoms, suggesting a diagnosis of MS, can be produced by a number of other disorders as well, not all of which involve demyelination. In fact, approximately 250,000 Americans have other disorders which are closely related to MS. Thus, patients experiencing symptoms similar to those which have been described should seek medical attention and advice to determine their cause.

MS diagnosis can be difficult to make

Patients with MS-like symptoms may be referred to a neurologist, a specialist in brain, spinal cord, and muscle disorders, who is skilled in looking for clinical evidence of involvement of parts of the central nervous system. For only when various parts of the central nervous system become involved, producing symptoms in different parts of the body, can a clinical diagnosis of MS begin to be developed.

Currently, a number of tests aid the diagnosis of MS, but none as yet yields an absolute answer. Diagnosis is based on the clinical determination that myelin damage has occurred in different parts of the central nervous system at different times. For when demyelination occurs in only one area of the central nervous system, doctors cannot rule out the possibility that some disorder other than MS may be responsible. This problem frequently is frustrating for physicians and patients alike. For example, when a patient has had only one episode, or a symptom occurring in only one part of the body, the most likely diagnosis may be MS. However, the physician cannot be sure, and must wait for additional signs to appear before making a positive diagnosis. Although realizing that obtaining a diagnosis is a source of great concern to the patient — anxious to pinpoint the cause of his or her difficulties — the physician, in good conscience, does not want to render a premature judgment.

Some laboratory tests may be useful diagnostic aids, particularly those involving removal of a sample of fluid which bathes the spinal cord. A spinal tap for removal of this fluid is a benign procedure which causes only minimal pain and *no* further MS damage. Spinal fluid samples are used primarily to measure levels of certain proteins and white cells (used by the body to ward off infection). Of particular interest is immunoglobulin G (IgG), a protein fraction which is elevated in approximately 75 percent of patients with MS. However, elevated IgG is not specific for MS, and not everyone with higher than normal levels has MS; moreover, 22 percent of MS patients do not have elevated levels of IgG. Another diagnostic tool examines visual evoked potentials. This painless test measures the time it takes for an electrical impulse to travel from the eye to the brain. An electrode placed on the skin at the back of the head records signals as the patient watches an alternating white and black checkerboard. This test can detect trouble in the optic nerves even when vision seems entirely normal.

Other similar experimental diagnostic procedures called auditory (hearing) and sensory (touch) evoked potentials are aimed at providing evidence of multiple areas of demyelination.

But despite these procedures, MS remains difficult to diagnose. When evidence of trouble in only one part of the central nervous system can be found, it is often necessary to do special X-ray tests to rule out other causes, particularly tumors. Thus, patients may be asked to participate in sophisticated X-ray tests using a CAT (computerized axial tomography) scan, or tests called myelograms or angiograms to be sure there are no other treatable causes of the symptoms.

The impact of diagnosis often is twofold. As expressed by one woman who was told she had MS, "I felt completely alone. Why was this happening to me?" But then, she wrote, "It's oh so much better to know. Then you know how to cope with it and what you can and can't do."

Once a diagnosis of MS can be established reliably, it often comes as a relief to the person with MS who has been struggling to find an explanation for the unpredictable and baffling appearance and disappearance of symptoms. For, once the MS diagnosis is made, the work of understanding its nature and of learning how to accept and deal with it can begin in earnest.

Unpredictable course

The immediate question following diagnosis is how will it affect my life? How mild or serious will it be? And will it limit activity, and if so, by how much? Currently, there is no foolproof method for making a long-range prediction. Some doctors feel that the MS pattern established during the first 3 to 5 years may be indicative of the long-range course. For instance, the disorder may cause fewer problems in the future if initial symptoms occur in the sensory rather than in the motor system. Thus, if initial exacerbations are sporadic, occur infrequently and not too closely together, and leave little remaining impairment, there is good reason to expect that the overall course may follow this trend.

Treatment

The nature of MS renders treatment difficult to evaluate. For, since remissions and exacerbations occur sporadically and unpredictably, it is difficult to prove that the experimental treatment — and not a naturally occurring remission — is responsible for improvement. Nonetheless, active research is pursuing means for developing effective methods for controlling MS.

To date, no treatments have proven effective in stopping MS, although many have been suggested over the years. Suggestions have included diets, certain drugs, electrical (dorsal spinal column) stimulation, substances which suppress the immune (defense) system responses (immuno-suppressants), and substances which stimulate the immune response. While many of these still are under investigation, including transfer factor (using donor immune white cells), none yet has been shown to alter the course of MS. And unless, or until, compelling evidence is discovered indicating that these proposed treatments are indeed helpful in MS, the reaction produced in many patients often is similar to that expressed by one woman with the disorder who wrote: "Other persons, well-meaning, but ill-informed, often plague patients with miraculous 'cures' of which they have read or heard. Inevitably, these tales produce guilt (I should be doing something more to help myself than I am already doing.) and frustration (the 'cures' by an odd coincidence, nearly always are hundreds, if not thousands, of dollars and miles away)."

Now, exciting new research techniques (discussed later) which may permit objective assessment of a treatment's efficacy may partially alleviate that problem.

Until effective treatment is found, however, many MS symptoms *can* be helped. Doctors agree that maintaining good general health, following a balanced diet, avoiding excessive overweight or underweight, getting sufficient rest and relaxation, and appropriate daily exercise can help the person with MS feel better. During periods of exacerbation of symptoms, doctors may advise bed rest.

In addition, specific measures benefit several symptoms in many MS patients. (Since each person with MS is unique, the patient's doctor is in the best advisory position concerning use of these measures.) For instance, many patients with incontinence problems often benefit from drug treatment of urinary infections and from regulating the amount of fluids they consume during each day; moreover, urinary frequency and urgency often can be controlled with drugs, such as propantheline bromide and amitriptyline, which relax the bladder. In selected instances, a bladder operation may be helpful. Many patients with muscle stiffness may be aided by physical therapy, as well as by moderate exercise. This keeps limbs supple and, although it cannot replace lost muscle strength, it can help the functioning of remaining muscular abilities. Electrical stimulation of the spinal cord to aid some muscle and bladder functions is being tried experimentally in a few centers. In addition, some patients have reported short-term benefit from steroids such as ACTH. This has been most useful in treating sudden worsening of symptoms.

Constipation can be helped by laxatives or bran. Spasticity or cramps often can be aided by muscle relaxants (such as diazepam, baclofen, and dantrolene sodium). However, spasticity can be helpful in some instances in compensating for lost muscle strength. Depression often can be helped by psychotherapy, antidepressant drugs, discussions with health professionals (including — in addition to the physician — nurses, social workers, occupational therapists, and psychologists). Often the patient's spouse and family members can be an invaluable resource of support and help.

Professional counseling can be a major help to both the patient and family in alleviating emotional concerns which actually may contribute to or result from the physical situation. Counseling referrals often are offered by the local chapters of the National MS Society. Sometimes referrals can be obtained from state or local health departments.

The patient's own physician is in the best position to offer advice on treatment for relief of symptoms and to coordinate management of the patient's problems. As medical research produces effective new methods of diagnosis or treatment, every effort will be made to see that the general medical community and the public are immediately informed. If questions arise concerning possible new methods of diagnosis or treatment or other MS research results, patients may wish, in addition to consulting their own physician, to contact either the NINCDS, the National Multiple Sclerosis Society, 205 East 42nd Street, New York, N.Y. 10017, or the Regional Health Administrator in one of the Department of Health, Education, and Welfare's 10 Regional Offices (see page 316 for a listing of these offices).

Furthermore, while demyelination is considered to be the primary cause of exacerbations, several factors which may accentuate MS symptoms can be effectively controlled. Among those considered to have a direct influence on symptoms are: heat, stress, emotional upset, anxiety and fatigue. Of course, tolerance to these factors varies greatly among patients. But when these conditions worsen symptoms, often their removal will lessen the symptoms' severity. Fevers and infections also can worsen symptoms.

Additional factors whose possible effects on MS symptoms are less well established include serious injury and mild physical trauma.

During pregnancy, patients may tend to have fewer MS attacks. However, following delivery, patients may experience an increase in attacks. Patients planning families should fully discuss the matter with their partner and should understand that physical limitations could attend raising children. Except in very severe instances, there are no contraindications to pregnancy, and no significant risk to the fetus. Moreover, MS is NOT a directly inherited disease, though there is a small percentage of familial incidence. These probably are due to similarities in environment and to inherited immune system characteristics. Consultation with the patient's physician regarding pregnancy can be particularly helpful in providing guidance and perhaps in allaying possible undue concern.

Many consider motivation to be the key in living with MS. One man with MS wrote, "Platitudes and encouraging words do little good for the MS patient until that patient has motivated himself." But family and friends can play an important part in encouraging self-motivation and determination to get on with life. In addition, sensitivity by family and friends to the needs and concerns of those with MS often can do much to enhance the quality of life. Professional counseling often can provide valuable guidance in this regard. As one woman with MS expressed, "I want understanding or help friends can give in any way. But I don't want pity. I've always been a person that has done for herself."

Research seeks the answers

MS research is devoted to finding the elusive cause of this disorder so that effective means of prevention can be developed, and to finding improved methods of diagnosis and treatment.

The NINCDS conducts a vigorous MS research effort at its Bethesda, Maryland, laboratories, and supports intensive MS studies at major medical centers throughout the country. In addition, the institute also supports several clinical research centers involving participation by a limited number of patients in studies seeking the cause of MS. A list of these centers can be obtained from the NINCDS.

These efforts are joined by those of the National MS Society, and its more than 160 local chapters and branches which help to support more than 70 clinics, clinical programs, and MS centers. The National MS Society has waged a tireless effort to support research and to maintain a valuable link between the scientists working on the problem and patients and their families, providing information on MS and on services available throughout the country.

Through the joint efforts of researchers, clinicians, patients and their families — with government, voluntary and private agencies — the reality of finding the answers to MS comes a bit closer every day.

In a disease of unknown cause, various scientific approaches are being pursued, some of which are diametrically opposed. For example, potential avenues of research include the possible role of either an underactive or overactive immune (defense) system response.

The most promising areas of research primarily center on viruses, the immune (defense) system, autoimmunity (a misdirected attack by the body against itself), the biochemistry of myelin, and population and genetic patterns of MS. Current scientific thought supports the possibility that MS may be caused by an interwoven combination of these factors or of others yet to be discovered.

The past several years have led to a tremendous advance in our knowledge of viruses and the body's defense system. Recent —

though inconclusive and unconfirmed — studies of possible viral involvement in MS are accelerating increased interest in this approach.

This interest stems in part from demonstration by NINCDS Nobel Laureate Dr. D. Carleton Gajdusek and colleagues of the existence of at least two human neurological disorders caused by slow viruses which lie dormant in the body for years before some event triggers them into action. Since MS usually does not occur until early adulthood, the possibility of a slow viral infection is particularly intriguing. Supporting this theory are the population and geographical studies of MS, which indicate that certain regions of the world with a temperate climate, such as the northern U.S., Canada and Europe, have a high prevalence of MS (and are thus called high risk areas) compared with tropical regions (low risk areas). Moreover, the age of 15 seems to be significant in terms of risk: well documented studies indicate that a person moving from a high to a low risk area before the age of 15 tends to adopt the risk of the new area; while other studies (although less well documented) suggest that those moving after age 15 maintain the risk of their homeland. These findings encourage speculation that predisposing events for MS may occur sometime during the first 15 years of life.

Research on how the body defends itself against disease has leaped ahead in the past few years, through use of new scientific tools, and now is one of the most exciting and promising areas of MS research. Scientists can take an MS patient's antibodies (formed by the body to ward off a particular invader) and observe their action in a test tube.

Scientists are particularly interested in one type of antibody, IgG (mentioned in the "diagnosis" section) which is found in blood and spinal fluid. Since many patients with MS have elevated amounts of this antibody, scientists are working to determine the antibody's target. They are using a test which exposes the antibody to a variety of agents to see if the antibody, like a magnet, is drawn to one particular agent.

Some studies are concentrating on the possibility that the defense system is unable to differentiate an MS-causing factor from a naturally occurring substance in the patient's body. Thus, a misdirected (autoimmune) attack by the body against itself may be taking place in persons with MS. This has been demonstrated in animals. For example, an NINCDS researcher, using a tadpole with a transparent optic nerve, has shown that spinal fluid from MS patients harms myelin surrounding the tadpole's nerve. Thus, the search is intensified to determine what property of MS patients' spinal fluid causes this myelin destruction.

There is also some evidence to suggest that MS patients may have too little immune system activity. This has been found to occur in another disease affecting myelin. But if a defective defense system is involved in MS, neither increasing nor decreasing the MS patient's immune response has proved to be a successful treatment for MS. However, definite conclusions regarding these approaches cannot be made until additional studies are completed.

Research also is continuing on an MS-like animal disease called experimental allergic encephalomyelitis (EAE) which can be induced in animals using a part of myelin, called myelin basic protein, isolated from CNS tissue material. EAE in animals produces demyelination, scar tissue formation, and, under certain experimental conditions, a remitting course. Studies of the mechanism responsible for this disorder in laboratory animals may provide important clues to the cause, and possibly to the treatment, of MS.

By using new laboratory techniques, scientists have identified myelin basic protein in the blood and cerebrospinal fluid samples of MS patients which, initial studies indicate, is not found in fluid of persons with other nervous system disorders. So this test has possible diagnostic potential. Furthermore, the test has implications for testing experimental MS treatment, for the scientists have found that levels of myelin basic protein in MS patients correlate with symptom levels. Patients experiencing an attack (and presumably demyelination) have higher levels of the protein than patients who are in a period of remission. Thus, any treatment which decreases myelin basic protein levels might reasonably be expected to decrease symptoms, possibly by containing demyelination.

Keeping informed through the NINCDS and the NMSS

Each year, the NINCDS prepares a summary of current research approaches and advances, which can be obtained by writing to the institute. In addition, as mentioned earlier, information on a variety of topics is available through the National Multiple Sclerosis Society. No one knows where the breakthroughs will emerge. They may come from one of these scientific approaches, or they may come from studies of some other neurological disorder, or from some as yet unknown and unexplored avenue of research. Every year, advances in scientific research and technology are being made. With the continued dedication, imagination, and hard work of scientists, and the continued cooperation, energy, and participation of patients, the answers to MS will be found.

In the meantime, it is often the courage and perseverance of the men and women with MS which can make the fight a winning one. As one patient wrote in an MS Society award-winning article published in the *New York Sunday News*: "I live with MS. My family lives with MS. What is there to say? We have our moments. I and many other MS patients in my area have discovered that we are not alone . . . that there is practical assistance available now while work is going forward to find the cause and cure for this mysterious disease."

Department of Health, Education and Welfare Regional Offices

Region I

Connecticut, Maine, Massachusetts, New Hampshire, Rhode Island, Vermont

Regional Health Administrator
John F. Kennedy Federal Building
Government Center
Boston, Massachusetts 02203
(617) 223-6827

Region II

New York, New Jersey, Puerto Rico, Virgin Islands

Regional Health Administrator
Federal Building
26 Federal Plaza
New York, New York 10007
(212) 264-2560

Region III

Delaware, Maryland, Pennsylvania, Virginia, West Virginia and District of Columbia

Regional Health Administrator
P.O. Box 13716
Philadelphia, Pennsylvania 19101
(215) 596-6637

Region IV

Alabama, Florida, Georgia, Kentucky, Mississippi, North Carolina, South Carolina, Tennessee

Regional Health Administrator
Suite 1203, 1001 Marietta Towers
Atlanta, Georgia 30323
(404)221-2316

Region V

Illinois, Indiana, Michigan, Minnesota, Ohio, Wisconsin

Regional Health Administrator
300 South Wacker Drive
Chicago, Illinois 60606
(312) 353-1385

Region VI

Arkansas, Louisiana, New Mexico, Oklahoma, Texas

Regional Health Administrator
1200 Main Tower
Dallas, Texas 75202
(214) 655-3879

Region VII

Iowa, Kansas, Missouri, Nebraska

Regional Health Administrator
601 East 12th Street
Kansas City, Missouri 64106
(816) 374-3291

Region VIII

Colorado, Montana, North Dakota, South Dakota, Utah, Wyoming

Regional Health Administrator
1961 Stout Street
Denver, Colorado 80202
(303) 837-4461

Region IX

Arizona, California, Hawaii, Nevada, Guam, American Samoa

Regional Health Administrator
Federal Office Building
50 United Nations Plaza
San Francisco, California 94102
(415) 556-5810

Region X

Alaska, Idaho, Oregon, Washington

Regional Health Administrator
Arcade Plaza
1321 Second Avenue
Seattle, Washington 98101
(206) 442-0430

Chapter 19

Neurofibromatosis

Neurofibromatosis

What is neurofibromatosis?

Neurofibromatosis is a genetic disorder of the nervous system. Characteristic signs in the adult are six or more flat, coffee-colored (café au-lait) skin spots; multiple, usually benign tumors, called "neurofibromas" when they appear on the nerves; and, sometimes, curvature of the spine.

How common is the disorder?

No formal system exists for collecting statistics on neurofibromatosis, but the National Neurofibromatosis Foundation estimates that approximately 100,000 Americans, of both sexes and all national origins or races, are afflicted. Each year the disease affects approximately 1 in every 3,000 babies born. This would place neurofibromatosis among the most common hereditary diseases.

What are its signs and symptoms?

Symptoms usually appear in childhood or adolescence, but can occur as late as age 50. Neurofibromatosis patients may develop any one or several of the following problems:

- Many small tumors (nodules) just under the skin;
- Nodules on the iris of the eye in adolescents and older individuals;
- Large pressure-sensitive tumors just under the skin;
- Severe curvature of the spine;
- Enlargement and deformation of bones other than the spine;
- Tumors on the auditory nerves, causing deafness;
- Tumors on the optic nerves, causing blindness in one or both eyes;
- Tumors of the brain or spinal cord;
- High blood pressure in younger people.

What causes neurofibromatosis?

Most cases of neurofibromatosis are inherited from one of the parents, but some result from the spontaneous change (mutation) of a gene. Once a mutation has taken place, neurofibromatosis can be passed on to succeeding generations. How the mutant gene produces neurofibromatosis is unknown.

How is it inherited?

Neurofibromatosis is an autosomal dominant disorder. Each child of an affected parent has a 50 percent chance of inheriting the defective gene and developing neurofibromatosis.

What are the early signs?

Children with neurofibromatosis can almost always be identified shortly after birth by the appearance of light-brown spots on their skin. Physicians generally consider that any young child with five or more such "café-au-lait" spots, each half a centimeter or more in diameter, has neurofibromatosis. Characteristic tumors may appear on the nerves and elsewhere in the body during childhood, but usually do not develop until early adulthood.

What forms does neurofibromatosis take?

Neurofibromatosis has been classified into two somewhat overlapping types: peripheral, and central with bilateral acoustic neuromas.

Peripheral neurofibromatosis — This type is characterized by six or more café-au-lait spots, many small tumors, and a network of larger tumors under the skin. Enlargement and deformation of bones and other parts of the body may occur. Severe left-right curvature of the spine (scoliosis) is common. Occasionally, tumors may develop in the brain, cranial nerve, or spinal cord.

Central neurofibromatosis with bilateral acoustic neuromas — This type is characterized by multiple tumors on the cranial and spinal nerves, and by other lesions of the brain and spinal cord. Tumors of both auditory nerves are the hallmark, with hearing loss, beginning about age 20, generally the first symptom.

Do benign tumors ever become malignant?

Yes, in about 3 to 5 percent of all cases.

Is there any treatment for neurofibromatosis?

Not for the disorder itself, but there are treatments aimed at controlling symptoms. Bone malformation, particularly scoliosis, is treated by surgery, a back brace, or both. Auditory or optic nerve tumors can be treated by surgery, but if nerves on both sides are affected, the risks may be greater than the benefits. Painful or disfiguring skin tumors can be removed by surgery, but there is some danger that they will grow back in greater numbers.

Do neurofibromatosis patients lead normal lives?

In most cases, symptoms are mild and patients live completely normal and productive lives. In its more severe forms, however, neurofibromatosis can be devastating and debilitating.

Is there a prenatal test?

For those who are affected by neurofibromatosis, the decision to have or not to have children can be a difficult one. There is currently no prenatal test to determine if an unborn child is affected by neurofibromatosis. A genetic counselor can offer support and guidance to couples faced with the childbearing decision.

What research is being done?

The National Institute of Neurological and Communicative Disorders and Stroke, a part of the National Institutes of Health (NIH), is studying genetics and cell growth in neurofibromatosis patients. In 1979, a weekly research clinic was begun at NIH to study patients and families with the disorder; referring physicians retain responsibility for the care and treatment of their patients. Research is also being carried on at several large medical centers in the United States. Scientists are conducting clinical studies on the diagnosis and treatment of neurofibromatosis. Investigators are also trying to locate the mutant gene that causes the disease. Other scientists are studying the role of hormones and growth factors in the development of neurofibromatosis.

How can I help research?

The National Institute of Neurological and Communicative Disorders and Stroke and the National Institute of Mental Health support two national human specimen banks, one at the Wadsworth Veterans Administration Hospital in Los Angeles and the other at McLean Hospital near Boston. These banks supply investigators around the world with tissue from patients with neurological and psychiatric diseases. Both banks need tissue from neurofibromatosis patients to enable scientists to study this disorder more intensely. Prospective donors should write to:

Dr. Wallace W Tourtellotte, Director
Human Neurospecimen Bank
VA Wadsworth Hospital Center
Los Angeles, CA 90073
Telephone: (213) 824-4307 (call collect.)

Dr. Edward D. Bird, Director
Brain Tissue Bank, Mailman Research center
McLean Hospital
115 Mill Street
Belmont, MA 02178
Telephone: (617) 855-2400 (call collect 24 hours a day.)

Where can I get medical care?

Physicians who specialize in diagnosing and treating neurofibromatosis may be contacted through university medical centers. In addition, the following centers have neurofibromatosis clinics;

- Massachusetts General Hospital, Boston, MA
- Mt. Sinai School of Medicine, New York, NY
- Children's Hospital, Philadelphia, PA
- Children's Hospital National Medical Center, Washington, DC
- Baylor School of Medicine, Houston, TX

Where can I get more information?

Information for patients, families, and physicians is available from:

National Neurofibromatosis Foundation, Inc.
70 West 40th Street
4th Floor
New York, NY 10018
(212) 869-9034

The foundation was chartered by the State of New York in 1978 as a nonprofit organization. Its purposes are to provide neurofibromatosis patients and their families with information about the disease and to help them find medical, social, and genetic counseling. The foundation also provides information on neurofibromatosis to health professionals and supports scientific research on the disease.

For information about the NIH Neurofibromatosis Clinic, write:

Coordinator, Inter-Institute Genetics Program
Building 10, Room 1D21
National Institutes of Health
Bethesda, MD 20205
(301)496-1380

Chapter 20

Parkinson's Disease

Parkinson's Disease

Mary found she had Parkinson's disease when she was in her late fifties. For a while, she continued to work as a housewife, but gradually her ability to walk and to do simple tasks decreased. By the time she was in her mid-sixties, she was bedridden. Luckily, her husband had reached retirement age by then, and he now takes care of her at home.

Jacob is in his late fifties and receiving drug therapy for Parkinson's disease. Most of the time the drugs — and the understanding of his students and the college administrators — enable him to teach in a Hebrew seminary. But, increasingly, he has to be helped to the classes, and sometimes in the middle of teaching he has problems speaking.

Tom, on the other hand, has received great benefit from taking standard antiparkinson drugs developed through scientific research. After 10 years of treatment, his disease shows no sign of worsening.

Amy has also been greatly helped in living with her parkinsonism but, in her case, the benefit came from joining a support group. "She was almost dead when I first saw her," says the nurse who directs the group. "Since she discovered other patients with Parkinson's, she swims every day and attends meetings regularly."

Four different people, four different courses of Parkinson's disease. Taken together, they emphasize several important facts about this neurological illness:

First, Parkinson's is a serious disease that, if left untreated, can disable the patient.

Second, treatment with drugs can help most parkinsonian patients to remain independent for many years. Some patients have been quite successful in maintaining the normal motor skills that we all take for granted. But current drug therapy does not cure the disease or even halt its progression. That is why scientists are continually looking for new medications to fight this debilitating illness. Several promising drugs are now being tested.

Third, the most effective therapy for Parkinson's disease includes, in addition to medications, an exercise program and a great deal of caring support from relatives and friends.

Research to improve treatment for Parkinson's disease and to find a cure is going on at many medical centers. Much of this work is supported by the National Institute of Neurological and Communicative Disorders and Stroke (NINCDS), a world leader in research on brain and central nervous system disorders and the focal point in the U.S. Government for the support of research in these areas.

In addition to a multimillion-dollar investment in research conducted through universities and medical institutions, the NINCDS also searches for answers to Parkinson's disease in its own laboratories and clinics at the National Institutes of Health in Bethesda, Maryland. Through this research, scientists hope to understand better the basis of Parkinson's disease, and ultimately to prevent the disorder's occurrence.

History

Before 1817, what we now know as Parkinson's disease was just one of a number of similar disorders of movement. Then a British doctor, James Parkinson, published a paper on what he called "shaking palsy." In it, he described the major symptoms of the disease that would later bear his name.

Dr. Parkinson's observations allowed the disease to be studied as a special illness for the first time. During the next century, scientists defined its distribution, symptoms and onset, and the prospects for recovery. But most important, in the early 1960s they identified the fundamental brain defect that is the hallmark of the disease. This information led to the first effective treatment for parkinsonism and suggested ways of devising new and more effective therapies.

A disease of later life

Very few persons with Parkinson's disease develop serious symptoms before age 40. The great majority of cases are diagnosed between ages 60 and 70, so that the average age of parkinsonian patients is 65 years. In one community studied, the frequency of the disease in those above 50 increased markedly with age. The increasing number of older persons in the U.S., therefore, would seem to foreshadow an increase in the number of people who will develop parkinsonism.

Both men and women appear to be equally affected. There are now perhaps 500,000 people with the disease in the United States, but this number is not exact, since many cases are not severe enough to need treatment.

Among many populations in the world, there is wide variation in the occurrence of Parkinson's disease. Some scientists believe that high disease rates in certain populations might be due to an increased genetic susceptibility; but other research findings suggest that heredity may not play a major role in determining who gets the disease. An NINCDS study of over 40 Parkinson's disease patients who had an identical twin uncovered only one case in which the twin also had the disease. This and other findings lend support to the likelihood that an environmental factor, rather than heredity, causes parkinsonism — an idea that is now being investigated.

Early symptoms

The first signs of Parkinson's disease may appear to be simply part of the normal aging process: a little shakiness, some difficulty in rising from a deep, comfortable chair. This is especially true since most symptoms of Parkinson's are first noticed when persons are in their sixties.

But the signs very gradually become more pronounced and extensive. The shaking or *tremor* that affects about two-thirds of parkinsonian patients begins to interfere with daily activities. It may be more difficult to hold utensils steady when eating. A newspaper may shake enough to make it hard to read.

The shaking may become worse when the patient is relaxed. This is characteristic of Parkinson's. A few seconds after the hands are rested on a table, for instance, the shaking is most pronounced.

Although tremor is usually the most obvious early sign of Parkinson's disease, a more distressing problem to the patient is the symptom known as *bradykinesia* — the gradual loss of spontaneous movement. A person with Parkinson's may sit in one position for a long time without moving. Or the patient may find it difficult to start walking.

Bradykinesia may lead to the loss of facial expression. This is not a sign of an emotional problem, but a loss of activity in the nerves that control the facial muscles. The link between emotions and facial expressions is instinctive: expressions don't require conscious thought. In Parkinson's, a patient may have natural emotional responses, and not be aware that his or her face is not showing those feelings.

A parkinsonian patient may also have flat, expressionless speech. About half of Parkinson's disease patients experience such problems as loss of volume, difficulty beginning to speak, or inability to speak clearly. Again, these are not emotional problems, but a loss of normally spontaneous activity of the nerves and muscles.

A third characteristic of Parkinson's disease is *rigidity*. This symptom may not be as obvious to patients as is tremor. They may be aware only of a certain amount of stiffness when they move their arms or legs. But if another person tells a patient to relax and then tries to move the patient's arm, the movements will be ratchetlike: resistance, followed by a quick short movement, then rigidity again.

The result is a series of short, jerky motions, as though the arm is being moved by a gear.

A major principle in the body is that all muscles have an opposing muscle. Movement is possible not just because one muscle becomes more active, but because the opposing muscle relaxes. It may be a disturbance of this dynamic balance that causes rigidity.

Parkinsonian patients may also experience other motor problems. For instance, the posture may become stooped with the shoulders bent forward. When the person is standing at rest, the arms may not hang down in the normal way, but may bend upward from the elbow.

Telltale signs

To an experienced neurologist the diagnosis of Parkinson's disease is usually obvious. Shakiness is part of several other diseases, but the special quality of the parkinsonian tremor — that it becomes worse after a few seconds of resting the hand — is very characteristic. By the time the patient has decided to seek medical help, other symptoms are usually also present. The neurologist can put the tremor together with the lack of spontaneous facial expression, flat speech, and the patient's unusual stillness while sitting, and arrive at a fairly certain diagnosis. Peculiar handwriting, which becomes smaller and more cramped after the first few written words, is also a strong clue.

The ability to make a diagnosis almost solely on the basis of clinical signs is fortunate, since there are no sophisticated tests for Parkinson's disease. In about 10 percent of the suspected cases of this illness, there may be some hesitation about making a diagnosis at the first visit. But, with time, the telltale signs of parkinsonism almost always appear.

As the disease worsens

Without treatment, Parkinson's disease becomes progressively more severe and disabling. But different patients experience different rates of disease progression. It is generally agreed, however, that with current treatments, many parkinsonian patients enjoy a normal life span.

The course of the disease is variable. With time, patients whose symptoms appeared only on one side of the body may have movement problems on the other side as well. On the other hand, cases of one-sided parkinsonism with no further development of movement problems are well known.

The patient may also begin to experience certain annoying problems, such as drooling. This comes from the difficulty in swallowing due to decreased function of the throat muscles. This swallowing problem can also make eating difficult, and can lead to choking if the patient is not careful. To some extent, the patient can control this problem by eating slowly and swallowing often.

There may also be overproduction of the normal oily coating of the skin, a condition called seborrhea. Its cause is poorly understood. The condition is not dangerous, but does require extra care.

The more serious symptoms of advanced Parkinson's disease are aggravations of the movement problems, such as a severe loss of the sense of balance, sometimes compounded by loss of the normal arm swing that we all use to maintain our walking rhythm. The short steps characteristic of a parkinsonian patient's walk are an attempt to compensate for lost stability.

With a failing sense of balance, the parkinsonian patient may develop a slight forward lean. This leaning causes a shift in the body's center of gravity, and the patient may take a series of quick, small steps forward to "catch up" with the changed gravity center. This stepping forward is the symptom called *festination*. Another problem — a backward lean — may also appear. When bumped from the front or when starting to walk, patients with this problem have

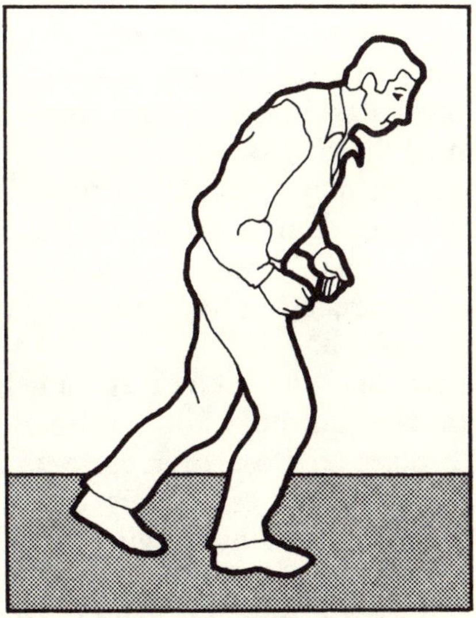

"Hurrying" gait of advanced Parkinson's disease is an adaptation to balance problems.

a tendency to step backwards. This is known as *retropulsion*, and usually accompanies only fairly advanced disease. When either one of these symptoms appears, the use of lifts on shoes or a tripod cane can be helpful.

Late in the course of Parkinson's disease, the patient's loss of spontaneous movements may worsen. When severe, such bradykinesia results in periods when the person is completely unable to start movements. These "frozen states" are called *akinesia*. This loss of voluntary movement affects walking most dramatically.

A peculiar feature of these frozen states is that they may be triggered by situations or objects, such as an open doorway or a line drawn on the floor. Or patients may "freeze" when caught in crowds. Since this difficulty is partly psychological, personal support can be of considerable help. A hand or arm quietly offered to a parkinsonian patient experiencing akinesia can be all he or she needs to get going again. On the other hand, if a companion becomes agitated or obviously embarrassed by the patient's condition, the frozen state may get worse.

It is important to remember that most patients with Parkinson's disease continue to think clearly. Late in the course of the illness, some patients do suffer loss of mental skills. They may become forgetful, have trouble calculating or counting money, and may lose their way when going between familiar places. These are symptoms of the disorder known as *dementia*. (Dementia does not mean wild behavior or emotional outbursts, as it is sometimes popularly understood, but only refers to loss of mental abilities.) How many parkinsonian patients undergo these losses is not clear, but it is interesting that James Parkinson did not include dementia in his original description of the disease.

Parkinsonian patients may also feel depressed. Some neurologists have suggested that depression is a result of the disease process, but this idea is still controversial. Another possibility is that the depression is simply "a realistic reaction to a progressive, crippling illness," as one clinician expressed it.

Parkinsonism symptoms themselves are not fatal. Patients most often die of an illness acquired while confined to bed during the latter stages of the disease. Loss of muscle tone makes coughing difficult, so the lungs are not effectively cleared and the patient becomes susceptible to pneumonia. Lying in bed also makes the patient susceptible to blood clots in the legs that can travel to the lungs and be fatal. Another problem is urinary tract infections, which can spread to the blood. Clearly, good nursing care of the bedridden parkinsonian patient is important.

Brain changes in Parkinson patients

In the early 1960s, research scientists were excited to discover several changes in specific areas of brains taken from deceased Parkinson's disease patients. These observations led to an important insight into the basis for Parkinson's disease: Parkinson patients cannot control their movements because of a deficiency in the part of the brain that produces smooth, directed muscle activity.

The scientists saw that certain pigmented nerve cells were lost from a region of the brain known as the basal ganglia, which appears to be responsible for the dynamic balance of opposing muscles mentioned earlier. This loss of nerve cells (or neurons) occurred in patients with longstanding Parkinson's disease, and was most evident in the substantia nigra ("black substance," so called because the cells in this area are dark), a part of the basal ganglia thought to adjust nerve signals passing to the muscles from the command centers of the brain.

In addition, all regions of the basal ganglia were deficient in a normal brain substance called dopamine, a chemical messenger that transmits signals from one nerve cell to another. Dopamine is made by the pigmented cells of the substantia nigra, the same neurons that are greatly reduced in parkinsonism. Since these cells send fibers throughout the basal ganglia, much like a tree sending out roots, loss of cells from the substantia nigra lowers the supply of dopamine in nearby areas as well.

Without dopamine, the nerve cells in the basal ganglia are like a team of astronauts with no radios in their spacesuits — they are ready for action, but they can't communicate. As a result, the nerve cells can't cooperate to fine-tune the signals flowing to the muscles.

This conclusion is supported by experiments in animals showing that dopamine loss in the brain leads to abnormal movement. An even more convincing observation is that the extent of loss of dopamine nerve cells found at autopsy is related to the severity of patients' symptoms, especially akinesia and tremor.

What causes Parkinson's disease?

In a small number of parkinsonism cases, a specific cause can be identified. Carbon monoxide and manganese poisoning may produce parkinsonism, as can certain drugs used to treat psychiatric illness. Parkinsonism caused by psychiatric drugs disappears when the drugs are withdrawn.

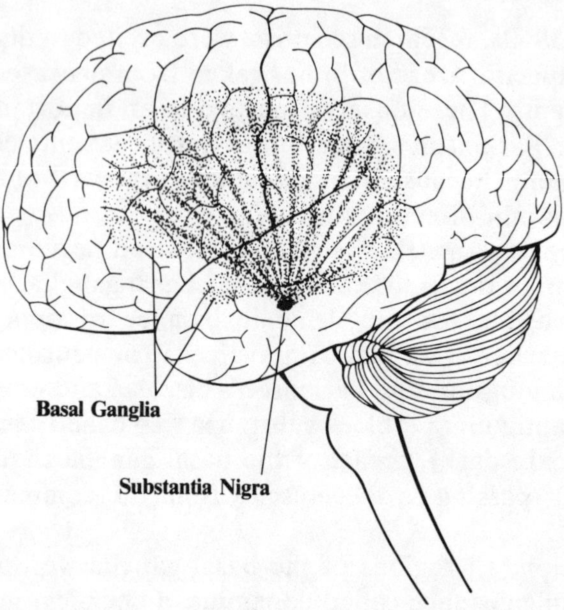

The loss of dopamine nerve cells from the brain's substantia nigra is thought responsible for the symptoms of parkinsonism.

But the vast majority of cases of parkinsonism are "idiopathic," meaning that no cause is known. Even the finding that specific nerve cells are lost in the brains of parkinsonian patients has not led scientists to the cause of the disease.

Brain research has provided one important clue, however. Even persons who die early in the course of Parkinson's disease have advanced damage to their dopamine-containing nerve cells. This implies that the disease is the result of a gradual decay process that starts long before symptoms appear. So the search for the first event in the course of Parkinson's disease must involve persons in their forties, thirties, or earlier, when the unseen stages of the disease probably begin.

Treatment

Therapy of Parkinson's disease has involved both surgery and drug treatment. Many patients also benefit from exercises, which may provide added strength to help combat movement problems.

The only operation that has been of value for Parkinson's disease was a procedure called cryothalamotomy, or "destruction of the thalamus by cold." In the most successful form of this procedure, a probe cooled with liquid nitrogen was placed into a part of the brain called the thalamus. Guided by a framework around the patient's head, the probe touched only very specific areas of the brain. Nerve cells in these areas were destroyed by the supercooled metal tip of the probe.

This operation successfully stopped the tremor in many patients. Unfortunately, it did little to help the rigidity and loss of spontaneous movement that are the more disabling symptoms of Parkinson's disease.

Cryothalamotomy had another drawback. When performed on both sides of the thalamus (which was necessary to stop tremor on both sides of the body), the surgery itself could produce neurologic damage. Today, with the development of effective drug therapies, cryothalamotomy is seldom performed except in severe cases of unstoppable tremor or movement disorder.

Drug therapy

After James Parkinson clearly delineated the illness that bears his name, many chemicals were tested against it. These included fish-poison bark, strychnine, arsenic, and turpentine. It is not surprising that several classes of drugs were found that had at least some mild benefit for parkinsonian patients. Extracts from the belladonna plant, for example, were used against Parkinson's disease until the 1940s. But effective control of all symptoms was not possible until the drug levodopa was introduced in the 1960s.

The success of levodopa — sometimes called L-dopa — in treating the symptoms of Parkinson's disease has been one of the triumphs of modern research. After dopamine nerve pathways were shown to be depleted in persons with parkinsonian symptoms, several scientists tried to restore normal function by administering levodopa, a natural brain chemical that nerve cells can use to make dopamine. (Dopamine itself could not be given because it does not enter the brain.)

In initial studies, levodopa caused many patients to vomit. But, in 1967, a New York neurologist showed that starting with small doses and slowly increasing the dosage overcame this problem. When doctors were able to gradually give higher doses of levodopa, their patients' conditions improved greatly.

Both rigidity and tremor were greatly reduced. But most important, levodopa reduced the most disabling symptom of the disease, bradykinesia, the difficulty in starting movements. No previous medication had controlled this problem.

Still, in the first few years of levodopa use, little more than half of the patients improved. In the other patients, side effects made it impossible to give a high enough dose to reduce the symptoms. Besides nausea, patients experienced movements called *dyskinesias*, which are undirected involuntary movements. Some also suffered heart problems and others had dangerous drops in blood pressure.

The next major advance was the development of drugs that stopped levodopa from changing to dopamine before it reached the brain. These drugs, called "extracerebral decarboxylase inhibitors," include carbidopa and benserazide. When levodopa is kept from changing before it reaches the brain, nausea is reduced. Low blood pressure and heart problems are also avoided. With a decarboxylase inhibitor, many patients can reduce the number of levodopa pills they need, and full doses of levodopa can be reached in weeks instead of months. Carbidopa or benserazide is now combined with levodopa in most medicines.

With today's levodopa treatment, symptoms are reduced in about three of every four parkinsonian patients. The patients also remain independent longer, and many live out a normal life span.

In some cases, however, patients experience involuntary movements from the levodopa treatment, and others have mental symptoms. Reducing the dosage sometimes lowers these side effects. But this means that the doctor must be very skilled in adjusting the levodopa amount to improve symptoms while avoiding bad effects. The doctor must also be aware that certain drugs given for other illnesses can defeat the effect of levodopa.

Eventually, however, the benefits of levodopa may wear off. In about half of the patients with Parkinson's disease, several troubling problems are likely to appear suddenly after 3 to 5 years of successful levodopa control.

One of these problems is called the "on-off" reaction. The patient may alternate between dyskinesia (uncontrolled movements) and akinesia (lack of movement), switching back and forth between these states every few seconds or minutes.

A second problem is "end-of-dose akinesia," or the quick return of parkinsonian symptoms 3 to 4 hours after taking a dose of levodopa.

Some doctors think that these problems are due to the relentless advance of parkinsonism. But not all agree. One doctor who treats parkinsonian patients determined how long each benefitted from levodopa therapy. If the reduced effectiveness of levodopa is due to progression of the disease, then the patients who had less severe symptoms at the start of treatment should have been helped by levodopa longer. But this was not so.

Instead, he found that patients who took the highest doses of levodopa lost the benefit of the drug soonest. The doctor suggested that giving high doses of levodopa may lower its effectiveness.

This theory is by no means proven. But it has led to two possible methods of prolonging the period of levodopa's effectiveness.

The first is to begin treatment with less powerful drugs, reserving levodopa for the more advanced stages of the disease. When levodopa is started, frequent small doses are given.

One class of drugs that is used first is called anticholinergic agents. These drugs were the main treatment for Parkinson's disease from the early 1940s until the introduction of levodopa. Some of the most common anticholinergic drugs are trihexyphenidyl (Artane®), benztropine mesylate (Cogentin®), and biperiden (Akineton®). They are helpful against tremor and rigidity, but do not affect bradykinesia. Antihistamines such as diphenhydramine (Benadryl®) are weaker anticholinergic agents.

Another drug that could be used for early parkinsonism is amantadine hydrochloride (Symmetrel®), which was first used to treat and prevent respiratory virus infections. Amantadine also produces modest improvement in tremor and rigidity, plus some reduction of bradykinesia.

A second method for coping with the problems of continued levodopa therapy is the so-called drug holiday. This is a period of 3 to 7 days or more during which the patient is hospitalized and taken off levodopa completely. This hospitalization may be preceded by a period of gradually decreasing doses of levodopa at home. Hospitalized patients must be watched closely, especially if their disease has progressed to the point of affecting their breathing muscles. During the drug-free period, some patients participate in physical, occupational, and speech therapy programs to reduce the hazards of stopping the medication.

A number of doctors have had success with the drug holiday. They find that many patients can resume levodopa therapy without on-off problems or end-of-dose akinesia. Some patients can even benefit from lower doses than they were taking before the drug holiday. This method is still being tested.

Physical therapy

Besides drug treatment, many doctors prescribe muscle-strengthening exercises for their parkinsonian patients. These include exercises for speaking, swallowing, and overall muscle tone.

Exercise will not stop disease progression, but may provide a stronger body so that the patient may be less disabled by movement problems. Exercise can also improve the emotional well-being of parkinsonian patients.

As one doctor puts it, "I include physical therapy with a professional therapist as a standard part of my prescription. You are not doing anything fundamental to the disease, but you are bringing the patient's motor function to an optimal level."

Needed: support and understanding

One of the most damaging aspects of Parkinson's disease is its demoralizing effect. The patient's world is completely changed. Emotional support and understanding are needed to encourage the patient to remain as active as possible.

Parkinson's disease can also separate patients from their families. "This disease puts a terrible strain on families," says one neurologist who has treated many parkinsonian patients. One problem is that normal family relationships are changed and traditional expectations are turned upside down.

A man used to supporting his family for years may find that he can no longer do his job. "I have to work two jobs to support us and pay for John's medical bills," said the wife of a parkinsonian patient. While the wife is working, the daughter must stay home to watch her partially disabled dad. These limitations and demands can create resentment in even the most closely knit families.

One older woman who lived alone after her husband died refused to accept the limitations of her Parkinson's disease. "I've had a terrible time with her," said her adult daughter. The patient refused to accept help even though her disease progressed and she fell and broke a hip. After some time in a nursing home, she is returning to her house, but still wants to live alone. Naturally, this causes the daughter intense worry.

This situation may not be uncommon. One doctor believes that falling has replaced pneumonia as the greatest danger to parkinsonian patients. Levodopa therapy allows patients to walk around, but does not completely reverse their impaired balance. If they are not cautious, they can easily fall.

For patients and their families, support groups can be a great help. At meetings, people learn ways of dealing with their problems. But, more important, they can talk to other people who understand the difficulties they are having.

Such an outlet can be important in relieving the frustrations that both patients and families feel. Parkinsonian patients can do many things for themselves, but they are often very slow. When a patient goes to a store or for a walk, the companion should not try to hurry the impaired person along. Even eating or speaking can be better managed if other people don't become impatient.

Another problem faced by families is the suspicion that a person with parkinsonism is "faking it." They may think, "Why is he so capable sometimes and so helpless at other times?" Talking with support groups will show them that this is a normal feature of the disease.

These groups can also help members learn about financial and support services. The parkinsonian patient with advanced disease may need custodial care, and support groups can help the family decide which options best suit its financial and personal situation.

Finding answers through research

Finding ways to treat, cure, and prevent Parkinson's disease requires carefully planned programs of scientific research. Subtle changes in parkinsonian brains must be uncovered, and new drugs to supplement or replace levodopa are needed.

One promising area of Parkinson's disease research involves studying the brain with a new imaging system called positron emission tomography (PET). PET produces pictures of chemical changes taking place in the brain or elsewhere in the body. For instance, PET can show how much sugar or oxygen various parts of the brain are using for energy, as a person performs an action like reading or listening to music.

According to Dr. Donald Tower, former director of the National Institute of Neurological and Communicative Disorders and Stroke, "With PET we will be able to see the development of brain lesions and look for functional differences in patients with neurological disorders." Such changes may be an early sign of the more obvious brain damage that shows up in the brains of Parkinson patients at autopsy.

Because the NINCDS believes so strongly in the research potential of this new technique, it established a national PET Research Program: major research centers around the country, including a center at its own research facility in Bethesda, Maryland, all working to perfect the technique and utilizing it to conquer neurological disease.

One group of NINCDS scientists is using PET to study parkinsonian patients who have symptoms only on one side of the body. The scientists hope to find differences between the two sides of the brain in these patients. This would further define which parts of the brain give rise to parkinsonism.

Studies like these may show other areas of the brain, besides the basal ganglia, that are not functioning correctly. This could provide new targets for drug therapy that can bring even greater benefit to parkinsonian patients.

Promising new drugs

Searching for new treatments for parkinsonism, NINCDS-supported scientists at the Illinois Institute of Technology have tried chemically attaching levodopa to the metals copper and zinc. In animal tests, these combinations sent more levodopa to the brain than the combination of levodopa with carbidopa or benserazide. If the same result is found in parkinsonian patients, the side effects of levodopa therapy could be reduced. It could also be possible to prolong the drug's period of effectiveness by allowing lower amounts to be used.

A second approach has been to combine levodopa with a specific type of drug that blocks the action of dopamine. Dopamine may act at several sites in the brain, perhaps reducing parkinsonian symptoms at the basal ganglia while causing dyskinesias at another site. One group of British doctors using the new L-dopa/ dopamine "blocker" combination has reported improvements in parkinsonian symptoms and reduced dyskinesias.

Improved delivery of dopamine to the brain has also been tried by a radical new technique: implantation of a small number of cells from the adrenal gland into the brain. The adrenal gland, located on top of the kidney, contains some cells that make dopamine. A group of Swedish doctors recently placed some of these cells into the brain of a parkinsonian patient. According to one NINCDS scientist, this is "a very exciting area," but the procedure is still experimental.

Perhaps the most promising group of new drugs is a class called dopamine agonists. Agonists are substances which produce effects similar to the effects of certain naturally occurring chemicals. Rather than increasing the amount of dopamine in the brain, as levodopa does, dopamine agonists mimic dopamine's activity in the brain. NINCDS scientists have taken the lead in selecting the dopamine agonists that are most promising for human trials and in evaluating the first treatment attempts. One of these drugs, bromocriptine, was introduced to clinical Parkinson's disease research in the United

States in 1981. Several others, including pergolide and lisuride, are now being tested in parkinsonian patients.

Whether dopamine agonists should be used as a first treatment or after levodopa has lost its effectiveness has yet to be worked out. It is also possible that the best course will be to combine low doses of a dopamine agonist with low doses of levodopa. However they are used, it seems clear that one or two of this new class of agents will have a large role in future treatment of parkinsonian symptoms.

Another experimental substance soon to be tested in parkinsonian patients is called tetrahydrobiopterin. This chemical occurs naturally in the human brain and is necessary for nerve cells to make dopamine. NINCDS scientists have found that tetrahydrobiopterin is reduced in parkinsonian patients. These investigators plan to find out if giving the chemical to parkinsonian patients improves dopamine production and reduces symptoms.

NINCDS scientists are also testing the element lithium in parkinsonian patients who have developed on-off reactions after taking levodopa for a long time. On-off reactions are thought to be due to extreme sensitivity of the sites where dopamine acts. In animal experiments, lithium lowered this sensitivity. If lithium also lowers sensitivity to dopamine in the human brain, it could possibly eliminate on-off reactions while allowing levodopa to relieve symptoms.

Hope for the future

Research progress in drug treatment and improving technologies for exploring the brain are encouraging advances for thousands of Parkinson's disease patients. The promise of research and the support of generous families, friends, and volunteers sustain them in their fight against Parkinson's disease, and give them hope.

Human tissue banks

The study of brain tissue from persons with neurological disorders is invaluable in research, especially in conditions like Parkinson's disease where the cause is obscure. NINCDS supports two national specimen banks, one in Los Angeles and one near Boston. For information about tissue donation and collection write:

Dr. Wallace W. Tourtellotte, Director
Human Neurospecimen Bank
VA Wadsworth Hospital Center
Los Angeles, CA 90073

Dr. Edward D. Bird, Director
Brain Tissue Bank, Mailman Research Center
McLean Hospital
115 Mill Street
Belmont, MA 02178

Voluntary organizations

The following organizations are devoted to research, care, treatment, and ultimate prevention of Parkinson's disease. They also work to increase public awareness of the disorder, and to provide Parkinson's disease patients and families with assistance and support. For information write:

American Parkinson Disease Association
116 John Street
New York NY 10038
(212) 732-9550

National Parkinson Foundation, Inc.
1501 N.W. Ninth Avenue
Miami, FL 33136
(305) 547-6666

Parkinson's Disease Foundation
William Black Medical Research Building
640 West 168th Street
New York, NY 10032
(212) 923-4700

United Parkinson Foundation
360 West Superior Street
Chicago, IL 60610
(312) 664-2344

Parkinson Support Groups of America
11376 Cherry Hill Road, Apt. 204
Beltsville, MD 20705
(301) 937-1545

Bibliography

Other booklets on Parkinson's disease are available from the following sources:

American Parkinson Disease Association
A Manual for Patients with Parkinson's Disease

Home Exercises for Patients with Parkinson's Disease

Speech Problems and Swallowing Problems in Parkinson's Disease

Aids, Equipment and Suggestions to Help the Patients with Parkinson's Disease in the Activities of Daily Living

National Parkinson Foundation, Inc.
What the Patient Should Know About Parkinson's Disease
Psychological Factors in the Management of Parkinson's Disease

Parkinson's Disease Foundation
The Parkinson Patient at Home
Parkinson's Disease: Progress, Promise and Hope!
Exercises for the Parkinson Patient With Hints for Daily Living

United Parkinson Foundation
One Step at a Time (an exercise manual)

Other:
Bourke-White, Margaret (1963): *Portrait of Myself* Simon and Schuster, New York, N.Y. (This now out-of-print book describes the famous photographer's life with parkinsonism.)

Dorros, Sidney (1982): *Parkinson's: A Patients View*. Seven Locks Press, Inc., P.O. Box 72, Cabin John, MD 20818. (A personal account of one man's 20-year struggle with Parkinson's disease.)

Duvoisin, Roger C. (1978): *Parkinson's Disease: A Guide for Patient and Family*. Raven Press, 1140 Avenue of the Americas, New York, NY 10036.

Stern, Gerald and Lees, Andrew (1982): *Parkinson's Disease: The Facts*. Oxford University Press, 200 Madison Avenue, New York, NY 10016.

Chapter 21

Shingles

Shingles

When the itchy red spots of childhood chicken pox disappear and the child goes back to school, the battle with infection seems won. But, for all too many of us, this triumph of the body's immune system over a virus is only temporary. The virus has not been destroyed, but lies low, ready to strike again later in life. This second eruption of the chicken pox virus is the disease called shingles.

"I was having exams at college and I got a rash in a band around my waist. I first thought it was chicken pox, but I'd had that years before and, instead of itching, this time the spots were very painful," recalls a young woman who had shingles in her twenties.

The young woman's memory was correct. She *had* had chicken pox as a child. You cannot develop shingles unless you have had an earlier bout of chicken pox. The woman was also typical in her symptoms: Shingles is often more painful than it is itchy. Her age was unusual, however. While young people do develop shingles, the disease most often strikes in later years. About 10 percent of normal adults can be expected to get shingles during their lifetimes, usually after age 50. The incidence increases with age so that shingles is 10 times more likely to occur in adults over 60 than in children under 10.

The chances of developing shingles are greatest for individuals whose immune systems are weakened. That holds for children as well as adults. The child who is suffering from a disease which damages the immune system, or who is taking anticancer drugs that suppress the immune system, is a prime candidate for an attack of shingles. At present, as many as 10 percent of children with leukemia and 52 percent of children with Hodgkin's disease develop shingles.

Still another group of children vulnerable to shingles are youngsters whose mothers had chicken pox late in pregnancy — 5 to 21 days before giving birth. Sometimes these children are born with chicken pox or develop a typical case within a few days. In any case, as many as a third develop shingles during the first 5 years.

A "girdle" of pain

The first sign of shingles is often pain in or under the skin. The individual may also feel ill with fever or headache. After several days, a rash of small fluid-filled blisters appears on reddened skin.

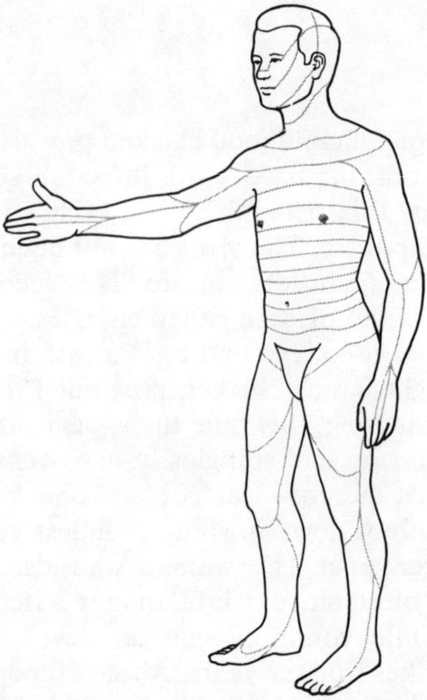

The lines on the drawing mark the areas of skin supplied by individual brain or spinal nerves. When shingles strikes, the rash is confined to one of the narrow bands or segments.

The blisters, or lesions, are usually limited to a band spanning one side of the trunk or clustered on one side of the face. This striking pattern gives the disease its name: *Shingles* comes from *cingulum*, the Latin word for belt or girdle. Similarly, the medical term for the disease, *zoster*, is the Greek word for girdle.

More importantly, the distribution of the shingles spots is a telltale clue to where the chicken pox virus has been hiding for all the years following the initial infection. Scientists now know that the shingles lesions correspond to the area of skin supplied by one of the major nerves that exits from the brain or spinal cord.

The assumption is that the chicken pox viruses that weren't wiped out in the original battle were able to leave the skin blisters and travel in the nervous system. There, the viruses settled down in an inactive form inside nerve cells (neurons) that lie in clusters adjacent to the spinal cord and brain. These neurons are called sensory cells because they relay information to the brain about what your body is

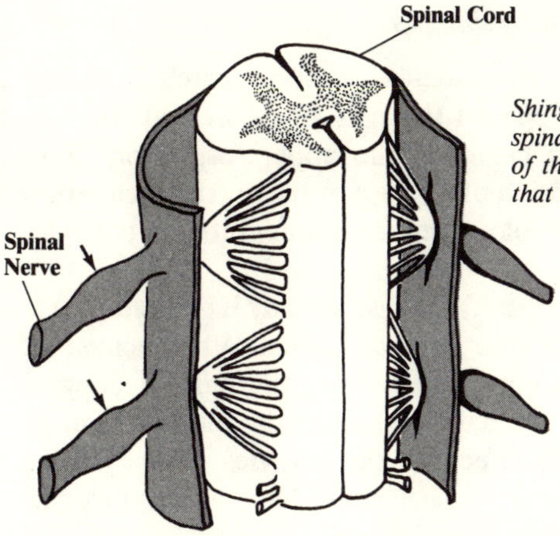

Shingles viruses hide inside nerve cells adjacent to the spinal cord and brain. The arrows point to the portion of the spinal nerve containing the sensory-cell bodies that house the virus.

sensing: whether your skin feels hot or cold, whether you've been touched or feel pain. Comparable nerve cell clusters in the head relay information about pain, temperature, or touch in that area, as well as information about what you're seeing, hearing, tasting, or smelling.

When the chicken pox virus reactivates, the virus moves down the long nerve fibers that extend from the sensory cell bodies to the skin. There, the viruses multiply and the telltale rash erupts. Now the nervous system is deeply involved, however, and the symptoms are often more complex and severe than those of childhood chicken pox. People with "optical" shingles (where the virus has invaded an ophthalmic nerve) may suffer painful eye inflammations that leave them temporarily blind. Infections of facial nerves can lead to paralysis or excruciating pain. People with lesions on the torso may feel spasms of pain at the gentlest touch or breeze.

Because of the nervous system involvement, the chicken pox/-shingles virus is of great interest to the National Institute of Neurological and Communicative Disorders and Stroke (NINCDS), the principal federal agency supporting research on the nervous system. The disease is of equal concern to the National Institute of Allergy and Infectious Diseases (NIAID). In addition, the National Cancer Institute and the National Institute on Aging support research on shingles because of the prevalence and severity of the disease among cancer patients and the elderly.

The aftermath

For the majority of normally healthy individuals, the second bout with the chicken pox virus is almost always a second triumph of the body's immune system. The shingles attack may last longer than

On catching chicken pox...but not catching shingles

Chicken pox is a highly contagious disease.. Most of us catch it during childhood because the virus can be spread through air as well at through contact with the rash. The infection begins in the upper respiratory tract where the virus reproduces over a period of 15 days or more (the incubation period). The virus then spreads to the bloodstream and migrates to the skin, giving rise to the familiar rash.

In contrast, you can't catch shingles. You must already have had a case of chicken pox and harbor the virus in your nervous system. When activated, the virus travels down the nerves to your skin causing the painful shingles rash. In shingles, the virus does not normally spread to the bloodstream or lungs, so the virus is not shed in air. Because the shingles rash contains active virus particles, however, a person who has never had chicken pox can contract chicken pox by exposure to the shingles rash.

chicken pox, and you may need medication for pain but, in most cases, the body has the inner resources to fight back. The lesions heal and the pain subsides within 3 to 5 weeks.

There are exceptions. Sometimes, particularly in older people, the pain and other symptoms persist long after the rash is healed. It is important to realize that these individuals no longer have shingles: Their infection is over. Instead, they are suffering a neurological disorder, the result of damage to the nervous system.

Investigators think that the virus attack has led to scarring or other lesions affecting the sensory cells and associated nerves. If the eye is involved, the damage from shingles can lead to blindness.

In other cases facial paralysis, headache, and persistent pain are the aftermath. Possibly because the nerve cells conveying pain sensations are hardest hit, or are exquisitely sensitized by the virus attack, pain is the principal complication of shingles. This pain, called *postherpetic neuralgia*, is among the most devastating known to mankind — the kind of pain that leads to insomnia, weight loss, depression, and that total preoccupation with unrelenting torment that characterizes the chronic pain sufferer.

Even in such severe cases, however, the paralysis, headaches, and pain generally subside, although it may take time. As one elderly sufferer recalls: "The worst thing was that the pain went on for months and months. Another bad part was reflecting on the 60 years since I had the chicken pox. Am I only a culture medium for viruses, for heaven's sake?"

Postherpetic neuralgia may be a nightmare, but it is not life-threatening. Doctors treating the pain currently employ a variety of

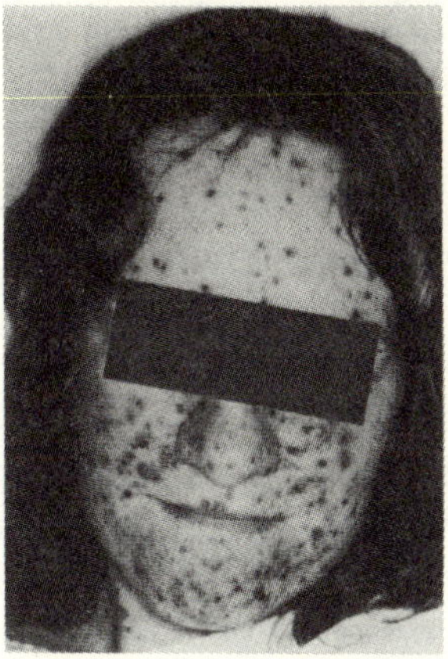

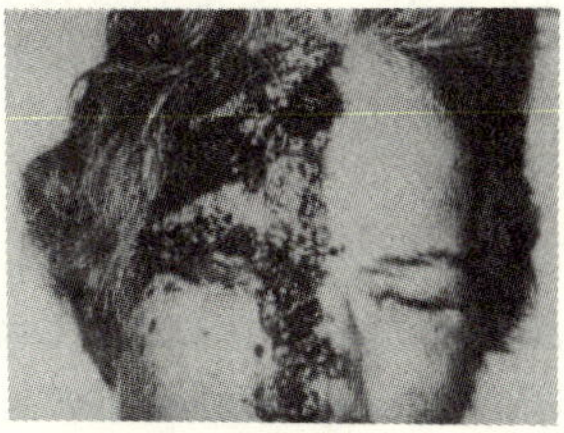

The woman on the left has a bad case of adult chickenpox. In contrast, note the sharply circumscribed region and closely spaced blisters of the shingles rash on the woman's face at right.

medications. They generally avoid the powerful narcotic pain relievers in favor of newer nonaddictive but, potent, painkillers. Studies have also shown that some anticonvulsant drugs used to treat epilepsy, such as carbamazepine (Tegretol®) are sometimes effective in relieving postherpetic neuralgia. Antidepressants can help, also. In addition to their effects on mood, the antidepressants appear to relieve pain. Some doctors report that patients occasionally benefit from some of the more controversial treatments for pain, such as acupuncture and electrical stimulation of nerve endings.

Shingles *is* a serious threat to life in immunosuppressed patients. The child or adult with leukemia, Hodgkin's disease, or other cancers is often treated by drugs or radiation to destroy cancerous tissue. Unfortunately, these treatments also damage cells of the immune system that normally fight invading organisms. Patients with kidney or other organ diseases who receive organ transplants are also vulnerable to shingles. These patients are given drugs that suppress the immune system to prevent the body from rejecting the foreign tissue. Should any of these patients contract shingles, there is a real danger that the disease will spread throughout the body, reaching vital organs like the lungs. If unchecked, such disseminated shingles can lead to death from viral pneumonia or secondary bacterial infection.

Shingles in pregnancy

Many mothers-to-be are concerned about any infection contracted during pregnancy, and rightly so. It is well known that certain viruses can be transmitted across the mother's bloodstream to the fetus, or can be acquired by the baby during the birth process. What about shingles? The chief of the NINCDS Infectious Diseases Branch notes that there have been a few isolated reports of maternal shingles leading to birth defects, but the cases are poorly documented. "It is controversial," he says, "but I do not think shingles in the mother increases the risk for the baby."

In contrast, maternal *chicken pox* poses some risk to the unborn child, depending upon the stage of pregnancy when the mother contracts the disease. During the first 30 weeks, maternal chicken pox may, in some cases, lead to congenital malformations. Such cases are rare and experts differ in their opinion on how great is the risk.

If the mother gets chicken pox from 21 to 5 days before giving birth, the newborn may have chicken pox at birth or develop it within a few days, as noted earlier. But the time lapse between the start of the mother's illness and the birth of the baby generally allows the mother's immune system to react and produce antibodies to fight the virus. These antibodies can be transmitted to the unborn child and thus help fight the infection. Still, a third of the babies exposed to chicken pox in the 21-to-5 day period before birth develop shingles in the first 5 years.

Suppose the mother contracts chicken pox at precisely the time of birth, however. In that case, the mother's immune system has not had a chance to mobilize its forces. The newborn may be infected at birth, but will have precious little ability to fight off the attack because the baby's immunological system is immature. For these babies chicken pox can be fatal. They must be given "zoster immune globulin," a preparation made from the antibody-rich blood of adults who have recently recovered from chicken pox or shingles.

The clever culprit

The virus responsible for shingles and chicken pox belongs to the *herpes* group of viruses. The group includes the virus that causes cold sores, fever blisters, mononucleosis, and genital herpes — a sexually transmitted disease. Like the shingles-causing virus, many herpes-viruses can take refuge in the nervous system after an individual has suffered an initial infection. The virus may remain latent for years, then travel down nerve cell fibers to cause a renewed infection.

Scientists call the chicken pox/shingles-causing agent the VZ virus, short for *varicella-zoster*. *Varicella* is a Latin word meaning "little pox" to distinguish the virus from smallpox, the scourge that once disfigured or killed its victims. (The word "chicken" conveys the same idea of weakness or mildness as in "chicken-hearted.") Like many viruses, the varicella-zoster virus looks as though it were designed by a mathematician. It is a microscopic sphere encasing a 20-sided geometric figure called an icosahedron. Inside the icosahedron is the genetic material of the virus, deoxyribonucleic acid (DNA). When activated, the virus reproduces inside the nucleus of an infected cell. It acquires its spherical wrapping as it buds through the nuclear membrane.

As early as 1909, a German scientist suspected that the viruses causing chicken pox and shingles were one and the same. In the 1920s and 1930s the case was strengthened. In an experiment, children were inoculated with fluid from the lesions of patients with shingles. Within 2 weeks, about half the children came down with chicken pox. Finally, in 1958, detailed analyses of the viruses taken from patients with either chicken pox or shingles confirmed that the viruses were identical.

Note what that means: A person with shingles can communicate chicken pox to a susceptible individual. But the opposite is not true: A person with chicken pox cannot communicate shingles to someone else. You must already harbor the virus in your nervous system before shingles can develop.

"It's a clever virus," notes the NINCDS virologist. "It doesn't kill its host, but lives for a long time in a suppressed state. And it can reactivate, given the opportunity," he adds.

Killing the opportunity

Shingles imposes two immediate challenges to medical research. The first is to develop drugs to fight the disease and to prevent complications. The second challenge is to understand the disease well enough to prevent it, especially in people known to be at high risk.

Only recently have scientists succeeded in developing antiviral drugs. In 1975 there were virtually no virus-fighting drugs available. Progress has been impressive since then, and now there are several antiviral agents in clinical use, with more on the way. While no medications have yet been approved for treatment of shingles, several candidates are being tested:

- Vidarabine. One drug in limited use is vidarabine (also known as Ara-A®). Vidarabine interferes with the virus's ability to make new genetic material and thus prevents the virus from reproducing and spreading in the body. Early treatment with vidarabine decreased the duration of shingles in a group of 87 patients with deficient immune responses. The patients treated early also had more rapid pain relief and a shorter period of lesion formation compared to patients who received the drug later in the course of their disease. This trial was conducted by the NIAID Collaborative Antiviral Study.

- Acyclovir. Another drug being tested on zoster patients is called acyclovir. It is administered to the patient in an inactive form. When the drug reaches a VZ virus-infected cell, a chemical produced by the virus activates acyclovir. Once activated, acyclovir is able to destroy a vital chemical that the virus needs to reproduce. This oddly self-destructive behavior on the part of the virus — cooperating in its own demise — has led some investigators to label acyclovir a "suicide promoter." Acyclovir has appeared promising in preliminary tests on cancer patients with shingles.

Newer, even more potent drugs are in earlier stages of testing. The chief of the Medical Virology Section of NIAID predicts that, within a few years drugs, taken by mouth or applied to the rash will effectively shut down VZ virus infections.

- Interferon. This disease-fighting substance is not a drug, but a compound naturally produced by body cells. It is currently being investigated as a cure for everything from the common cold to cancer — and shingles. In studies at Stanford University, some 150 immuno-suppressed patients were given a particular type of interferon. The compound not only reduced the pain and extent of the shingles lesions, but also lessened complications. Currently, not enough interferon is available for clinical use. By using the newer genetic engineering techniques that enable interferon to be produced in specially treated bacteria (instead of having to isolate interferon from human blood), scientists expect to have enough on hand for future treatment.

The goal of prevention

The second major challenge to investigators is to protect susceptible patients from a shingles attack. To do that, scientists will need to know much more about the VZ virus, especially how it remains latent in the body for so long, and what induces it to become active again.

While the virus is presumed to hide in the nervous system between bouts of chicken pox and shingles, it has never been recovered from nerve cells at autopsies unless the patient had shingles at the time of death. In contrast, herpes *simplex*, which causes recurrent infections of cold sores and fever blisters, has been identified in spinal nerve cells during its latent periods.

If the whole VZ virus does not remain intact in nerve cells, perhaps its core genetic material — the DNA — survives. Scientists suspect that the viral DNA may be inserted into one of the chromosomes of the nerve cell — the larger units that house the cell's own genetic material. The chief of the Virology Section at NIAID is using new gene-splicing techniques to produce copies of parts of the viral DNA. To find out if the viral DNA is built into a nerve cell's chromosomes, he plans to label the viral DNA with a radioactive substance. Such labeled DNA will bind to matching strands of DNA in a cell and the radioactivity given off will pin down its precise location. The virologist hopes by this method to locate viral genes in human nerve cells.

The technique is expected to show how many people carry latent VZ virus in their nerve cells. The number may be as high as 90 percent of the adult population — the people who have had chicken pox.

What keeps the VZ virus quiet during its long latency? Probably the immune system, scientists think. A healthy immune system protects against all kinds of diseases, but people with depressed immunity are vulnerable to many illnesses, and have a high incidence of shingles. Even among normal individuals, temporary depression of the immune system because of stress, a cold, and even sunburn, may be associated with an attack of shingles.

Antibodies, one of the immune system's major defense mechanisms against infection, are not very helpful against shingles. Studies have shown that patients with shingles produce VZ antibodies: They just don't check the infection. Similarly, injections of antibody-rich blood serum do not prevent the dissemination of shingles in cancer patients or others whose immune systems are depressed. (This is in contrast to the protection conferred by the serum when given to newborns with chicken pox.)

The components of the immune system that do appear to combat shingles are two types of white blood cell: the T lymphocyte, and a scavenger cell called a macrophage. Scientists are trying to find ways of boosting the activity of these cells — especially in patients at high risk for severe or disseminated shingles.

A human disease

The development of preventive measures and treatment for shingles has been hindered by scientists' difficulty in working with the VZ virus in the laboratory. The virus grows very poorly in laboratory cells and does not infect animals other than man. A leading investigator says that less is known about the biology of VZ virus than about any other herpesvirus.

Current research is aimed at finding better methods for growing the VZ virus and identifying animal models of the disease. So far, the best animal model is the patas monkey. NINCDS scientists working with these monkeys note that the animals succumb to a disease resembling chicken pox when injected with a virus very similar to the VZ virus. Indeed, the two viruses are so closely related that a vaccine made from the human virus can be used to protect the monkeys from their version of chicken pox.

But the monkey studies are aimed at learning more about the behavior of the VZ virus in the body, not at developing a shingles vaccine. A successful vaccine against shingles is considered unlikely because the disease typically develops in people who have naturally built up an immune response. Remember, if you have had chicken pox, you have developed the same antibodies against the VZ virus as a vaccine would induce — but those antibodies do not control shingles.

On the other hand, there is considerable interest and experimental work in developing a vaccine for chicken pox. Japanese investigators have produced a vaccine containing live VZ virus which has become inactivated by growing it in tissue culture in the laboratory. More than 2,000 healthy people and more than 500 hospitalized or chronically ill children have received the vaccine in Japan. There were few side effects, and most of the recipients not only developed antibodies to the virus, but also did not succumb to chicken pox when exposed to it under test conditions.

Whether the vaccine is truly protective will depend on continued experience with the vaccine in high-risk patients. If those vaccinated do not get chicken pox when exposed to the natural disease in the community, the vaccine may be of enormous benefit, a true lifesaver for many leukemic children and other high-risk patients.

There is a catch, however. If you inject a vaccine that contains an altered but still living VZ virus, might not the virus take refuge in the nervous system and later give rise to shingles? To resolve that question, the National Institute on Aging is currently supporting trials of chicken pox vaccine at New York University in New York City.

The NYU scientists plan to observe children with acute leukemia — a group that is particularly vulnerable to shingles. The investigators will note the incidence and severity of shingles occurring in children who have received the chicken pox vaccine in comparison with children who have had natural cases of chicken pox. The data from Japan suggest that shingles will not be a problem among the vaccinated.

Investigators at the University of Texas (San Antonio), as well as at Children's Hospital in Philadelphia, are also conducting vaccine experiments with leukemic children. In addition, the Philadelphia group thinks that a chicken pox vaccine might provide a general boost to the immune system for people who have had chicken pox, helping them ward off shingles. They plan to inoculate elderly volunteers who have had chicken pox and note if they have a lower than normal incidence of shingles for their age group. If that is so, the VZ virus vaccine might confer immunity to shingles as well as to chicken pox — double protection.

But maybe not. "In the long run, the VZ virus will be more difficult to eliminate than the smallpox virus," says the NINCDS Infectious Diseases Laboratory chief. "Because the virus is so widespread and because it can reactivate at any time, even an effective vaccine would need to be administered indefinitely." Currently, physicians are uncertain whether it will ever be desirable to vaccinate whole populations of normal children routinely against chicken pox.

So it looks as if shingles will continue to afflict people in the years to come. The greatest practical hope lies in the measures rapidly being developed to decrease the discomfort and risk of shingles. In the course of that work, scientists expect to uncover important information to use against other diseases, learn more about the body's immune system and ultimately outwit the clever viruses that evade that system.

For further information

A number of institutes of the National Institutes of Health support research on shingles and related herpes viruses. For details on current programs or other inquiries write:

Office of Scientific and Health Reports
National Institute of Neurological and
Communicative Disorders and Stroke
Building 31, Room 8A06
National Institutes of Health
9000 Rockville Pike
Bethesda, MD 20205

or

Office of Research Reporting and Public Response
National Institute of Allergy and Infectious Diseases
Building 31, Room 7A32
National Institutes of Health
9000 Rockville Pike
Bethesda, MD 20205

Chapter 22

Smell and Taste Disorders

Smell and Taste Disorders

How do smell and taste work?

Smell and taste belong to our chemical sensing system, or the chemosenses. The complicated processes of smelling and tasting begin when tiny molecules released by the substances around us stimulate special cells in the nose, mouth, or throat. These special nerve cells transmit messages to the brain where specific smells or tastes are identified.

Olfactory, or smell, nerve cells are stimulated by the odors around us — the fragrance from a rose, the smell of bread baking. These nerve cells are found in a tiny patch of tissue high up in the nose, and connect directly to the brain.

Taste cells react to food or drink mixed with saliva. These surface cells send taste information to nearby nerve fibers. The taste cells are clustered in the taste buds of the mouth and throat. Many of the small bumps that can be seen on the tongue contain taste buds.

Taste and smell cells are the only cells in the nervous system that are replaced when they become old or damaged. Scientists are examining this phenomenon while studying ways to replace other damaged nerve cells.

A third chemosensory mechanism, called the common chemical sense, contributes to our senses of smell and taste. In this system, thousands of free nerve endings — especially on the moist surfaces of the eyes, nose, mouth, and throat — give rise to sensations like the sting of ammonia, the coolness of menthol, and the "heat" of chili peppers.

We can commonly identify four basic taste sensations: sweet, sour, bitter, and salty. Certain combinations of these tastes — along with texture, temperature, odor, and the sensations from the common chemical sense — produce a flavor. It is flavor that lets us know whether we are eating peanuts or caviar.

Many flavors are recognized mainly through the sense of smell. If you hold your nose while eating chocolate, for example, you will have trouble identifying the chocolate flavor — even though you can distinguish the food's sweetness or bitterness. That's because the familiar flavor of chocolate is sensed largely by odor. So is the well-known flavor of coffee.

What are the smell and taste disorders?

The most common chemosensory complaints are a reduced ability to detect odors (*hyposmia*) or to taste sweet, sour, bitter, or salty substances (*hypoqeusia*). Some people can detect no odors (*anosmia*) or no tastes (*aqeusia*)

In other disorders, the nervous system may misread and distort an odor or a flavor. Or a person may detect a foul odor or taste from a substance that to the normal individual is pleasant smelling or tasting.

Smell and taste disorders sometimes occur together. Overall, smell disorders are more common.

What causes smell and taste disorders?

Some people are born with chemosensory disorders, but most patients develop them after an injury or illness. Upper respiratory infections are blamed for some chemosensory losses, and injury to the head can also cause smell or taste problems.

Chemosensory disorders may result from polyps in the nasal or sinus cavities, hormonal disturbances, or dental problems. Loss of smell and taste can also be caused by prolonged exposure to certain chemicals such as insecticides, and by some medicines.

Many patients who receive radiation therapy for cancers of the head and neck later complain of chemosensory disturbances.

How common are smell and taste disorders?

One study estimates that more than 10 million Americans have chemosensory disorders. The predominant problem is a natural decline in smelling ability that typically occurs after age 60.

Another estimate suggests that more than 200,000 persons visit a physician for a smell or taste problem each year. Many more smell and taste disturbances go unreported

Are smell and taste disorders serious?

A person with faulty chemosenses is deprived of an early warning system that most of us take for granted. Smell and taste alert us to fires, poisonous fumes, leaking gas, and spoiled foods. Chemosensory problems may also be a sign of sinus disease, growths in the nasal passages, or, in rare circumstances, brain tumors. Because taste triggers many digestive processes, a malfunction of this sense may upset normal digestion. Smell and taste losses can also lead to depression, especially in persons whose occupations (fireman, chef) depend upon these senses.

How are smell and taste disorders diagnosed?

The extent of a chemosensory disorder can be tested by measuring the lowest concentration of a chemical that a person can accurately detect and recognize. A patient may also be asked to compare the smells or tastes of different chemicals, or to note how the intensities of smells or tastes grow when a chemical's concentration is increased.

Scientists have developed an easily administered "scratch-and-sniff" test to evaluate the sense of smell. A person scratches pieces of treated paper to release different odors, sniffs them, and tries to identify each odor from a list of possibilities.

In taste testing, the patient reacts to different chemical concentrations: this may involve a simple "sip, spit, and rinse" test, or chemicals may be applied directly to specific areas of the tongue.

Can smell and taste disorders be treated?

If a certain medication is the cause of a smell or taste disorder, stopping or changing the medicine may help eliminate the problem. Some patients — notably those with serious respiratory infections or seasonal allergies — regain their smell or taste simply by waiting for their illness to run its course. In many cases, nasal obstructions such as polyps can be removed to restore airflow to the receptor area. When there is a more serious cause for the disorder — a brain tumor, for example — correcting the larger medical problem can also correct the loss of smell and taste. Occasionally, chemosenses return to normal just as spontaneously as they disappeared.

What research is being done?

Within the federal government, the focal point for research on the chemosenses is the National Institute of Neurological and Communicative Disorders and Stroke (NINCDS). A unit of the National Institutes of Health, the NINCDS supports fundamental studies and clinical investigations of chemosensory disorders at grantee institutions across the nation. Some of these studies are conducted at several institute-supported chemosensory research centers, where scientists working in different laboratories and clinics unravel the secrets of smell and taste.

In a study of 2,000 volunteers at the NINCDS supported chemosensory research center at the University of Pennsylvania, scientists have found that the sense of smell is most accurate between the ages of 30 and 60 years. It begins to decline after age 60, with a large proportion of elderly persons having lost their smelling ability. The study also showed that women of all ages are generally more accurate than men in identifying odors, and that smoking adversely affects the ability to identify odors.

The University of Pennsylvania scientists have discovered that some patients with a range of normal smelling abilities have different levels of certain chemicals in their cerebrospinal fluid. The investigators are comparing these chemical levels to the patients' olfactory profiles. This work could eventually lead to a drug treatment that would improve smelling ability by correcting a chemical imbalance in the central nervous system.

Although certain medications can cause chemosensory problems, others — notably anti-allergy drugs — seem to improve the senses of taste and smell. Pennsylvania investigators sponsored by NINCDS are also working to find medicines similar to allergy drugs that can treat chemosensory losses with few side effects.

With NINCDS support, scientists at the University of Connecticut's chemosensory research center are conducting studies to understand better how smell and taste work. In one project, the responses of taste nerve cells in the tongue to taste, touch, and temperature are being analyzed to see how these stimuli interact. Investigators are also mapping the pathways that take these messages to the brain.

The Connecticut scientists are using new taste tests to study genetic variations in tasting ability and to evaluate taste function in individuals who are pregnant or have certain diseases. Other research projects are aimed at sharpening the diagnosis of even small olfactory losses, so that occupational exposure to smell-damaging substances can be assessed.

Patients who have lost their larynx, or "voice box," commonly complain of poor ability to smell, a problem some investigators have attributed to the nerve damage caused by the laryngectomy. However, in an NINCDS-supported smell research center at the State University of New York's Upstate Medical Center, scientists found that in spite of nerve damage, the sense of smell is greatly improved when laryngectomy patients use a special "bypass" tube to breathe through the nose again rather than through an opening in the neck. This finding emphasizes the contribution of adequate nasal air flow in olfactory perception. The investigators are now using sophisticated machines to "map" the normal flow of air through the nose.

What can I do to help myself?

If you experience a smell or taste problem, it is important to remember that you are not alone: thousands of other patients have faced the same situation. Proper diagnosis by a trained professional can provide reassurance that your illness is not imaginary. You may even be surprised by the results. For example, what you may think is a taste problem could actually be a smell problem, since much of what you think you taste, you really smell.

Diagnosis may also lead to treatment of an underlying cause for the disturbance. Many types of smell and taste disorders are reversible, and for those that are not, counseling is available to help you cope.

Smell and taste research centers supported by the NINCDS often need research patients to help their scientists study the chemosenses more intensely. Prospective research patients should have their physicians write to:

Dr. James B. Snow. Jr.
Clinical Smell and Taste Research Center
Hospital of the University of Pennsylvania
3400 Spruce Street, G1
Philadelphia, PA 19104
Telephone: (215) 662-2653

Dr. Marion E. Frank
Department of Oral Biology
Connecticut Chemosensory Clinical Research Center
University of Connecticut Health Center
Farmington, CT 06032
Telephone: (203) 674-2459

Dr. Maxwell M. Mozell
SUNY Upstate Clinical Smell Research Center
766 Irving Avenue
Syracuse, NY 13210
Telephone: (315) 473-5591

NINCDS Information
For additional information about research supported by the NINCDS, contact:

Office of Scientific and Health Reports
National Institute of Neurological and
Communicative Disorders and Stroke
National Institutes of Health
Building 31, Room 8A-06
Bethesda, MD 20892
Telephone: (301) 496-5751

Chapter 23

Developmental Speech and Language Disorders

Developmental Speech and Language Disorders

Eliza, age 2½, toddies around her nursery school classroom, the straps of her purple overalls slipping off her shoulders. She watches and smiles, and, generally, she follows directions, but Eliza is silent. The only words she utters are *dog* to describe a wooden plaything and — when it's time to go home — *bus*.

Ben is older, nearly 5, and as sweet-faced as little Eliza. But his only "words" — used sparingly in two word phrases — are all but unintelligible to a stranger. Ben wants to join in the activities of his class, but he cannot understand his teacher's instructions about putting a beanbag on his head, on his shoe, on his shoulder. He simply holds on to the beanbag and smiles, waiting to imitate the other children's responses.

Eliza and Ben are in a special program for preschoolers with speech and language disorders. Eliza is language disordered and has a brain dysfunction: she is delayed primarily in her ability to translate thoughts into language, even though she understands almost everything that a child her age is expected to. Ben is disordered in both speech and language. His problems involve the neurological motor skills that produce speech, as well as the brain function of understanding language. The treatment he requires is more complex. And if Ben has normal intelligence — which can be determined by specialized testing — then this intelligence is masked by his halting, stumbling phrases.

What causes speech and language disorders in children like these? How can the problems be treated? Will children who are slow to speak and understand what is said to them also be slow to read, to write, to think logically? Evidence suggests that the answer to the latter question may be yes for some children, but scientists continue to search for causes and effective treatments that will give parents and professionals a basis for hope. Encouraged by the National Institute of Neurological and Communicative Disorders and Stroke (NINCDS), the primary source of federal support for research on the brain and disorders of speech and language, investigators around the country are developing new techniques for studying normal disordered speech and language acquisition as well as treatments for speech and language impairments.

Eliza and Ben have a chance of being helped because their problems have been discovered and are being treated early in life. But many questions will remain unanswered for years. The children will be watched closely when they enter school — Ben probably in a special classroom, Eliza perhaps mainstreamed into a regular school — to see whether their speech and language delays show up later in other guises, particularly as reading disabilities. And as they reach adulthood, another question looms: Will they pass their speech and language difficulties on to their own children?

The scope of the problem

A child with a language disorder has difficulty understanding language or putting words together to make sense, indicating a problem with brain function. A child with a speech disorder has trouble producing the sounds of language, often resulting from a combination of brain-coordination and neurological motor dysfunction. Either child will lag significantly behind the level of speech and language development expected of a playmate of the same age, environment, and intellectual ability.

Language impairment may show itself in several ways:

- Children may have trouble giving names to objects and using those names to formulate ideas about how the world is organized. For example, they cannot learn that a toy they play with is called *car*, or that a toy car of another color, or a real car, can also be called *car*.
- They may have trouble learning the rules of grammar. Such children might not learn, for example, how to use prepositions and other small words like *in* or *the*.
- They may not use language appropriately for the context; for example, they might respond to a teacher's question by reciting an irrelevant jingle heard on television.

Speech problems seem to be more prevalent than language problems. Both disorders appear to decline as children get older. Speech disorders affect an estimated 10 to 15 percent of preschoolers, and about 6 percent of children in grades 1 through 12. Language disorders affect about 2 to 3 percent of the preschool population and about 1 percent of the school-age population. In all, nearly 6 million children under the age of 18 are speech or language disordered. Two-thirds of them are boys.

It is difficult to be more precise about just how prevalent the problem is, because the definition itself is so unwieldy. How delayed must a child be to qualify as "disordered"? How does one recognize the delay in the first place?

When is there a problem?

Experts use phrases such as *developmental language disorder, delayed speech, impaired language, motor disorder,* and *idiopathic* (no known cause) *speech* and *language disorders* to describe a variety of speech and language difficulties in children. In this text, delayed speech or delayed language means a problem that appears in the course of the child's development and for which there is no apparent cause. Eliminated from this discussion are speech or language problems that can be traced to deafness, mental retardation, cerebral palsy, or autism.

Speech-language pathologists generally define children as disordered if they lag significantly behind their age peers in reaching certain speech and language milestones. The significance of this lag is determined by a thorough professional examination. British studies show that the range of normal for early language acquisition is enormous. Normal children speak the first word at anywhere from 6 to 18 months, and combine words into phrases for the first time at anywhere from 10 to 24 months. It takes a skilled practitioner to distinguish between a slow child who will eventually catch up and a child with a true delay.

Speech and language professionals have devised a general outline of what speech sounds should have been acquired by a certain age. A child who is not quite on schedule, of course, is not necessarily delayed or disordered; it may just be that the child's individual time table is different from most children's.

An understanding of what constitutes normal language development is helpful when parents try to evaluate whether their child is abnormally slow. The most widely accepted speech and language milestone for children age 1 to 7 years are outlined in the chart at the end of this text.

Language problems are most obvious among 2- to 3-year-olds, whose language skills are usually developing very rapidly. Many of these problems subsequently resolve themselves; others require the aid of therapy.

Among older children, speech and language disorder might emerge in a different guise. A 5- or 6-year-old might have caught up in language and social skill sufficiently to communicate with others, but not sufficiently for good reading or thinking. Such a child could be considered reading- or learning-disabled.

The physical tools of speech

Speech has four components: *articulation*, *phonation*, *resonance*, and *rhythm*:

- *Articulation* is the ability to make specific sounds: the *g* in gum, the *b* in bear, the *s* in snake. Articulation is the component most often affected in children with speech disorders of unknown cause.
- *Phonation* is the utterance of vocal sounds — the voice — produced in the larynx, or "voice box."
- *Resonance* is the modification of the voice after it leaves the larynx. The voice is modified by the cavities inside the mouth, nose, and pharynx (the throat).
- *Rhythm*, or what scientists call *prosody*, involves the rate and timing of speech.

For speech to begin, the brain and the vocal and auditory systems must be in good working order. The human vocal system components are perfectly adapted for speech. Our teeth, for example, are usually evenly spaced and equal in size (unless there are dental problems), and our top and bottom teeth can get close enough to pronounce such sounds as *s*, *f*, *sh*, and *th*. Our lips have more developed muscles than the lips of other primates, and our relatively small mouths can open and shut rapidly to form sounds such as *p* and *b*. The size of our mouth opening can be varied to pronounce a range of vowel sounds.

The location of the larynx is perhaps the most important feature of the human vocal system. In the adult human, the larynx, where the vocal cords are located and voice sounds originate, is located farther down in the throat than is the larynx of any other primate. This extra room allows humans to modulate speech and to pronounce such sounds as the consonants in *g*ut and *c*ut.

Defects in the structure of the lips, palate, or teeth can interfere with a child's ability to make speech sounds correctly. A hole in the palate — the "cleft palate" seen in some newborns — is the most common such problem. A cleft palate can usually be corrected surgically but, even after surgery, affected children may have too much nasal resonance and difficulty producing certain speech sounds. Other children with growths in the larynx or vocal cords may have voices with a harsh, husky sound.

The auditory system comprises the three parts of the ear — the outer ear, the middle ear, and the inner ear — and the connections between the inner ear and the auditory center of the brain. The middle ear is prone to infection during childhood because of the angle of the eustachian tube, which connects the middle ear to the throat. When a child has a cold, the short eustachian tube cannot

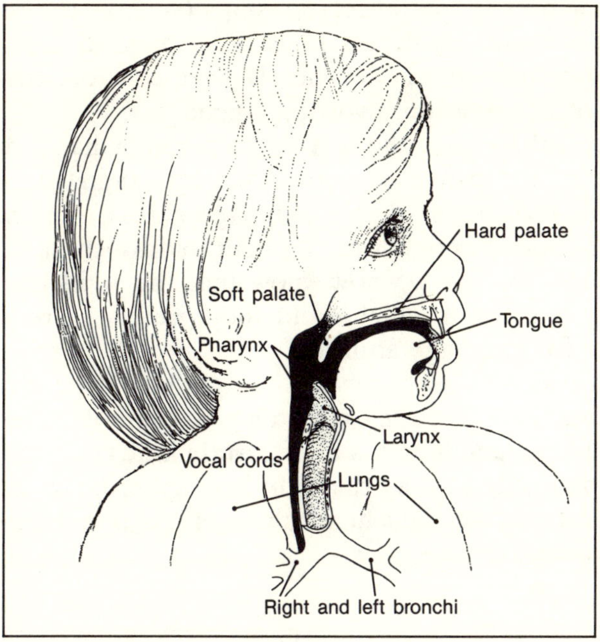

The structures of the vocal system.

drain excess mucus properly, and the fluid that builds up becomes a breeding ground for bacteria. The resulting condition is called otitis media.

If the auditory system is not in good order and a hearing loss exists as a result of continual ear infections and fluid buildup, the child may mishear adult speech and produce it incorrectly. To avoid this problem, an otolaryngologist, a physician who specializes in ear, nose, and throat disorders, should be consulted at the first sign of a hearing loss. The otolaryngologist may refer the child for testing to an audiologist, an expert on the hearing process.

The role of the brain

If scientists were asked to identify the most important feature of the brain that enables humans to speak, they would point to the brain's functional division into left and right hemispheres. This characteristic appears to be related in most people to the brain's asymmetry. Even at birth one can see evidence of this asymmetry: the left hemisphere tends to be larger than the right in most newborns.

Although most complex functions involve both sides of the brain to some extent, certain functions can be traced to one hemisphere or the other. In approximately 90 percent of us, the right hemisphere controls how we see spatial relationships (such as the recognition of faces) and recognize patterns (such as a musical melody). In that same 90 percent of us, the left hemisphere controls how we process sequences of information involving language.

Neuroscientists once thought that a person's handedness showed which side of the brain was dominant for language: right-handed people were thought to derive language skills from the left hemisphere, left-handed people were thought to draw these skills from the right hemisphere. But we now know that the tendency is for most individuals, no matter which hand they prefer, to rely on the left hemisphere for language abilities.

In certain situations, however, the right hemisphere can take over language function. In young children, for example, the loss of left-hemisphere language function after certain kinds of brain surgery can be well compensated for by the right hemisphere. But in adolescents and young adults, the right hemisphere is less able take language or speech production.

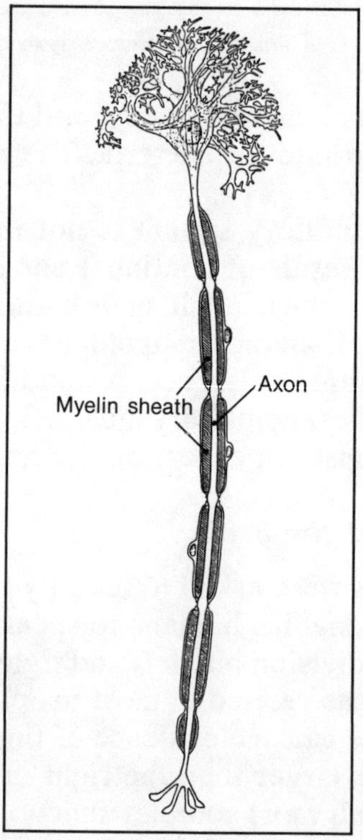

The axon of a neuron is covered by a myelin sheath, a fatty casing that facilitates the transmission of brain messages.

The maturing nervous system. The development of the brain's asymmetry is part of the overall maturation of the system which occurs before birth. Scientists believe that sometime in the middle of gestation, nerve cells, or neurons, migrate from germinal zones — areas where cells reproduce — to the regions of the brain in which they will reside. This brain cell migration usually begins at about the 16th week and ends by the 24th week.

If the migration of cells to the brain is incomplete, or interrupted by something in the fetus' environment (perhaps an antibody developed by the body in response to a foreign substance), the fetus could die before or shortly after birth. If migration occurs, but with errors, the result could be language delay.

After mid-gestation, and probably through the first decade of life, the neurons of a child's brain begin to mature. As neurons develop, they grow axons: long connecting arms linking one brain cell to another. As neuronal development continues, these axons are covered by a myelin sheath, a fatty casing that protects the axons and helps them transmit messages more efficiently. This myelinization of message pathways in the brain occurs at a rapid rate until about age 2 and continues at a slower pace until puberty. The process is crucial

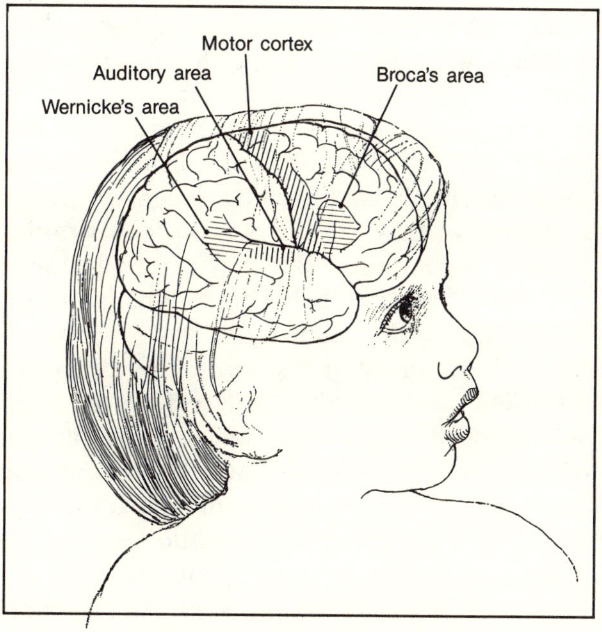

The areas of the brain involved in speech and language.

to the child's growing capacity for understanding and expressing language.

The brain's language centers. Two areas in the brain are known to be involved in speech and language. Broca's area, named after the French surgeon Peirre-Paul Broca, is in the left frontal lobe, close to the part of the brain that controls movements of the tongue, larynx, and other structures involved in speech. Broca's area is responsible for translating thoughts into speech.

Wernicke's area, named after the German neurologist Karl Wernicke, is located behind Broca's area, just around the temples. It contributes to the understanding of the spoken and written word and, in most individuals, is larger in the left hemisphere than in the right. Wernicke's area is quite close to the auditory cortex, the brain region that controls the input and analysis of sound.

The difference in function of the two language regions is apparent when either area is damaged. *Aphasia* is the loss of language after a brain injury. An adult aphasic with damage to Broca's area has reduced speech that sounds like a message in a telegram: asked about the weather, he might respond "rainy" or, if pressed, "rainy day." An adult with damage to Wernicke's area may articulate well and form grammatically correct sentences, but provides very little coherent information his speech. Such a patient might answer a question about the weather by saying, "I think it's not good. I don't like it when it's like that." Many aphasic patients may have other language problems as well.

Translating sounds into meaning. Some children may have language difficulty because of a problem with the brain's ability to analyze speech. Research scientists have studied dozens of language-delayed children and found that they are unable to process rapid speech-like signals produced by a computer. But they can be trained to differentiate among sounds if the time between sounds is prolonged.

Scientists now know that soon after birth, babies are able to detect differences between speech sounds. Investigators have found that infants as young as 1 month can detect the minute differences between closely related speech sounds such as *p*at and *b*at.

Most children develop a phonological system, an internal sense of how different categories of speech sounds are used, by about age 3. This system differs according to the child's native language. An English-speaking child, for instance, does not have within his phonological system the same *s* sound as a Spanish-speaking child, a sound that is somewhere between the English *s* and *th*, or the guttural *kh* sound of a German-speaking child.

Children must first perceive the unique characteristics of a sound in order to be able to repeat it. But many sounds in the English language differ only minutely — and sometimes the differences are a matter of timing. The difference between the initial sounds for the words *b*in and *p*in, for example, is a function of something called voice onset time. To utter the *b* sound, the vocal cords begin to vibrate almost as soon as the speaker releases air by opening the lips. For the *p* sound, there is a delay of about 20 extra milliseconds between the time the lips first open and the time the vocal cords start vibrating.

Even though these differences are very small, most persons can discriminate between *b* and *p*, or *d* and *t*, or *g* and *k* — consonants distinguishable by short differences in voice onset time. Speech-language pathologists believe that when children consistently fail to make these distinctions, they may have incorrectly established the sounds in their phonological systems.

Think of what happens to an adult trying to learn a foreign language. The adult can generally imitate the sounds of that language after hearing a word about 50 to 100 times, but still does not know the phonology — the range of possible sounds of the language and the rules for their order. Similarly, a child can imitate the sounds his speech pathologist urges him to make, but to him they're like a foreign tongue. A little boy who speaks like Elmer Fudd, the cartoon character who calls Bugs Bunny a "scwewy wabbit," may be capable of making an *r* sound the way he's told to, but to him the *r* sound isn't supposed to sound like an *r*. He thinks it should sound like a *w*.

Other influencing factors

The normal development of speech and language depends largely on the health of the brain and the vocal and auditory systems. But children who are abnormally slow in speech or language acquisition may show no signs of physical problems that could explain the delay. In such cases, certain other factors may be slowing things down.

Ear infections. Controversy exists about the relationship between chronic otitis media and the rapidity with which a child learns to speak. Most studies investigating the question have found no clear association between otitis media and language disorder, unless a hearing loss is present. The prudent course of is to treat ear infections promptly and to be alert to signs of poor hearing — inattentiveness, failure to respond, requests to have words repeated or to have the television volume raised — in a child with frequent otitis media. Treatment may include antibiotic therapy and the insertion of a tube into the middle ear to drain the fluid. Recent NINCDS-supported studies found that decongestant and antihistamine compounds are ineffective for otitis media, but that the antibiotic amoxicillin is effective.

Poor models in the home. The role of the environment in language acquisition has never been fully explained. For example, a normal child whose parent suffers from a language problem may reach full language competence despite an environment in which language models are scant. Psycholinguists, who study psychological and biological roots of language, believe most children have an innate drive to learn the language of the community no matter what the environment.

But children whose brain structures are abnormal, even in quite subtle ways, may be born with a tendency toward language problems and, if their environments are language-deficient, they just don't have the inner resources to compensate. In addition, a vicious cycle of silence is all too easy to establish in the home of a language-impaired child. Parents react to the cues their babies give them. If a baby does not respond with sounds and words, the parent is unlikely to know that the baby is indeed ready for conversation. According to one scientist, the communication difficulties of language-impaired children have a direct impact on the parent's efforts to talk to them.

A collection of disorders

Speech and language disorders wear many faces. Common speech disorders include:

- ***Phonological impairment***, also called misarticulation. Here, the child says the sounds wrong, or omits or duplicates certain sounds within a word. The problem may reflect poor neurological motor skills, a learning error, or difficulty in identifying certain speech sounds. Examples of common errors are *wabbit* for *rabbit*, *thnake* for *snake*, *dood* for *good*, and *poo* for *spoon*.

Another phonological impairment is unstressed syllable deletion, in which a child simply skips over a syllable in a long word, as in *nana* for *banana* or *te-phone* for *telephone*. Many of these misproductions are a part of normal development and are expected in the speech of very young children, but when they persist past the expected age they are considered abnormal and usually indicate brain dysfunction.

• *Verbal dyspraxia*. This term is used by some scientists and clinicians to describe the inability to produce the sequential, rapid, and precise movements required for speech. Nothing is wrong with the child's vocal apparatus, but the child's brain cannot give correct instructions for the motor movements involved in speech. This disorder is characterized by many sound omissions. Some verbally dyspraxic children, for instance, speak only in vowels, making their speech nearly unintelligible. One little boy trying to say "My name is Billy" can only manage "eye a eh ee-ee." These children also have very slow, halting speech with many false starts before the right sounds are produced. Their speech errors may be similar to those of children with phonological impairment.

• *Dysarthria*. Here muscle control problems affect the speech-making apparatus. Dysarthria most commonly occurs in combination with other nervous system disorders such as cerebral palsy. A dysarthric child cannot control the muscles involved in speaking and eating, so the mouth may be open all the time or the tongue may protrude.

A child with a language problem has difficulty comprehending, or using language, and several different types of errors may result. Three of the more common are:

• *Form errors*. These are present when the child can understand or use the rules of grammar. A child with this problem might say "We go pool" instead of "We went to the pool."

Language-disordered children seem to have particular difficulty with complex sentence constructions such as questions and negative forms. This is exemplified below:

EXAMPLES OF FORM ERRORS

Corrected sentence	Disordered sentence
They won't play with me.	They no play with me.
I can't sing.	I no can sing.
He doesn't have money.	He no have money.
When will he come?	When he will come?
What is that?	What that?

• *Content errors*. This language disorder is involved when the semantics, or what the child understands or talks about, is limited or inaccurate. The child may have a limited vocabulary or may fail to understand that the same word — *match*, for example — can have multiple meanings.

• *Use errors*. This term concerns what linguists call pragmatics, the ability of the child to follow the rules of communication: when to talk, how to request information, how to take turns. A child with a use error might be unable to ask an adult for help, even though he knows that help is needed and the adult can provide it. Autistic children who have difficulty communicating with people may have use errors.

Categorizing patients

If children with a speech or language problem are to benefit from different treatment approaches now available, they must be accurately subgrouped according to type of impairment. In categorizing speech- and language-impaired children, experts tend to ask two questions. First, is the disorder expressive, receptive, or a mixture of both? Second, is the child simply delayed in speech or language development, or is the child not only delayed, but abnormal in speech and language when these skills begin to develop?

Expressive or receptive? Some language-impaired children have primarily expressive (speaking) disorders; others have mainly receptive (understanding) disorders. Most have a combination of both.

Clinicians often encounter children who may be unable to communicate effectively, but nonetheless show signs of understanding others quite well. Consider Becky, a 6-year-old girl seen at a speech clinic. Her conversation with a clinician goes like this:

Clinician: What is your favorite game?
Becky: Doctor.
Clinician: How many can play that game?
Becky: Two four.
Clinician: Two or four?
Becky: Or three.
Clinician: How do you play doctor?
Becky: One has to be doctor.
Clinician: Anything else?
Becky: One operation man.
Clinician: Anything else?
Becky: No.
Clinician: What do you want to be?
Becky: A nurse.
Clinician: Oh, you need a nurse?
Becky: No, you don't.

Becky has an expressive language disorder. Her responses are limited to incomplete sentences that may be inappropriate to the question, and they reveal Becky's inability to use verbs, conjunctions, or any of the subtleties of language. Like some children with expressive language problems, Becky has a good vocabulary, but she has difficulty connecting words. Even though she is 6, she talks like a 2-year-old.

Children with expressive language problems may or may not have articulation problems. But even if their speech is perfectly articulated, communication is impaired because language remains ungrammatical, reduced, babyish.

Paul, who is 7 years old, is Becky's opposite, a child with a receptive language disorder who has difficulty understanding language. Receptive language problems rarely occur alone; usually they are accompanied by at least some degree of expressive language disorder. The condition often is misdiagnosed as attention problem, behavioral problems, or hearing problems. Standardized language tests may reveal, though, that a child with receptive language disorder is trying to cooperate but simply cannot understand the instructions.

Paul, for instance, cannot point to a picture that best reveals his understanding of single vocabulary words or grammatical associations between words. When asked to point to a picture of "the ball under the table," Paul might just as readily point to a picture of a ball *on* the table. When asked to point to the picture of "the boy running after the girl," he might instead choose the one of a girl running after a boy.

Delay or disorder? Scientists have not agreed whether language-impaired children acquire language normally — but more slowly — than other children, or whether they develop language in an abnormal way when they begin to talk and understand. If a consensus has been reached in the past decade, it is that both sides may be right. There may be two quite separate conditions, one in which speech or language is delayed and another in which speech or language is not only delayed, but also incorrect.

In the 1970s, several groups of scientists tackled the problem. Generally, children had been categorized according to certain measures of language development, such as the average length of spontaneous sentences. One study found that language-impaired children used simpler grammatical sentences and fewer questions than other children. Another study found that language-impaired children understood the meanings and relationships of words in much the same way that other children did. Language-impaired children seemed to develop the ability to express themselves in the same progression as normal children, but only after they had reached a higher-than-normal level of language comprehension.

The general consensus from research of recent years is: Many language-impaired children seem to be merely delayed, but a sizable number also develop language in an abnormal way. The distinction is important, because it can help clinicians recognize that some children should be treated aggressively and others left alone.

A visit to the doctor

A child whose parents suspect a speech or language disorder will probably enter the health care system through the pediatrician's office. Before referral to a speech-language pathologist for assessment, the physician will try to determine if there are underlying conditions that might be the indirect cause of the speech or language delay.

A child is likely to be tested to rule out the following conditions:

• *Hearing problems*. Language acquisition is a continual process of hearing, imitating or spontaneously trying a word or phrase, hearing one's own productions, and refining them. Scientists have observed that infants who have impaired hearing from birth tend to be delayed in their instinctive babbling and produce fewer different sounds.

A physician faced with a child over 2 years old who does not speak often will refer that child for complete audiological testing. Such tests involve the use of tones delivered through headphones: as soon as the tone is heard, the child responds by raising a finger or performing some other behavior or gesture. Occasionally, children with hearing problems may unintentionally hide their conditions from their parents because they become so adept at using environmental cues — facial expressions, vibrations, and what little hearing they have — to get by. These cues fall short of helping the children learn the complex sounds of language.

• Mental retardation. The developmental language disorders described in this chapter occur in children of normal or above-normal intelligence. However, language problems are also common among the mentally retarded. Experts estimate that nearly half of all mildly retarded children, 90 percent of severely retarded children, and 100 percent of profoundly retarded children have language disorders of some sort.

A pediatrician may suspect mental retardation if the delay in achieving speech and language milestones is accompanied by a delay in other mental and physical milestones. Gross neurological motor development — sitting, standing, crawling, and walking — and fine motor development — reaching, grasping, building towers of blocks — are often interpreted as clues to whether a child's mental capacities are normal. If mental retardation is a source of concern, tests are available to see just where a child ranks with his or her age peers in mental and physical areas of development. These tests involve such tasks as having the child imitate an examiner's arrangement of blocks or copy geometric shapes.

• ***Autism.*** One of the hallmarks of the disorder called autism is the inability of the child to communicate. Autism begins before age 2½ years; it includes particular speech and language problems; total lack of language, a pervasive lack of responsiveness to people, and peculiar speech patterns. The latter include immediate or delayed echoing of another's comments, speaking in metaphors, or reversing pronouns. In addition to having communication problems, autistic children may be resistant to change, may be overly attached to objects, and may have bizarre and unexpected responses to their environments. A child neurologist will ask about the child's behavior to rule out autism.

• ***Cerebral palsy.*** The muscle control problems characteristic of cerebral palsy can sometimes interfere with speaking. When this happens, children may understand language better than they can speak. They may have trouble expressing themselves because of difficulty moving their lips or tongue.

• ***Acquired aphasia.*** Children are considered aphasic when the brain injury that causes loss of language occurs after speech and language have begun to develop. Aphasia can occur after severe head trauma or a brain infection. Some acquired aphasia is an unfortunate consequence of surgery, as in those rare cases when children undergoing a heart operation suffer a stroke after blood flow to the brain is blocked.

Children who suffer damage to the left half of the brain exhibit many of the symptoms that adult aphasics do. Their problems are predominantly expressive, but also may be receptive. They may have speech articulation problems or make errors in syntax. They may also speak in reduced, incomplete sentences, just as adults do when there is damage to Broca's area.

But a child with acquired aphasia is different from an adult aphasic in one important way — the child is better able to recover. Because the brain continues to reorganize itself until adolescence, neurons seem to be capable of compensating for an injury that happens early in life.

• ***Other conditions.*** A handful of genetic conditions also are characterized by language or speech problems. These include *cri du chat syndrome*, which leads to mental retardation and a tendency to make catlike mewing sounds, and *Tourette syndrome*, a neurological disorder characterized by involuntary sounds such as barking, clicking, and yelping.

A team of experts

Once a child has been identified as having a speech or language disorder, most successful diagnosis and treatment involves a team of experts. The audiologist, an expert in the process of hearing, evaluates and assists those with hearing disorders. The audiologist may work in consultation with an otolaryngologist, a physician who specializes in ear, nose, and throat disorders. These two health professionals determine which hearing conditions can be treated — and perhaps corrected — medically or surgically, and which require rehabilitative techniques such as hearing aids or lip reading.

The speech-language pathologist, also called a speech therapist, studies the normal and abnormal processes of speech and language and measures and diagnoses speech and language problems. The pathologist can also enhance early learning of language, teach the correct production of speech and language, and help a child learn to understand words and sentences.

The neurologist is a physician with expertise in the workings of the brain and nervous system. The neurologist may use modern brain imaging techniques to "see" through the skull and detect brain abnormalities in a child with speech or language delay. A range of pencil-and-paper and physical tests has also been devised to help diagnose any underlying brain disorder that might account for the language problem.

The psychologist studies the science of human development and personality, and can administer tests to evaluate the child's cognitive capabilities. Such tests can help determine how the child's language age compares to his or her mental and chronological ages.

The new therapy

In the 1970s, language-delayed children were taught to repeat sentences in a robot-like fashion. As one NINCDS scientist puts it, "These children could say, 'We went swimming today' perfectly, but they couldn't change it to say the same thing with different words."

Today, the emphasis in therapy is less on imitation than on grasping the context of language. Children play with toys and are taught to translate their activities into words — a mode of learning that is more meaningful for them and that gives them the tools to construct their own sentences.

For the child whose speech is impaired or delayed, treatment may focus on one sound group at a time, starting with the sounds that babies naturally learn first. Young clients are encouraged to use the sounds in a variety of contexts, to watch the clinician make the sound — even putting their hands on the clinician's throat or mouth while the sound is spoken — and to watch themselves make the sound, putting their hands on their own mouths and watching themselves in a mirror.

The most important and continuous help comes from parents. Guided by speech and language pathologists, parents can do a great deal to improve the language environment in their home.

Parents can learn better ways to respond to their children's utterances so that language skills improve. When a child says, "more milk," a parent may respond several ways. The least helpful are silently to refill the milk glass, or to say, "here milky in cuppy," or some other form of nongrammatical baby talk. But adults are tempted to give such answers with youngsters who never seem to benefit from more sophisticated replies such as, "Do you want more milk?" A better response would be the simple statement, "More milk for Sam."

If the parent peppers responses with what linguists call *expansions* — new words, new sentence constructions, new rules of grammar — the child can eventually learn new bits of language as noted below. Expansions introduce new information or help the parent develop the child's words into a grammatically correct sentence.

WAYS ADULTS CAN HELP A CHILD LEARN LANGUAGE

1. Expand the statement, preserving the child's intent.
   a. Expand the statement using the same noun.
      Child: kitty jump
      Adult: The kitty is on the chair.
   b. Replace the noun with a pronoun.
      Child: kitty jump
      Adult: She is jumping.
   c. Expand the statement adding new information.
      Child: kitty jump
      Adult: The dog is jumping, too.

2. Respond by indicating the truth value of the child's utterance, rather than its linguistic accuracy (or inaccuracy).
   Child: kitty jump
   Adult: Yes, the kitty is jumping.

The long-term outlook

How do speech- and language-impaired children fare in adolescence and adulthood? Most followup studies indicate that speech disorders tend to be outgrown by adolescence, but that difficulties involving language use production, or understanding, can persist into adulthood.

One study from the University of Iowa examined 36 adults, 18 of whom had been diagnosed as speech-disordered and 18 as language-disordered when they were children. Nine of the language-disordered children still had communication and learning difficulties in adulthood, compared to only one in the speech-disordered group.

A Cleveland-based study of 63 preschoolers with speech and language disorders found that 5 years after initial diagnosis, 40 percent of the children still had speech and language problems, and 40 percent had other learning problems, such as below-normal achievement in reading and in math. NINCDS-supported scientists at the University of California at San Diego are now conducting a study of 100 language-impaired 4-year-olds to see how they fare up to 5 years after identification of their language problems. Preliminary results suggest that children with only expressive language losses have a lower risk of long-term problems than do children with both expressive and receptive impairments.

The promise of research

Scientists are pursuing research leads that promise improved therapy for children with speech and language disorders. Studies of these disorders are supported by NINCDS, other federal agencies including the National Institute of Mental Health and the National Institute of Child Health and Human Development, and private and medical institutions.

The brain's organization. Studies of cell structure of the brains of dyslexic individuals — otherwise normal people who have extraordinary difficulty learning to read — show that speech and language disorders may be caused by abnormal development of the brain's language centers sometime before or soon after birth.

"From the middle of gestation until about the first or second year, the actual floor plan of the brain is being laid down," says one of the NINCDS grantees who conducted these studies at Boston's Beth Israel Hospital.

Using a technique called cytoarchitectonics, in which the actual structure and arrangement of cells is revealed, the investigators examined the brains of seven adults who had been diagnosed as dyslexic. They found a series of abnormalities in the cerebral cortex. These included *ectopias*, neurons found in the language centers of the brain that seem to have arisen elsewhere and migrated to the wrong area; *dysplasias*, or misshapen neurons; and so-called brain warts, neurons that are nodular in appearance. The brains also failed to show the normal degree of asymmetry.

Other methods are being used to study how the brain may be abnormal in children with speech or language disorders. Some scientists are using brain-imaging techniques to try to locate the site of auditory processing in the brains of children with expressive and receptive language impairments. These investigators hope to pinpoint regions where speech sounds are processed and to see how those regions differ between language impaired and normal children.

The genetic connection. Speech and language problems seem to run in families. This could be accounted for by environmental influences: a home in which language is misused is a home where children develop poor language skills. But most scientists think there may be a large genetic component. Investigators are now studying families with speech and language problems to find out how these disorders are inherited.

Speeding things up. Some language disorders may originate in the abnormally slow rate at which the child's brain is able to process information. To test this theory, scientists are experimenting with ways to train language-impaired children to process speech and language more rapidly. NINCDS grantees at the University of California at San Diego are using computers to teach children to hear the most subtle sound shifts — such as those that differentiate *ba* from *da* — by exaggerating those differences. The computer produces and gradually speeds up speech sounds until the children can hear the *ba/da* distinction at the rate at which it occurs in ordinary conversation.

Some language-delayed children avoid words that are hard to pronounce. In an NINCDS-supported study of word avoidance, scientists at Purdue University are asking both normal and language-delayed children to say the hard-to-pronounce nonsense names assigned unusual objects and toys. By characterizing the patterns of word avoidance in the two groups, the scientists hope to devise improved treatment methods for the language delayed children.

As scientists learn more about how the normal brain controls language and initiates speech, they will also discover just what goes wrong in brains when problems arise. After the underlying mechanisms are detected, investigators hope to develop new treatment techniques to help the millions of children whose thoughts and feelings are poorly expressed.

Where to get help

A number of private organizations have been set up to help people with speech and language disorders. These organizations distribute educational material and, in some cases, provide lists of treatment experts. For more information, call or write to the following organizations:

American Speech-Language-Hearing Association
10801 Rockville Pike
Rockville, MD 20852
(301) 897-5700

The Council for Exceptional Children
Division of Children with Communication Disorders
1920 Association Drive
Reston, VA 22091
(703) 620-3660

National Association for Hearing and Speech Action
Suite 1000
6110 Executive Boulevard
Rockville, MD 20852
(301) 897-8682

National Easter Seal Society, Inc.
2023 West Ogden Avenue
Chicago, IL 60612
(312) 243-8400

The Orton Dyslexia Society, Inc.
724 York Road
Towson, MD 21204
(301) 296-0232

Tourette Syndrome Association
42-40 Bell Boulevard
Bayside, NY 11361
(718) 224-2999
(800) 237-0717 (toll free)

NINCDS information

For more information about the research programs of the NINCDS, contact:

Office of Scientific and Health Reports
National Institute of Neurological and
Communicative Disorders and Stroke
Building 31, Room 8A-16
National Institutes of Health
Bethesda, MD 20892
(301) 496-5751

Language Milestones*

Child's age	Speech behavior the child should have mastered
1 year:	Says 2 to 3 words (may not be clearly pronounced)
	Repeats same syllable 2 to 3 times ("ma, ma, ma")
	Carries out simple direction when accompanied by gestures
	Answers simple questions with nonverbal response
	Imitates voice patterns of others
	Uses single word meaningfully to label object or person
2 years:	Says 8 to 10 words by age 1½, 10 to 15 words by age 2
	Puts two words together ("more cookie," "where kitty?")
	Points to 12 familiar objects when named
	Names 3 body parts on a doll, self, another person
	Names 5 family members, including pets and self
	Produces animal sound or uses sounds for animal's name (cow is "moo-moo")
	Asks for some common food items by name when shown ("milk," "cookie," "cracker")

* (Adapted from the Portage Guide to Early Education, 1976, cooperative Educational Service Agency.)

3 years: Produces two-word phrases combining two nouns ("ball chair"), noun and adjective ("my ball"), or noun and verb ("daddy go")

Uses *no* or *not* in speech

Answers *where*, *who*, and *what* questions

Carries out a series of two related commands

Consistently uses *ing* verb form ("running"), regular plural form ("book/books"), and some irregular past tense forms ("went," "did," "was")

Uses *is* and *a* in statements ("This is a ball.")

Uses possessive form of nouns ("daddy's")

Uses some class names ("toy," "animals," "food")

4 years: Uses a vocabulary of 200 to 300 words

Uses *is* at beginning of questions when appropriate

Carries out series of two unrelated commands

Expresses future occurrences with *going to*, *have to*, *want to*

Changes word order appropriately to ask questions ("Can I?" "Does he?")

Uses some common irregular plurals ("men," "feet")

Tells two events in order of occurrence

5 years: Carries out series of three directions

Demonstrates understanding of passive sentences ("Girl was hit by boy.")

Uses compound and complex sentences

Uses contractions can't, don't, won't

Points out absurdities in picture

Tells final word in opposite analogies

Names picture that does not belong in particular class ("one that's not an animal")

Tells whether two words rhyme

6 years: Points to some, many, several

Tells address and telephone number

Tells simple jokes

Tells daily experiences

Answers *why* question with an explanation

Defines words

Chapter 24

Spina Bifida

Spina Bifida

Laurie Baxter likes to amaze people — something she usually does when she "pops a wheelie" with her wheelchair or water skis. Laurie, who has a disabling birth defect called spina bifida, works as hard as she plays. Four years ago she was hired as a secretary-receptionist for a home improvement company; today, she's the vice president.

Laurie was born with a lump on her back — the most common sign of spina bifida. In spina bifida, literally "split spine," the spinal cord forms abnormally and the arches of the vertebrae, the bones that surround the cord, fail to develop. The tissue covering the spinal cord, or the cord itself, may be displaced outside the spinal canal. Nerves supplying the legs, bladder, and bowel are incompletely developed or damaged.

This nerve damage can result in varying degrees of muscle paralysis, bladder and bowel problems, loss of skin sensation, and spine and limb deformities. Most babies with spina bifida develop an associated condition called hydrocephalus — a potentially dangerous buildup of fluid and pressure within the brain.

Spina bifida is one of the most prevalent birth defects. It occurs in 1 to 2 out of every 1,000 babies born in the United States.

The promise of research

Laurie, now 31, was born during a time when many babies with spina bifida died of hydrocephalus or infections of the nervous system soon after birth. With research advances in neurosurgery and with better control of infections by antibiotics, an estimated 80 to 95 percent of babies born today with spina bifida survive and grow to maturity. Like Laurie, many will go on to lead productive lives.

The quality of life for patients has also improved with the development of devices to control hydrocephalus, techniques to control bladder and bowel function, and new surgical and bracing procedures.

Many of the scientists who developed these life-enhancing and life-saving procedures have been supported by the National Institute of Neurological and Communicative Disorders and Stroke (NINCDS), a world leader in neuroscience research. The NINCDS is a unit of the National Institutes of Health, and is the focal point within the U.S. Government for research on disorders of the central nervous system.

NINCDS-funded research projects on spina bifida range from the possible role of diet in causing this defect to the normal and abnormal formation of the fetus's spinal cord during the first weeks of pregnancy. Scientists are hopeful that the fast pace of research established in the last 30 years will continue. They forecast improved treatment and, perhaps, prevention of spina bifida.

The developing nervous system

Spina bifida develops during the first month after conception — usually before a woman even knows she is pregnant. Although scientists have not identified the precise cause of this birth defect, they believe it results from a combination of environment and genetic factors.

Spina bifida is classified as a defect of the neural tube, the embryonic structure that evolve the brain and spinal cord.

Spina bifida develops during the time when the neural plate, a sheet of cells along the back of the fetus, forms the neural tube. As a normal fetus grows, the edges of the neural plate begin to curl up toward each other to form the tube. Once the tube has developed into a spinal cord, bone and muscle form a protective barrier around it.

In fetuses with spina bifida, parts of the neural plate fail to form a tube. Bone and muscle cannot grow around the incompletely

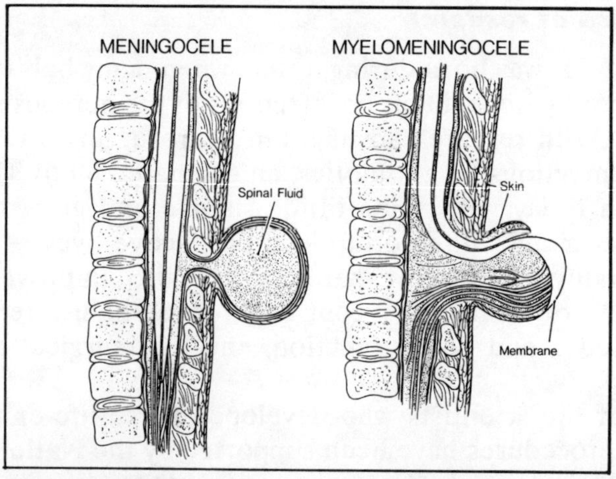

There are several forms of spina bifida manifesta. In meningocele, the spinal cord develops normally but the membranes bulge out of the back through an incompletely developed vertebra to form a sac filled with cerebrospinal fluid. Myelomeningocele occurs when a portion of the undeveloped spinal cord protrudes through the back.

developed area, and the cord or the meninges, the membrane that covers the cord, may herniate through the resulting gap. In certain forms of spina bifida, the cord develops normally, but the vertebrae fail to fuse completely.

There are two main types of spina bifida:

• ***Spina bifida occulta.*** This is the mildest form of spina bifida. *Occulta*, which means "hidden," indicates that the defect is covered by a layer of skin.

With some types of spina bifida occulta, the patient has a small cavity (called a dermal sinus) between two adjacent vertebrae. This defect indicates that the vertebrae of the spine have not fused properly. A hairy patch or birthmark may be above the defect.

In another type of spina bifida occulta, the spinal cord ends in fatty tissue which extends through the bony spinal column to bulge beneath the skin.

When the only abnormality in spina bifida occulta is the failure of a single vertebra to fuse, the patient usually has no symptoms. But when several vertebrae are involved and when a fatty area, a hairy patch, or a dimple in the skin over the defect is noticeable, the patient may eventually develop bowel, bladder, or motor problems.

• ***Spina bifida manifesta*** (also called *aperta* or *cystica*). In the two forms of spina bifida manifesta, a sac is immediately noticeable — or "manifest" — on the newborn's back.

In the disorder's relatively rare and mild form, the spinal cord develops normally but the membranes or meninges bulge out of the baby's back through incompletely developed vertebrae. The resulting sac is called a *meningocele*. (*Meningo-* refers to the membranes; *cele* indicates a swelling or cavity.) The sac may be covered by skin and contains cerebrospinal fluid that normally circulates over the brain and along the spinal cord. If nerves also herniate into this sac, the baby may have minor muscle paralysis or be unable to control bowel and bladder function.

In the most common and severe form of spina bifida, a portion of the undeveloped spinal cord itself protrudes through the back to form a *myelomeningocele*. (*Myelo-* refers to the spinal cord.) Some of these sacs are covered with skin; in others, tissue and nerves are exposed.

Generally, a person talking about "spina bifida" means the severe myelomeningocele form. In this text, unless otherwise indicated, "spina bifida" will stand for myelomeningocele.

When nerves fail

Nerve damage in patients with myelomeningocele occurs while the spinal cord is evolving and as the sac grows. Nerves may not develop properly or may be destroyed by pressure from the expanding sac. Furthermore, the abnormal spinal cord in the spina bifida patient is unable to transfer messages to and from the brain along existing nerves.

The nerves affected in spina bifida, called *spinal nerves*, extend out from the spinal cord at intervals along its length. When functioning properly, these nerves transmit messages to the brain from the sense organs, and from the brain to the muscles. It is through these messages that we are able to contract and flex our muscles, and to feel pain, heat, and cold.

There are 31 pairs of spinal nerves:

- ***Cervical nerves*** — eight pairs of nerves at the top of the spine that carry messages between the spine and the upper part of the body, including the arms and hands.
- ***Thoracic nerves*** — twelve pairs of nerves that supply the middle of the body, from the breastbone to the abdomen, and part of the arms.
- ***Lumbar nerves*** — five pairs of nerves that innervate the hips, the front of the legs, and the tops of the feet. These are the nerves most commonly affected in spina bifida.
- ***Sacral nerves*** — five pairs of nerves that supply the lower legs, feet, back of the legs, bladder, rectum, and genitals.
- ***Coccygeal nerve*** — one pair of nerves that supplies the skin and supporting muscles around the anus.

The types and severity of a patient's symptoms are determined by the particular spinal nerves involved. All nerves below the defect are usually affected. Therefore, the higher spina bifida occurs on the back, the greater the amount of nerve damage and loss of muscle function and sensation. If a child's upper thoracic cord and nerves are affected, for example, the lower limbs may be totally paralyzed and normal walking will be impossible. But a child with a lesion at the low sacral nerve level will have relatively mild paralysis and bladder and bowel problems. These patients would be able to walk without braces — although foot deformities might prevent them from going long distances.

Scientists are studying the various problems caused by nerve disruption in spina bifida. They are developing new techniques to control bladder and bowel function, and new surgical and bracing procedures that help patients walk better.

Searching for a cause

The cause of spina bifida is unknown. But scientists have found clues that suggest that a person's genetic makeup may combine with environmental factors to produce this birth defect.

Investigators offer these findings as evidence of spinal bifida's genetic connection: parents who have one child with spina bifida have

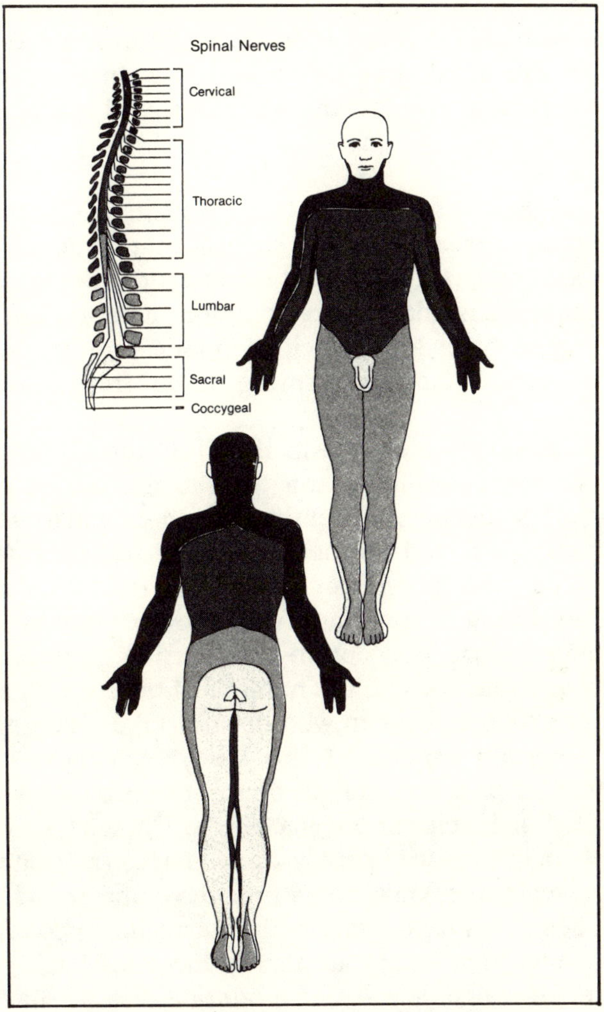

Thirty-one pairs of nerves originate in the spinal cord. The five color-coded groups of these nerves, ranging from the cervical nerves at the top of the spine to the coccygeal nerve at the bottom, serve the different areas of the body with the corresponding colors. The severity of spina bifida symptoms is determined by which nerves are affected.

an increased risk of bearing another child with the same problem; more female than male babies are born with spina bifida; and blacks, Asians, and Ashkenazi Jews have lower rates of spina bifida than do other whites or Egyptians.

Because spina bifida rates are higher in certain geographic areas than in others, some scientists believe that the environment may somehow contribute to the disease. A higher rate may also reflect increased genetic risk for spina bifida in certain populations. In the United States, where 1 to 2 out of 1,000 newborns have spina bifida, more babies with this defect are born in the eastern and southern states than in the West. But the defect is even more common in western Great Britain and Ireland where about 4 out of every 1,000 newborns are affected. At one time, 8 out of every 1,000 newborns were affected.

Since the highest rates of neural tube defects in Great Britain are found in the poorer areas, scientists suggest that inadequate maternal diet may be an important trigger of spina bifida. Some studies have suggested that spina bifida is more common in babies born to poorly nourished women from lower socioeconomic groups and in babies conceived in winter and early spring when fresh foods are less available.

Improved maternal nutrition in the U.S. and Great Britain has been cited as one possible reason for the decline of neural tube defects in the last decade. Recently, British scientists studied how prenatal vitamins affected the occurrence of spina bifida in babies born to women who previously had delivered a child with the disorder. They found that women who took a vitamin supplement with folic acid before conception and during part of pregnancy subsequently had one-seventh the number of babies with spina bifida than a similar group of women who did not take vitamins.

Although certain aspects of this study have been questioned, other scientists suspect there might be a connection between vitamin and folic acid deficiencies and spina bifida. Chemicals or drugs that decrease a woman's natural supply of folic acid (a B vitamin found in leafy green vegetables) may trigger the development of spina bifida in her baby. Scientists report that epileptic women who take valproic acid, an anticonvulsant drug that also reduces folic acid, during the first trimester of pregnancy are at moderate risk for having a baby with spina bifida.

Some investigators suggest that spina bifida may occur because the fetus lacks enough zinc. Others speculate that several vitamin shortages could work together to interfere with neural tube development, or that such deficiencies might permit other chemicals to disrupt neural tube development. Research will help determine the precise role of vitamins and other factors — including genetics — in the development of spina bifida.

Life-saving surgery

Babies with spina bifida are usually evaluated by a neurosurgeon, a physician who specializes in surgical repair of the damaged brain and spinal cord. The neurosurgeon generally will close the newborn's back within its first 24 to 48 hours of life to minimize the risk of infection. Possible infections include *meningitis*, affecting the meninges or tissue covering the spinal cord, and infection in the ventricles, the spaces in the brain that contain cerebrospinal fluid, a problem known as *ventriculitis*.

Additional surgery for hydrocephalus may also be required during a baby's first days. Between 70 and 90 percent of spina bifida babies either have hydrocephalus at birth or develop it soon after. In this condition, cerebrospinal fluid accumulates in the brain because of an obstruction that prevents the fluid's normal drainage from the brain and spinal cord. This accumulation creates pressure that may cause the skull to expand.

Hydrocephalus is caused also by the Arnold-Chiari malformation, a deformity in which the lower parts of the brain protrude into the spinal canal and block the flow of cerebrospinal fluid.

A baby who develops hydrocephalus may be irritable and vomit. Other symptoms include an unusually round and rapidly enlarging head, a bulging forehead that pushes the eyeballs downward, and tight stretching of the skin over the scalp giving it a shiny appearance.

Neurosurgeons do not have to wait for the appearance of these symptoms to diagnose hydrocephalus. Early, even prenatal, detection of this condition is now possible with diagnostic ultrasonography that relies on sound waves to produce an image, and with computerized tomography (CT) scanning, a technique that creates an x-ray image of the brain. If either test shows evidence of hydrocephalus, neurosurgeons will consider implanting a shunt in the patient's head. This tube drains excess cerebrospinal fluid into the abdominal area or a heart chamber. Without shunt surgery, the baby's brain could be damaged and the child might die.

As recently as 10 years ago, the insertion of a shunt was associated with a 30 percent chance of developing meningitis or ventriculitis. But with today's improved procedure developed by research scientists, the chance of infection is minimized: between 2 and 5 percent.

If infection develops, if the shunt malfunctions, or if the child outgrows it, a new shunt may have to be implanted. One pediatric neurosurgeon estimates that a shunt may need to be replaced after about 10 years' use. CT scans can provide early evidence of a shunt problem, but parents also should be alert to a malfunction. Signs include headache, vomiting, swelling over the implant, personality change, declining school performance, and seizures.

Stridor or noisy breathing is a relatively rare condition associated with shunt malfunction. Stridor occurs when the pair of nerves that supplies the vocal cords is paralyzed. When a shunt malfunctions, increased pressure can be placed on those nerves. Stridor caused by a shunt problem is characterized by increased breathing difficulty and anxiety. Breathing may become so difficult that a tracheostomy — insertion of a breathing tube in the windpipe — may have to be performed. A mild form of stridor may occur as a result of respiratory infections, crying, or other causes of rapid breathing.

Patient care: A team effort

In many cities, teams of physicians and other health professionals provide care for young spina bifida patients in clinics that offer a variety of medical services in a single location. The care is often coordinated by a pediatrician. The result is a less fragmented approach to treatment. One neurosurgeon calls this team approach "the most significant advance in the management of spina bifida in the last 20 years."

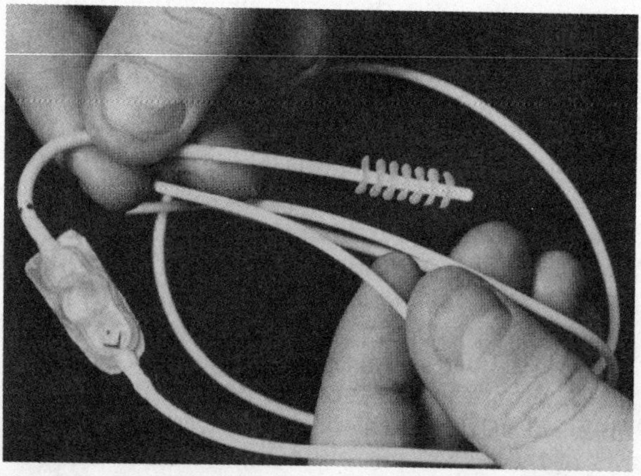

This shunt, implanted in the brain of a spina bifida patient, can prevent damaging hydrocephalus.

In addition to neurosurgeons, the team includes urologists, who treat kidney and bowel problems, and orthopedists and physical medicine specialists, who deal with problems of the spine, muscles, bones, and joints. These team members evaluate the newborn and predict probable surgery and other forms of treatment. During the child's first weeks of life, specialists may also recommend stretching exercises for hip, leg, and foot deformities. Such exercises are performed by a nurse or trained therapist while the child is in the hospital, and continued by the parents at home. Depending on the level of the defect, specialists may also recommend a hip splint or brace to foster development of the hip socket.

The team includes physical and occupational therapists who help the child make the most of his or her physical abilities. Psychologists may be consulted regarding a child's mental status and emotional adjustment. Orthotists fit splints to help straighten limbs. Medical social workers help parents by providing family support and advice about the use of community resources. Nurse clinicians are also important team members. Sometimes they serve as clinic coordinators.

Parents of a newborn with spina bifida are advised to bring their baby to a clinic or to the child's own pediatrician once or twice a month for the first 6 months. Visits may then be scheduled every 2 to 3 months. Beginning at age 1, depending on the child's orthopedic and urologic needs, visits are scheduled two to four times a year. The cost of health care is usually highest during the child's early years.

Bladder and bowel problems

Chronic bladder infections and kidney deterioration pose the greatest potential danger after age 1.

The kidneys serve a vital function: they filter waste products from the blood to form urine and return salts and other important substances to the blood. Urine flows from the kidneys to the bladder for storage. Retention and elimination of urine is controlled by the sphincter, a muscle at the neck of the bladder. When the bladder is full, nerves direct the sphincter to open and the bladder to contract in a coordinated process that releases the accumulated urine through a tube called the urethra.

Children with spina bifida are usually unable to control this process. Because of nerve damage, some children may not be able to feel when their bladder is full. Some patients cannot relax their sphincters enough to let all the urine flow out, while in others the sphincter is always open so that urine dribbles from the urethra. Many children have both incomplete emptying and leakage.

In a dangerous consequence of incomplete emptying, urine accumulates in the bladder and backs up into the kidneys. Unchecked, the pressure of this *reflux* can cause life-threatening kidney deterioration. Or bacteria may grow in the urine that collects in the bladder, and the infection may travel to the kidneys.

In recent years, improved methods of diagnosis, treatment, and prevention of bladder problems have greatly reduced the number of infections and their severity. These same techniques have also allowed children to exert greater control over leakage problems — important for both self-esteem and acceptance by others.

A urologist will examine the newborn with spina bifida to identify the baby's potential for such conditions as reflux. In one test — the intravenous pyelogram — a dye visible on an X-ray is injected into the baby's blood. The X-ray shows how well the material moves through the kidneys to the bladder. A second X-ray, called a cystogram, is taken when the baby urinates the dye. This test shows the operation of the sphincters. Urine cultures are also taken to check for infection.

Children who are found to have a nonrelaxing sphincter are at the greatest risk for reflux and infection. In the 1950s and 1960s, such patients had a ureteroileostomy, an operation in which a part of the small intestine was brought out through the abdomen and a bag was placed over the stomach to collect urine. Scientists found that this operation could cause kidney damage, kidney stones, or other problems. The procedure was replaced during the 1970s by a technique called *clean intermittent catheterization* (CIC).

In CIC, a clean — but not sterilized — catheter or drainage tube is temporarily inserted into the urethra to drain the urine from the bladder. The parents or school nurse can perform this procedure until the child can do so — sometimes as early as age 3 or 4. In 1984, the Supreme Court ruled that schools must provide CIC services as needed to handicapped children.

Clean intermittent catheterization requires the patient to empty the bladder every 3 to 4 hours. With such frequent emptying, there is little danger of bacterial buildup and infection — even though the catheter is only washed in soap and water. A child who practices CIC may also take medication to relax the bladder muscle and to increase the bladder's capacity between catheterizations.

The technique's effectiveness and low rate of complications have made it the treatment of choice for most spina bifida patients who cannot control urination. In one study conducted at Children's Hospital National Medical Center in Washington, D.C., 80 percent of the children using CIC were totally dry between catheterizations.

When CIC fails, children may benefit from the artificial sphincter. This surgically implanted device is usually recommended for more mature children whose bladders are large enough to store a moderate amount of urine. The entire mechanism of this silicone device is within the body. The patient presses through the skin to squeeze an implanted pump that helps release the urine. Urologists at St. Luke's Episcopal Hospital in Houston recently reported that of 132 children who had the sphincter implanted, 90 percent showed a significant improvement in controlling urination.

Another approach to urinary control is electrical stimulation of the bladder and nearby muscles through a catheter inserted into the urethra. This still experimental procedure has had mixed success.

In addition to urinary incontinence, children with spina bifida also have difficulty controlling bowel function. They are unable to sense when their bowel is full. The stool moves from the bowel to the rectum and outside the body without the child's awareness. Furthermore, the anal sphincter, the muscle that allows voluntary control of the stool's movement, may be weak.

Constipation is also a problem. Because of nerve damage, the patient's stool progresses too slowly from the bowel to the rectum; water is lost and a hard stool results.

Techniques that help manage bowel function include special diets, specific times for elimination, and medication. In children with spina bifida, a successful bowel control program depends on the patience and support of parents, teachers, and friends. Accidents should be accepted, but dealt with promptly.

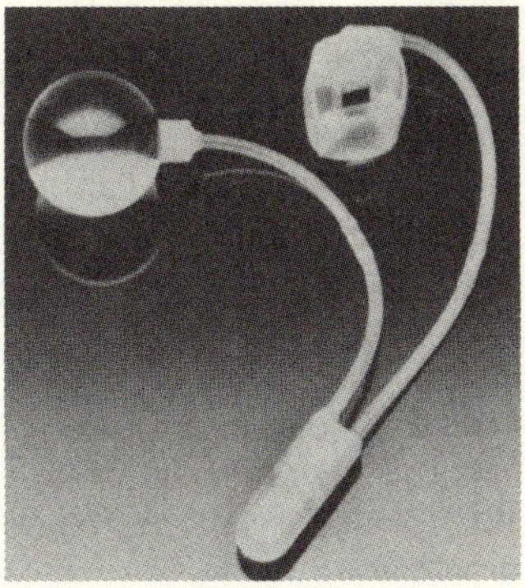

This artificial sphincter can be surgically implanted to help control urination.

A lack of sensation

"I could walk on a tack all day and not know it," says spina bifida patient Laurie Baxter. "In fact, I did once and didn't know it until the blood started coming out of my shoe. When I was 18, I burned my foot with a heating pad. I didn't feel the pain until blisters formed."

The lack of sensation characteristic of spina bifida places patients at risk of infection from cuts and burns. It also makes them prone to develop pressure sores. These sores occur when there is continuous heavy pressure on an area of skin, reducing blood flow to the area and causing tissue to erode and die. The healthy person senses pressure and shifts the body before a sore develops. But a person with spina bifida does not feel that pressure. A sore might appear on the buttocks or thighs of a patient who sits or lies in bed for long periods of time. Obese patients who put more pressure on their skin and incontinent patients with frequent soiling are likely to develop sores. Pressure sores can also result from improperly fitted braces or shoes.

Untreated, pressure sores can turn into deep ulcers that may require surgery. By shifting position frequently, ensuring that braces and shoes fit properly, and watching for warning signs such as redness, swelling, and blisters, spina bifida patients can prevent pressure sores. If a sore develops, it should be kept clean and dry.

Orthopedic problems

The ability to move from one place to another provides more than independence and freedom. Mobility affects educational achievement, the development of social skills, the ability to find and keep work, and enjoyment of recreational activities. How freely a spina bifida patient can move depends on several factors, including the level of the defect, the extent of orthopedic deformities, age, body build, weight, and motivation. These factors will influence, for example, whether a patient must use a wheelchair or will be able to walk with braces.

Through splinting, bracing, stretching and strengthening exercises, and surgical procedures, orthopedic and physical medicine specialists try to correct a patient's bone and muscle deformities and increase the ability to sit, stand, and move.

Hips, knees, and feet. Deformities of the hip, knee, and foot joints are caused by long-term improper positioning of that body part or by muscle imbalance. One of the two muscle groups that enable the ankles, knees, and hips to work may be absent or weak from paralysis. Because weak muscles grow more slowly than normal ones, the imbalance becomes more pronounced as the baby gets older. The stronger muscles pull the joint out of position and a deformity eventually results.

Some children with spina bifida are born with deformities, most commonly twisted or "club" feet and dislocated hips. Foot deformities are sometimes corrected by applying a soft brace or a cast; other cases may require surgical release of tendons and joints to realign the bones. This surgery is performed when the child would normally stand — between 1 and 2 years of age.

Hip dislocation occurs when muscle imbalance causes the hips to come out of their sockets. Some cases may be surgically corrected around age 2 to 4 by transferring working muscles to balance the hip.

Some deformities that occur during childhood can be prevented or their severity reduced if the child does not stay in one position too long, regularly moves the joints through a full range of motion, and uses braces or splints.

Spinal deformities. Between 8 and 15 percent of patients with spina bifida are born with kyphosis of the lower spine, a forward bending of the backbone that creates a hunchbacked appearance. Ulcers may form over the bony prominence created by the spine's abnormal curve. Children with severe kyphosis may have trouble breathing when they sit because the stomach is pushed upward into the lung area. Kyphosis can be treated and its progression delayed by surgery to reduce the bony hump and straighten the spine.

Some patients are born with scoliosis, a sideways bending of the spine, although it more commonly develops later in childhood. One cause of developmental scoliosis is weakened trunk muscles that fail to support the back. Spinal braces are sometimes used to treat mild scoliosis. Moderate to severe cases are usually corrected through surgery to reduce the spinal curve and fuse the bones so they no longer bend.

Scoliosis can also develop in hydrocephalic children whose shunt malfunctions. As the hydrocephalus worsens, cerebrospinal fluid accumulates in the brain and in the spinal cord. The abnormal concentration of fluid in the cord, a condition called *hydromyelia*, causes increased pressure on the nerves and muscle weakness that allows the vertebrae to shift, and produces scoliosis. Repair of the shunt or surgical drainage of the hydromyelia usually prevents the scoliosis from advancing.

Another cause of scoliosis is tethering or binding of the spinal cord to the surrounding tissue at the bottom of the spine. Tethering, which can develop at any age, occurs if the initial surgery to close the baby's back failed to free the spinal cord from this tissue, or if scars form at the site of the original spinal repair.

Because a tethered cord is bound, it stretches abnormally as the baby grows. This stretching causes further cord damage which weakens the spine's supporting muscles. The result: increased spinal curvature or scoliosis. A tethered cord can also cause bladder malfunction and walking difficulties in older children and adults. Surgery to free the cord can eliminate symptoms and may stop the progression of scoliosis.

Striving for mobility

Physicians recommend that a child with spina bifida be encouraged to progress as normally as possible with the development of motor skills. Between 6 months and 1 year, all children should sit; by 12 to 18 months, they should begin to crawl and explore their surroundings. Around age 1½, children should be encouraged to stand — even those with high thoracic damage who will eventually have to use a wheelchair. Standing reduces osteoporosis (a thinning of the bones that results from inactivity and increases the risk of fractures), improves bladder and bowel function, and strengthens the heart and upper body. Parents should also encourage 18-month-olds to walk.

There are a variety of devices to help spina bifida patients attain these developmental milestones. A wheeled device called a chariot, which moves when the sitting child rolls wheels by hand, helps patients who have trouble crawling. Standing appliances provide total body support so a child can be upright without crutches. The swivel-walker allows a child to shift weight from side to side in a movement that propels the patient forward. A recently developed long-leg brace helps children walk by propelling their legs forward.

Mobility varies according to the level of the child's defect. While some children do better or worse than expected, the following developmental patterns generally apply:

- *Upper thoracic lesions*. These children have poorly developed spinal, abdominal, and leg muscles and often have some weakness in their arms. They need support to sit. They should be able to walk around the house with a brace that supports the hips, knees, ankles, and feet until about age 12 to 15 when increased height and weight will require them to use more extensive bracing. After age 15, children who keep their weight down and are highly motivated should be able to continue a limited amount of walking at home with a brace and crutches. When away from home, these children will use a wheelchair.

- ***Lower thoracic lesions.*** The abdominal muscles of these patients are usually strong enough so they can sit without support. Up until age 12 to 15, they will use the same walking brace as children with upper thoracic lesions. After 15 years, they may continue limited household walking, but will use a wheelchair for getting around the community.
- ***Upper lumbar lesions.*** With some strength in the hip muscles but weak quadriceps, the muscles in the front of the thighs, these children should be able to get around the house with long-leg braces. Outside, they will need braces and crutches, and usually, a wheelchair for long trips. Some will use wheelchairs full time beginning in their 20s.
- ***Lower lumbar lesions.*** Children with a low lumbar lesion tend to have muscle imbalance around the hips, knees, and feet, and thus develop deformities. If these are corrected, however, the patients have a good chance of walking with braces because they have strong quadriceps. Children and adults can usually walk with an ankle-foot brace and forearm crutches.
- ***Sacral lesions.*** Children and adults with sacral lesions can walk, but may need an ankle-foot brace. Surgery may be needed for foot deformities that interfere with walking.

Because of decreased mobility, all children with spina bifida have a tendency to gain excess weight. Children who use a wheelchair most of the time are most likely to become obese. Ironically, obese children are often forced to rely on a wheelchair because they lack the strength to walk while carrying excess weight, or because their obesity makes braces hard to fit. Obesity also increases the occurrence of pressure sores and makes it difficult for the children to do their own clean intermittent catheterization. Parents should work with a nutritionist or dietitian to establish a diet for their children.

Trying to learn

"Will our baby have normal intelligence?" is one of the first questions that parents of a child with spina bifida ask. Recent studies show that about 70 percent of such children will have a normal I.Q. The rest will be slightly to severely retarded. Scientists have found that mental retardation in spina bifida patients is associated with hydrocephalus, meningitis, and ventriculitis.

To help young children reach their intelligence potential, many spina bifida clinics now offer infant stimulation programs in which therapists show parents how to improve their child's motor and visual skills, as well as ways to foster social development.

When the children reach school age, they may experience some learning difficulties, perhaps due to problems with fine motor control or poor visual or perceptual skills. Parents who suspect a problem should have their child tested at about age 3.

A consultation with an ophthalmologist is recommended, since some children with spina bifida are born with cross-eye, or *strabismus*. In this condition, weakness in one eye muscle prevents the eyes from looking in the same direction. If strabismus is not corrected early, a child could become blind in one eye.

Because children who have fine motor problems may not be able to write quickly or accurately, they could fail to complete a test in the allotted time or finish their homework. These problems may remain undetected until third or fourth grade when there are more writing assignments. Fine motor problems can also influence a child's ability to manipulate scissors or assemble a collage in art class.

If children have visual or perceptual problems, they might look up from a book for a second and have trouble finding their place again. Some children have difficulty with visual-motor integration: they are unable to copy letters, numbers, and shapes. Copying from a blackboard may also be a struggle.

Today, most children with spina bifida go to regular schools. If neither parents nor teachers realize that a youngster has learning disabilities, the child may be misjudged as stubborn or lazy. "Parents can help by understanding the problem," says a psychologist who specializes in child development and learning disabilities. "They should explain the problem to the teacher and assist in coming up with ideas about what is reasonable in the classroom."

Once the problem is recognized, solutions can be worked out. "We need to separate thinking from mechanics," says the psychologist. She suggests that children with fine motor problems learn to type in the third or fourth grade. Another option is the use of a cassette tape recorder. Children can speak their homework into the machine. Later they can play the tape back and write the words down — taking as much time as needed. For school tests, the psychologist suggests making arrangements for oral exams.

Some learning disabilities will improve as the child matures. Until then, the psychologist advises schools and teachers to "be sensitive, flexible, and creative."

Federal legislation supports this sentiment. States that receive federal education funds must provide disabled students with a free public education from ages 6 to 17, setting up individualized programs when necessary.

Growing up with spina bifida

Although 8-year-old Jimmy Randolph uses a wheelchair, he plays baseball, bowls, and swims. Wheelchair racing, however, is this spina bifida patient's favorite sport.

"I love to race," says Jimmy. "I go real fast, not faster than my girlfriend, though. She has spina bifida too — but not as much. That's why she's faster."

Like most children with spina bifida, Jimmy has adjusted to his disabilities. He's active, enthusiastic, and he has dreams. But the toughest time for Jimmy — and other children with this birth defect — is ahead.

"From mid to late adolescence they're rebellious about their situation," says the neurosurgical director of a spina bifida clinic. "The teenagers tend to deny the condition and the need for special care. They'll drop intermittent catheterization, for example. They won't want to come for their visits because they don't like to face the fact that there is an abnormality. They seem to grow out of this if they survive, which most do. Then they'll come back for care, but only for specific treatment — not for preventive care."

Concerns about sex. For a teenager with spina bifida, the typical concerns of adolescence — peer acceptance, sexuality, independence, and a future vocation — are even more troubling than usual.

"Junior high was the toughest," remembers Laurie Baxter. "Everybody was going steady with a new person every week. There was a big push for the boy-girl scene. Also, they're only looking at the body and not the mind. I had lots of crying fits."

Junior high heralds the onset of puberty, a time when young people are particularly concerned about their sexuality. For adolescents with spina bifida, it is a time to wonder if their physical handicaps include sexual problems. They may be concerned about their sexuality earlier than the average teenager. One study conducted at the Alfred I. Dupont Institute in Delaware found that children with spina bifida mature sexually an average of 2 years earlier than ordinary.

People with spina bifida have normal hormone levels and sexual drives. Most men and women with spina bifida can have orgasms. Women with spina bifida are able to have intercourse and bear children. However, during pregnancy they may find it harder to walk with braces or to transfer to and from a wheelchair. A woman with spina bifida has a 4 to 5 percent chance of having a child with the same defect, and may wish to seek genetic counseling if she is contemplating pregnancy.

About 60 percent of men with spina bifida can function sexually and are fertile. The other 40 percent have a variety of problems. Because of nerve damage, some men may be unable to achieve erections, a problem that might be resolved by penile implants.

Because a person's sexual identity begins before puberty, psychologists advise parents not to forget that a child with spina bifida is a sexual being. Parents are encouraged to discuss sexuality and sexual function with their children.

Adolescence is also a good time for a spina bifida patient to discuss future college and career plans with vocational and educational counselors. Around this time, social workers can also advise young patients about their future options for independent living — including group homes.

To foster independence, parents should encourage their children to take responsibility for urinary and bowel control and personal hygiene, and to perform household chores. "There's no reason why you can't vacuum the floor from a wheelchair," advises Laurie Baxter.

Although some teenagers with spina bifida may have difficulty learning to drive or actually driving a car, earning an operator's permit can add to a feeling of self-reliance. "It gives you a feeling of independence," says Laurie, "and for a disabled person, having those wheels makes you more normal than anything in the world."

The family copes. "The status of the family before the birth of a child with spina bifida has a lot to do with their ability to cope afterwards," says the director of a spina bifida clinic.

A sociologist who has studied parents of children with spina bifida agrees. "Having a child with a problem doesn't change the functioning of the family," she says. "Families that would have fallen apart anyway will fall apart, and strong families stay together."

Even a strong family, however, will feel the stresses that are part of having a baby with a birth defect. The parents must first cope with their failed expectations of having a normal baby. This can be particularly difficult when the baby is their first child.

Feelings of confusion and disbelief are common during the first weeks after birth. "My first reaction was mainly shock," remembers Betty Johnson, mother of an 8-year-old boy with spina bifida.

After the initial shock has passed, parents may wonder if they will be able to take care of their child. But caring for a newborn with spina bifida is, in many ways, the same as caring for any infant. All babies need loving, cuddling, diapering, bathing, and feeding. Later, when the parents have had time to adjust, they can learn such tasks as clean intermittent catheterization without feeling overwhelmed.

"Think of it as a baby first," Betty Johnson advises parents. "Then, well, everybody has problems one way or another and you can cope that way."

To help them cope, parents can talk to other parents of children with spina bifida and to sympathetic physicians, nurses, and social workers. Social workers offer support, practical advice on how to care for a baby with a birth defect, and information about sources of financial assistance.

If there are other children in the family, problems can develop. Older children may resent being asked to help with their sibling's care. Younger children may feel left out, envious of all the attention focused on the brother or sister with spina bifida. Usually, these problems can be worked out by the family, with the siblings adjusting to their disabled brother or sister and the parents learning to cope.

"I think the majority of parents who have raised a child with spina bifida become advocates and are fairly positive about their experiences," says the chief neurosurgeon of a children's hospital.

Prevention and diagnosis

After adjusting to life with a child who has spina bifida, many couples find that they want more children. A woman who has given birth to a baby with spina bifida has a 2½ to 5 percent risk of having a second child with the defect. A certain number of women may have a higher risk, depending on their medical history. If the spina bifida, for example, accompanies an inherited condition called Meckel's syndrome, which involves growth deficiencies and facial deformities, the mother is at higher risk of bearing another child with spina bifida. Diabetic women, too, are at increased risk of having children with neural tube malformations, as are patients with spina bifida manifesta.

A pregnant woman with a family history of spina bifida should discuss with her obstetrician and a genetic counselor her risk of having a baby with this defect. She may also seek advice on the benefits of prenatal diagnostic testing.

A genetic counselor may first advise a pregnant woman at risk for delivering a baby with spina bifida to take a blood test early in the second trimester of pregnancy to measure her level of alpha-fetoprotein (AFP). AFP is excreted in the fetus's urine, which crosses the amniotic sac into the mother's blood. Scientists have found that abnormally high levels of AFP either in the mother's blood or in the amniotic sac can indicate that a fetus has a neural tube defect such as spina bifida or anencephaly — incomplete brain development.

Since a high AFP level can also mean that a woman is carrying twins or that her baby has another problem like kidney disease, the test is used for screening, not diagnosis. Patients should know that the AFP test can give false results.

If a patient has a positive AFP blood test, other procedures are performed to explain the finding. A second blood test is usually scheduled along with a sonogram. Sonograms are produced by a technique called ultrasound in which inaudible high-frequency sound waves are bounced off a pregnant woman's uterus. As the sound waves touch the fetus, they bounce back and are recorded on an oscilloscope; the result is a picture of the fetus's anatomy.

Sonograms can offer clues about the development of a fetus's nervous system. They can also determine if a woman is carrying twins.

When a sonogram is inconclusive, a woman may elect to have amniocentesis. In this procedure, a fine needle is inserted into the mother's abdomen to obtain a sample of amniotic fluid. A portion of the amniotic fluid will be tested for AFP and an enzyme called acetylcholinesterase (AChE). When a fetus has a neural tube defect, AChE from the fetal brain and spinal cord oozes into the amniotic fluid. If abnormal levels of both AFP and AChE are found in the amniotic fluid, a second sonogram will often be performed to check for further evidence of spina bifida.

Answers through research

The possibility of preventing spina bifida intrigues many scientists. Among the prevention-oriented research projects supported by the National Institute of Neurological and Communicative Disorders and Stroke are studies of the development of the neural tube. Several investigators are examining the neural tube's cell structure and the events that control its metamorphosis into the spinal cord.

The developing spinal cord. Animal models play an important role in many neural tube investigations. Mutant mice with a naturally high incidence of neural tube defects, and chick embryos, which have a spinal cord similar to humans, are commonly studied.

At the University of Michigan in Ann Arbor, NINCDS-supported scientists are looking at the cell structure of the mouse neural plate as it forms into a tube. Using high-powered microscopes, the scientists are studying the role of the *basal lamina*, a carbohydrate-rich zone which supports the neural plate, in the development of spina bifida. The Michigan scientists find that neural tube defects occur when they give mouse fetuses chemicals that interfere with the formation of the basal lamina. Continued research should yield answers about the formation of the basal lamina in humans and its role in the development of neural tube defects.

NINCDS grantees at the University of California in San Diego are studying spina bifida in the loop-tail mouse. This breed of mouse has a high incidence of neural tube defects: about 25 percent of each litter is affected. The grantees are studying the cell structure of the neural plate as it forms into a tube and are looking for differences between healthy and defective mice. So far, the scientists have found that the surfaces of cells in abnormal neural tubes are flattened, while the cell surfaces in normal tubes are rounded. The basal lamina are also defective in the abnormal neural tubes.

With continued research, the investigators hope eventually to use these findings to help understand cell changes that may cause spina bifida in humans.

In another study of the neural tube's cell structure, NINCDS grantees at the University of Utah in Salt Lake City are looking at the role of microtubules in helping cells change shape and form a tube. Microtubules are small cylindrical bodies that help cells divide and that transport nutrients within cells. Using drugs and extreme cold, the investigators damage the microtubules of chick embryo cells, then gauge how the damage affects the neural tube's formation. Scientists know that as the neural plate folds up into a tube, the plate normally narrows and the cells elongate. Preliminary results from the Utah study indicate that destroying the microtubules makes the plate widen abnormally.

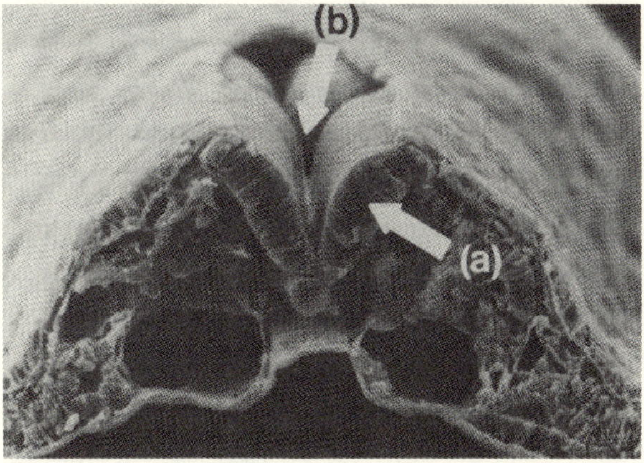

The neural plate (a) in this drug-treated chick embryo has failed to fold over and close, leaving an open neural tube defect (b).

Some investigators suggest that one or several chemicals may signal the cell changes that allow the neural tube to close. The theory is that a decreased production of such chemicals would prevent the tube from closing completely. At the University of New Mexico School of Medicine in Albuquerque, NINCDS-supported scientists are studying several chemicals that may be associated with the closure of the chick's neural tube. One of them, serotonin, is also a brain neurotransmitter, a chemical that transmits signals from one nerve cell to another.

The grantees found that areas of the chicken's neural tube contained serotonin for a brief period of time. To prove that serotonin has a role in neural tube closure, the scientists are giving chick embryos drugs that interfere with serotonin production. If these drugs cause neural tube defects, then the scientists will try to reverse the process by giving the chickens another chemical that blocks the effects of the first drug. "If we can go back and reduce the incidence of spina bifida, it will show us that this defect is truly related to serotonin," says the principal investigator.

Restoring nerve function. Many scientists hope for a day when they will be able to restore nerve function in defective spinal cords. One team of NINCDS grantees at Case Western Reserve University School of Medicine in Cleveland is working toward this goal. They have already developed a technique that may allow nerve fibers broken by spina bifida to grow across the gap in the spine — restoring nerve function and eliminating paralysis.

The new technique was first used to treat a birth defect in which the corpus callosum, a bridge of neural tissue that unites the two hemispheres of the brain, does not extend across these areas. The scientists implanted a paper-like substance in the brains of newborn mice whose corpus callosums had been cut. The implant was coated with glial cells, which provide a supporting structure for nervous tissue. New nerve fibers grew across the implant and connected with the appropriate nerve cells in the other side of the cut area.

The scientists now plan to create thoracic-level spina bifida in the mouse and rat fetus and to insert the implant coated with glial cells. "We hope to attract some nerve fibers across the lesion," says the investigator, "and, we hope, cure the spina bifida."

Preventing birth defects. In recent years, advances in diagnostic and microsurgical techniques have prompted some scientists to suggest that prenatal or *in utero* surgery may help correct spina bifida or associated hydrocephalus. Although research is still in its early stages, hydrocephalus has already been successfully treated in rhesus monkey fetuses. In these cases, scientists inserted a tiny shunt into the monkey fetus's skull through an incision in the mother's abdomen. Excess brain fluid then drained into the amniotic sac. More than 30 cases of hydrocephalus in humans have also been managed *in utero*.

Spina bifida has not yet been repaired *in utero*, but collaborating scientists at Georgetown University, Children's Hospital National Medical Center, and the National Institutes of Health (NIH) are taking the first step toward this goal. After inducing spina bifida in rhesus monkey fetuses, the investigators are testing a fetal bone paste developed at the NIH as a way to correct spinal deformity. If the surgery is successful in animals and if the scientists can produce enough bone paste, they may be able to correct human spina bifida *in utero* within the next decade.

Another prevention-oriented study is under way at Boston University's Center for Human Genetics. NINCDS-supported scientists there have begun a 5-year investigation of the influence of prenatal nutrition and other factors on the birth of a baby with a neural tube defect. The scientists are administering a questionnaire to 27,500 pregnant women undergoing amniocentesis because they are considered to be at high risk of delivering a baby with a birth defect. The questionnaire covers the women's intake of vitamin A, folic acid, and trace elements such as zinc. All of these substances have been associated with neural tube defects. Blood samples will provide additional information on the women's nutritional status.

Scientists will also evaluate the effect of hyperthermia (abnormally high blood temperature, as in fever), previous spontaneous abortions, and the use of spermicidal contraceptives on the development of neural tube defects.

A year after the women have given birth, a follow-up questionnaire will determine the status of the children.

The National Institute of Child Health and Human Development, another unit of the National Institutes of Health, is also sponsoring a study on the prevention of neural tube defects. Scientists at Northwestern University Medical School in Chicago and at the California Public Health Foundation in Berkeley are interviewing 1,500 new mothers by phone to determine their vitamin use around the time of conception. Vitamin use by mothers of infants born with neural tube defects will be compared with use by two other groups: mothers of infants born with other types of birth defects, and mothers who delivered a normal child.

A magnetic image. Both the CT scan and ultrasound have had a major impact on the management of spina bifida. But a new diagnostic technique called magnetic resonance imaging (MRI) may one day challenge the CT scan in providing images of the spine.

A patient who is placed in a magnetic resonance imager is surrounded by a powerful static magnetic field. The nuclei of the atoms of the patient's body line up in the direction of this field. A second, alternating field is then applied at right angles to the first, causing certain nuclei to move to a new alignment. When the second field is turned off, the realigned nuclei return to their original positions, releasing signals. A computer then converts these signals into an image displayed on a screen. Unlike computed tomography, an MRI scanner can "see through" bone to distinguish blood vessels, nerves, and soft tissue.

MRI is "the best method to demonstrate the anatomical detail of various forms of spina bifida," says an NINCDS neuroradiologist. MRI may also be useful for detecting hydrocephalus.

The most exciting MRI images, says a pediatric neurosurgeon at the University of Michigan, are those of the Arnold-Chiari malformation. The quality of these images, she says, has led to better understanding and improved surgical management of this abnormality.

Spina bifida is being studied with MRI at research centers around the country. At the NINCDS and the University of Michigan, scientists are evaluating MRI's ability to detect tethered cord. In another project, University of Michigan scientists using MRI scans are searching for a possible association between tethered cord and an orthopedic problem called *knee flexion contractures* — bent knees caused by tightened muscles in the back of the legs.

Treating physical problems. Many of the techniques now used to treat the orthopedic problems of spina bifida are derived from operations developed during the 1940s and 1950s to treat polio. In the last 30 years, scientists have been reviewing these operations for their usefulness in managing spina bifida. "We're keeping what works and throwing out what doesn't," asserts one orthopedic surgeon.

One procedure that works is muscle transfer operation developed during the 1950s to help polio victims with weak hips. Today, a modified version of this operation is used to strengthen the hip muscles of spina bifida patients. Muscle from the patient's abdomen is transferred to the hip, where it helps balance unequal muscle forces that can cause displacement. One recent study at the Indiana University Medical Center found that 60 percent of the children who had this procedure were eventually able to walk without their crutches. The operation can be performed on patients age 15 months to 26 years.

Special braces may help improve the results of the muscle transfer operation and also reduce hip dislocation. At the University of Michigan, scientists are studying the effects of a brace that helps the hip socket develop correctly. The brace is worn for the first 12 to 18 months of life, a time of rapid growth of the hip socket.

Scientists at Children's Memorial Hospital in Chicago are studying a brace to help children with high-level lesions walk more normally. The Reciprocating Hip-Knee-Ankle-Foot Orthosis extends from the chest to the feet and includes a cable system that connects the two hip joints. As the child moves, a hip joint extends and one leg goes forward; the cable then helps the other hip and leg to extend. (Previous braces kept the hip locked and the child had to swivel the entire body in order to walk.) The investigators are finding that 60 percent of the patients using the new device improve their walking ability.

Both walking and sitting are difficult for children with spina bifida who have severe scoliosis. At the University Michigan, scientists are taking a new look at the timing of spinal fusion, a surgical procedure that involves realigning and fusing the bones of the spine to reduce the curve and prevent it from worsening. Two procedures are performed to correct first the front and then the back of the spine. But orthopedic surgeons note that the surgery is difficult and is sometimes associated with infection.

Currently, children with scoliosis have these operations around age 12 to 14. However, the Michigan scientists believe that children with spina bifida mature physically about 2 years earlier than other children and might benefit from surgery performed at a younger age. Before the timing of spinal fusions is changed, however, the investigators will complete a pilot study on the development of scoliosis. They are now taking yearly X-rays of the spines of spina bifida patients, beginning at age 2 and continuing into adulthood. By observing the onset of scoliosis and the spine's growth, the scientists hope to pinpoint the best age for surgery.

Help for the incontinent. Research on incontinence includes the study of biofeedback, a technique that gives people control over body functions like muscle tension. Biofeedback, research has shown, can be used by children with spina bifida to improve sphincter control.

NINCDS-supported scientists at The Johns Hopkins University in Baltimore recently conducted experiments on the effectiveness of biofeedback and behavior modification in controlling bowel incontinence. Thirty-three children were taught to contract their sphincter muscles to apply pressure on balloons; as the children responded, a line on the biofeedback monitor started to rise. In addition to biofeedback sessions in the laboratory, the children practiced squeezing their sphincter muscles 50 times a day at home. Training continued until the patients were able to contract their muscles in response to simulated rectal fullness.

As part of the behavior modification program, parents placed their child on the toilet for 10 minutes immediately after dinner. This procedure was designed to teach the children to have bowel movements on their own. Successful bowel movements were rewarded with praise and treats. Parents also rewarded their children for accident-free days. The children were not punished for bowel accidents.

The scientists found that a combination of biofeedback and behavior modification enabled a third of the children to achieve continence; another third reduced their incontinence by at least 50 percent. Biofeedback was particularly effective in children with lower spinal cord lesions who had been having two or more bowel movements a day. Children who suffered from frequent constipation before the study were more likely to benefit from behavior modification techniques.

Children who achieve limited success with biofeedback or behavior modification may become continent by using an electrical stimulator that closes the anal sphincter. Scientists at the University of Michigan report that, over time, electrical stimulation appears to increase the sphincter's muscle tone so that the device is no longer needed.

In another area of spina bifida research, scientists are studying ways to detect urinary tract infections before they affect the kidneys. Early detection is often difficult because impaired sensation prevents patients from noticing painful urination and other signs. To screen for infections, most clinics require even symptom-free patients to visit a laboratory every 3 months for a urine culture. But this can be a burden for children who live far from a medical facility, and the visits may not be frequent enough to catch all infections.

To solve this problem, some physicians recommend regular home screening of urine specimens. With home screening, specially treated strips of paper or sticks are inserted into a urine sample. Changes in color could indicate an infection. The home tests are used only to screen — a follow-up lab test is always recommended.

A note of caution: these tests can give false negative results. Investigators at the University of Rochester recently reported that home screening devices do not pick up all infections.

Despite these results, the scientists contend that the potential benefits of accurate home screening warrant further research with a larger group of patients.

The future

"We've made significant progress in keeping children with spina bifida alive, and in preserving their intellect," says a neurosurgeon, "and I see no reason why the rate of progress shouldn't continue."

This physician and other scientists envision that the future will bring even better methods of diagnosis, treatment and, perhaps, prevention of this crippling birth defect. For Laurie Baxter, however, the focus is on today — and how she can help young people growing up with spina bifida. When she counsels young patients, her advice is clear: have a positive attitude, work hard, and try to be independent.

Voluntary organizations

The Spina Bifida Association of America offers support and educational material to parents of children with spina bifida. The association also refers parents to spina bifida clinics around the country and supports research on all aspects of this disorder.

Spina Bifida Association of America
343 S. Dearborn, Suite 310
Chicago, Ill. 60604
(312) 663-1562

The National Easter Seal Society supports rehabilitation and camping facilities throughout the United States for children with spina bifida and other birth defects. Physical and occupational therapy and vocational training are offered at these facilities.

The National Easter Seal Society, Inc.
2023 West Ogden Avenue
Chicago, Ill. 60612
(312) 243-8400

The March of Dimes Birth Defects Foundation answers queries about spina bifida and supports genetic counseling centers. The organization also funds research on spina bifida and other birth defects.

March of Dimes Birth Defects Foundation
1275 Mamaroneck Avenue
White Plains, N.Y. 10605
(914) 428-7100

NINCDS information

For information about the research programs of the NINCDS, contact:

Office of Scientific and Health Reports
National Institute of Neurological and
Communicative Disorders and Stroke
Building 31, Room 8A-16
National Institutes of Health
9000 Rockville Pike
Bethesda, Md. 20892
(301) 496-5751

Chapter 25

Spinal Cord Injury

Spinal Cord Injury

When the cat teetered on the brink of the balcony, the woman who owned him leapt to the rescue but fell three floors, landing on her back. The cat was all right, but the woman, a young doctor, was paralyzed from the waist down. Now in a wheelchair, she expects to complete her medical training at Johns Hopkins Hospital in Baltimore, Md., on schedule.

The bearded videotape producer at the helm of a sailboat in San Francisco Bay has been lowered into a captain's seat he himself had designed. Since 1967, he has been paralyzed from the chest down as a result of a head-on motorcycle collision.

The young husband and father of four liked doing repairs around the house. He fell off a ladder while working on the roof. He, too, is now paralyzed.

Heroic rescues, war wounds, traffic accidents, mishaps at work or play — these are the common causes of a not uncommon tragedy: the paralysis and loss of sensation that results from spinal cord injury. Some 200,000 Americans are now confined to wheelchairs because of spinal cord injuries. Each year, 10,000 new injuries occur. The lifetime cost of caring for one victim can exceed $250,000. The total cost to the nation is an alarming $2 billion a year.

The enormous financial burden of spinal cord injury may pale, however, beside the profound social and emotional costs to patients and their families — the disruptions to education, career, marriage. The sad truth is that spinal cord injuries usually happen to the young. An estimated two-thirds of the victims are 30 years old or under, the majority men. So, each year, thousands of young Americans who are newly independent — or yearn to be — suddenly become dependent on others.

The source of their problems is injury to a 2-foot long bundle of nerve cells and fibers that extends from the brain to the lower back: the human spinal cord. Together, the brain and spinal cord constitute the central nervous system, the command-and-control center that governs all human performance and behavior. The spinal cord acts as the brain's two-wave communications cable. It carries messages from the brain to the body's muscles, internal organs, and skin. The messages tell the body what to do — which muscles to relax, contract, and also what not to do — what information to ignore. Back to the brain, through the messages reporting on what's

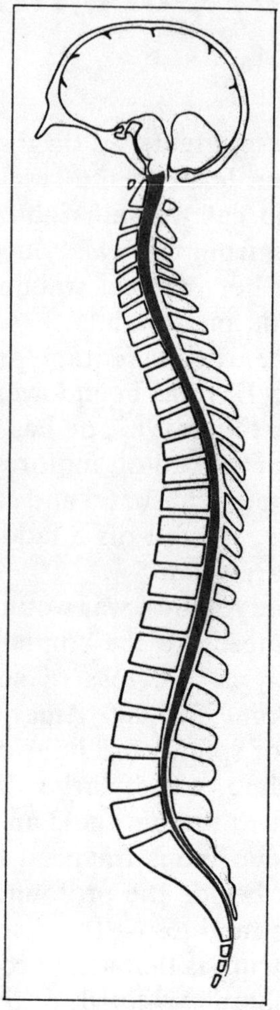

The spinal cord extends from the brain to the lower back. The detail shows the snug fit of the cord inside the spinal column. Both incoming and outgoing nerve signals are carried in the spinal nerves which exit from the sides of the cord through the spaces between the vertebrae.

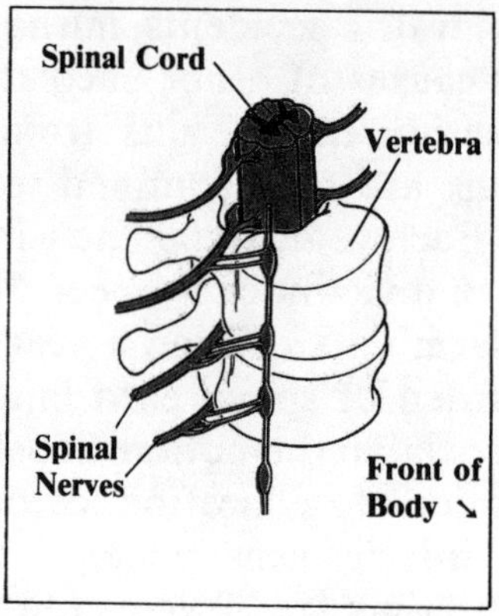

happening whether the skin is hot or cold, what the hands may be touching, whether the body is hurt. Injury to the spinal cord means that messages don't get through. Depending on the severity and location of the injury, the communications breakdown may be mild, serious, or fatal.

Generally the higher the level of injury, the greater the disability. An injury at the neck (cervical) level may cause paralysis in both arms and legs, called *quadriplegia* or *tetraplegia*. Injury at the chest (thoracic) level affects the legs and lower parts of the body. These patients are *paraplegics*. The woman doctor and the roof repair victim are both paraplegics; the sailing videotape producer, a quadriplegic.

However, the word paraplegic is often used to describe all victims of spinal cord injury.

The human spinal cord does not lack protection. Both the cord and the brain lie deep within the body, encased in tough membranes, cushioned by shock-absorbing fluid, and surrounded by the strong bones of the skull and backbone. Those defenses are enough to protect the cord from the bumps and minor falls of everyday life. They may not be enough to protect the cord from the impact of automobile accidents, or injuries incurred in sports or in operating heavy-duty equipment.

Unfortunately, nerve cells (neurons) in the brain and spinal cord are extremely sensitive. Unlike most body cells, damaged neurons in the brain and spinal cord rarely recover from severe injury. They either die without replacement or else they do not recover sufficiently to resume normal operations. The consequence is that the human spinal cord does not heal itself.

Scientists are beginning to question that last statement, however. "The view that there is no hope of restoring nerve pathways — the view you would have heard from virtually every scientist not long ago — is no longer held," says the director of the National Institute of Neurological and Communicative Disorders and Stroke (NINCDS), the leading federal agency supporting neurological research. "The mammalian nervous system does show evidence of attempts to regenerate itself. The machinery for regeneration seems to be there," he adds. Behind this optimism is a wealth of new information about the human nervous system made possible by ingenious tools and techniques. To be sure, the new findings may not help today's patients, nor are future benefits at all certain. Still, some scientists are predicting that answers to the mysteries of spinal cord injury and regeneration may come before the end of the century.

An acute problem

One mystery doctors would like to see solved quickly is why — far from healing itself — the spinal cord self-destructs following injury. Usually the spinal cord is not severed in an accident, but only crushed or bruised. However, in the next few hours (the acute stage) the injury gets worse. First the spinal cord swells. Then blood pressure drops off sharply in the damaged area, starving cells of their precious blood supply. Hemorrhaging begins in the center of the cord and spreads outwards. Nerve cells die, and their dying produces a gap in the cord with scar tissue forming on either side of the gap. Now the connections in the cord are well and truly broken, and the result is paralysis and loss of sensation below the break.

Many investigators, including scientists at Spinal Cord Injury Clinical Research Centers supported by NINCDS at Yale, New York, and Ohio State Universities, and at the Universities of South Carolina and Texas are trying to solve this problem. One of the intriguing leads they are following involves drugs.

- ***Steroids***. One family of drugs that may help prevent the cord's self-destruction is the steroids. These drugs have been used effectively to reduce the redness and swelling associated with a variety of illnesses or injuries. But their benefit in the case of spinal cord injury is not clear: Researchers at several NINCDS-supported Spinal Cord Injury Clinical Research Centers noted that small doses of steroids have little or no effect. On the other hand, larger doses may reduce the cord swelling, but may retard healing. A collaborative study of the effectiveness of the steroid methylprednisolone is now under way at the five NINCDS Spinal Cord Injury Clinical Research Centers and at the Universities of Miami and Puerto Rico.
- ***DMSO***. NINCDS-supported research scientists are also examining the properties of the controversial chemical, dimethyl sulfoxide (DMSO), a common industrial solvent thought to have healing and pain-relieving effects. DMSO is being tested on animals in experiments at five universities in the United States. As with all experimental drugs, the investigators are concerned with the safety and side effects of the drug as well as with determining its effectiveness.
- ***Endorphin blockers***. A major discovery in the past decade concerns a class of brain chemicals called endorphins — referred to as "the brain's own opiates" because they relieve pain. Now it appears that the endorphins are also involved in the production of shock. In shock, there is a sharp drop in blood pressure that can be life-threatening. During the acute stage of spinal cord injury, the cord also undergoes "spinal shock" — when blood pressure drops off sharply. Some investigators now think that endorphins are released by the brain at the time of injury — probably to relieve the victim's pain — but unwittingly cause more damage by contributing to shock. Suppose you injected a drug that blocks the actions of endorphins, the investigators reasoned. Would that treatment prevent spinal shock in laboratory animals with induced spinal cord injuries? Simulating the course of events in a real-life accident, the scientists injected an endorphin-blocking drug about 45 minutes after the spinal cords had been severed in laboratory animals. Not only did most of the animals avoid shock, but they also recovered from injury.

Many were able to walk again — some with no trace of injury. It is too soon to tell whether these results are applicable to human spinal cord patients, but the research is considered highly promising and is being followed closely.

Besides drugs, some specialists have tried cooling the injured cord to prevent secondary damage. If initiated soon after injury, the cooling should slow down metabolism and so might forestall tissue destruction.

Surgery during the acute stage may also be necessary to relieve pressure on the cord or reduce swelling. Damage to the bones of the spinal column — the vertebrae — might also need to be repaired, and the spinal column fixed in place around the cord.

Cool heads and efficient hands

Spinal cord injury represents a major medical emergency that demands knowledgeable handling at the scene of the accident and rapid specialized transport to medical facilities designed to treat trauma patients. The United States is considered the world leader in research on spinal cord injury, and the clinical research conducted at the five NINCDS-supported Spinal Cord Injury Clinical Research Centers reflects this expertise.

It is not unusual for a spinal injury victim to be taken first to a nearby hospital emergency room for immediate care of bleeding or other life-threatening condition, and later be moved to an appropriate medical facility. Treatment might be at one of over 300 regional trauma centers, for example, special spinal cord injury units, or major medical centers equipped to treat spinal cord injury. In some cases, patients may qualify for participation in clinical research projects conducted at the NINCDS-supported Spinal Cord Injury Clinical Research Centers. In any case, a multidisciplinary team at the center will be alerted to the arrival of a patient and prepared to make a rapid, but meticulous, diagnosis. First steps will include an evaluation of lung function — especially important in the case of injuries in neck and chest regions. An anesthesiologist stands by ready to provide emergency respiratory aid.

An examination of the injury will determine what measures will be employed to relieve pressure on the cord, and how to stabilize the spinal column so that it does not move and is properly aligned around the cord. Traction and weights may be used, as well as special bed frames, to prevent movement.

A neurological examination will determine the extent of nervous system damage. All efforts will be made to preserve whatever movements the patient can make or sensations he or she can feel. Neurologists will test reflexes and question the patient, but also rely on a battery of electrical and other tests to determine the extent of damage to spinal cord nerves. At the Medical College of South Carolina, NINCDS-supported specialists are refining electrophysiological tests to aid diagnosis and also to determine rapidly whether the cord has been partially or completely severed.

It is during this stage that drugs, cooling, surgery, or other techniques may be used to help prevent secondary damage to the cord. If, after 48 hours, the patient is unable to move or feel sensations below the level of injury, the resulting paraplegia or quadriplegia is considered "complete."

Man-made aids

Once the patient is out of danger, long-term treatment and rehabilitation can begin. Of growing importance in treatment are electronic aids that allow patients to regulate vital organs like the lungs or bladder, whose nerve supply may be impaired. Man-made devices that work by direct stimulation of nerves and muscles are one approach to the problem. NINCDS currently supports the development of a wide range of such devices, technically known as *neural prostheses*.

A Yale University research scientist has reported success with a new electronic device — the *Diaphragm Pacer* — designed to help paraplegics who have lost automatic control of their breathing muscles. Normally these patients have to be maintained on mechanical respirators. The system consists of an external radiotransmitter and antenna, a receiver implanted under the skin, and an electrode placed on the phrenic nerve. The phrenic nerve controls the diaphragm, the main breathing muscle. The transmitter's signals are picked up by the antenna, beamed to the receiver, and converted to electrical impulses which are sent to the phrenic nerve. The signals are beamed in an on-off pattern designed to match the normal breathing cycle. Electrophrenic electrodes have been implanted in over 200 patients so far. In clinical tests over a period of 8 years, the system has been found to be safe and effective.

Other neural prostheses designed to make life safer and more manageable for spinal cord injury patients are being developed:

- ***Bladder control***. Urinary tract problems are a frequent complication of spinal cord injury, and serious infections are a major cause of death. At the University of California at San Francisco, a device designed to enable a patient to empty the bladder voluntarily is being tested on animals. This prosthesis involves electrical stimulation of the sacral nerve roots at the base of the spine. If the bladder device proves safe and effective, bladder infections could be reduced, and perhaps eliminated.

• ***Hand control.*** At Case Western Reserve University in Cleveland, investigators report that electrodes implanted in paralyzed finger and thumb muscles have enabled patients to grasp and hold pens, pencils, spoons, forks, and other small objects. Plans call for further experiments aimed at the control of wrist and elbow muscles.

Paraplegic patients face other complications besides breathing difficulties and loss of bladder and bowel control. There may be painful muscle spasms, and bone and joint problems. Common illnesses present serious hazards. Flu or pneumonia, for example, can be fatal.

Pressure sores are a common problem. Sensations that ordinarily signal danger from heat, cold, or pressure may be lost below the level of injury. That loss, combined with reduced mobility, poor blood circulation, and inadequate nutrition, can give rise to troublesome skin ulcers. Careful daily inspection of the skin is necessary to prevent the sores and detect other problems.

The overall adjustment to a new life style is the overwhelming problem for the paraplegic, however. As one paralyzed veteran put it:

"The impact on the patient is traumatic, to say the least. There is the realization that a once whole and healthy body is no longer fully functional and is plagued with a myriad of secondary disabilities. The psychological/emotional problem of learning to accept this condition and learning how to cope with it is devastating in itself."

It is a tribute to human resourcefulness and strength that the great majority of paraplegics do adjust. They return to work, drive their own cars, and have fulfilling family and social lives.

Aiding and abetting them on their route to recovery are facilities designed to provide follow-up treatment once patients have passed the acute stage. Such treatment is available at regional spinal cord injury centers, rehabilitation institutes, veterans hospitals, departments of physical medicine or rehabilitation medicine in medical centers, and in clinics operated by nonprofit organizations such as the National Easter Seal Society.

The aim of a spinal cord injury rehabilitation program is to teach patients how to become independent. A variety of services and therapies are offered. Patients are often provided with self-care handbooks. An excellent example is one used at the New York

University Institute for Rehabilitation Medicine, "Spinal Cord Injury — A Guide For Care." No aspect of everyday living in a wheelchair is omitted. Here, for instance, are a few of the handbook's instructions on protecting skin and preventing pressure sores:

- Bathe daily and dry thoroughly, especially between toes and in the groin area. Make sure soiled skin is cleansed and dried thoroughly after bowel and bladder accidents . . .
- When sitting, buttock pressure should be relieved every 15 to 30 minutes by doing one-minute pushups or by shifting your weight from side to side. If you are unable to do this, ask for assistance . . .
- If you recline on a couch for long periods, use your air mattress or sheepskin under you.

The booklet tells patients what they need to know about nutrition, medication, foot care, and prevention of kidney and bladder complications. The assumption is that the patient *will* be independent. Tips range from how to negotiate a wheelchair to what to do about colds, asthma, allergies, or smoking.

Physical therapy is a major part of the treatment program in rehabilitation centers. If the patient is not yet permitted out of bed, a therapist will start bedside treatment. The degree of healing of fractured bones, the presence of pressure sores or infection, and the patient's general strength may limit the amount of exercise possible. But physical therapists will encourage patients to do as much as they can. A full physical therapy program often includes:

Progressive resistive exercises. These are exercises done with weights, pulleys, and special exercise machines. They are part of a vigorous advanced program to strengthen muscles.

Tilt table. A table that can be positioned at various angles to the horizontal helps the cardiovascular system readjust to upright position after a patient has been in bed for extended periods.

Mat class. Working on a mat, the patient relearns and practices the skills needed for independent living: changing position in bed, getting dressed, moving from one place to another.

Wheelchair class. The patient learns to handle a wheelchair, especially on curbs, ramps, stairs, and in a car. A patient's ability to negotiate these obstacles depends, of course, on the extent of impairment.

Driver evaluation and training. Most patients ask "Will I ever be able to drive my own car?" The center says, yes — in the vast majority of cases.

At most rehabilitation centers, treatment is coordinated by a team that includes neurosurgeons, urologists, internists, physical therapists, and vocational rehabilitation specialists. Some patients may be ready to leave after a month's stay in a center. For others, rehabilitation takes longer, because a great deal more is involved than just physical problems.

There are days during rehabilitation when most spinal cord injury patients feel hopeless and helpless, unable to see much point in living. At the New York University Center, when a patient has these feelings, a volunteer, perhaps a successful advertising agency executive, is likely to wheel in for a visit. The executive tells the despondent patient that he, too, was once consumed with anger. In a rage, he demanded: "Why me? Why did this have to happen to me?" He talks about how he overcame despair. He says, "I made it; you can, too." The executive himself was once a patient at the center.

A major factor in successful rehabilitation is motivation. It requires motivation, first, to accept irreversible facts. It takes still more motivation to make the most of what has not been injured — talent, creative energies, intellectual resources. In addition, rehabilitation experts say that three factors always seem to be present:

The patient has some definite activity — a job, a career, plans for an education — waiting to be undertaken as soon as he or she leaves the center. Just going home to idleness is demoralizing. The doctor with the cat refused to be frustrated in her career plans. "From the first day, I never thought of not coming back to finish my training," she says. And she acknowledges that some good has come from her experience: "As a doctor, you often don't realize how much control you lose over your own life when you're a patient. I'm a lot more sensitive to this now than I was."

The videotape producer had been a school dropout. He went back to school, studied art and communications, and now specializes in making films to teach paraplegics self-care and to educate the general public. The patient's family is genuinely interested in the rehabilitation. Family members get involved and actively support the patient's efforts. So important is this aspect of rehabilitation that some centers ask family members to attend formal counseling programs in which they meet weekly with staff professionals to discuss problems and exchange information.

The family doesn't coddle the patient, but encourages independence. After the home handyman's roofing accident, his wife made sure that he continued to play a central role in family decision-making and plans. She refused to treat him like an invalid when he struggled with his first attempts to cope with knives and forks, or with drinking from a cup. His rehabilitation — in spite of complications requiring repeated surgery — is considered so successful that the rehabilitation center, where he was a patient, routinely calls him any time they send a patient home in his area so he can provide encouragement and support.

The new research

Putting the injured human spinal cord back together again — achieving regeneration so that patients can once again control movements and enjoy sensations — is the ultimate goal of spinal cord regeneration research today. It is a goal that has eluded scientists for so long that investigators simply accepted the fact that the spinal cord in man — indeed, in all mammals — could not recover from injury. Even when simpler forms of life were studied, scientists remained skeptical on hearing that some experiment had shown an animal could move again after its spinal cord had been cut in half.

Recently, however, two investigators at Yale University employed a special dye technique that enabled them to trace individual nerve cells in an experimental animal. They chose an eel-like creature, the sea lamprey, interesting because it has large nerve cells and is capable of complex behavior: The lamprey has a backbone, making it a vertebrate. This places it relatively high up on the evolutionary scale, closer to mammals and man.

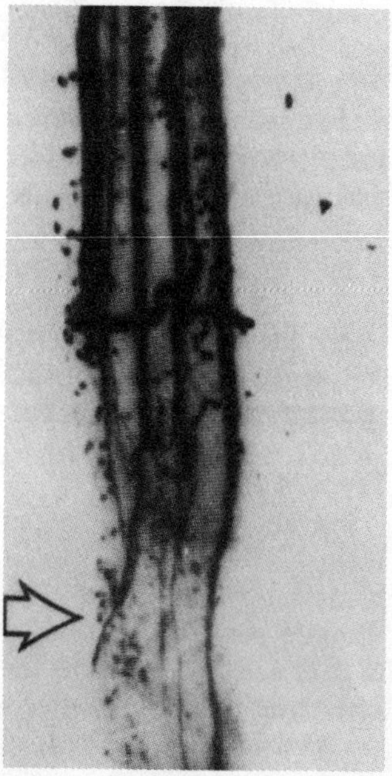

Regenerated spinal cord of sea lamprey: The long black lines on the right are dye-marked nerve cell fibers that have regenerated, crossed a gap in the spinal cord (at arrow), and made new connections below the break.

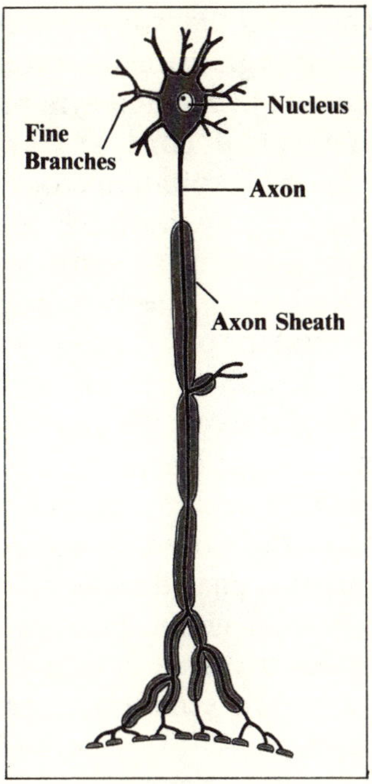

A typical nerve cell found in the spinal cord. Neurons of this type send their long branches (their axons) out of the cord to control the body's muscles.

The investigators operated on the lampreys to sever their spinal cords. Months later, they observed that some of the lampreys could swim again. To make sure that regeneration had actually taken place, they reoperated on the animals and injected their marker dye into the brain.

Long fibers descending from brain cells are among the nerves cut when the spinal cord is severed. If the cut ends can regenerate, the dye should eventually filter down and mark them out. Follow-up studies of the lampreys showed that that was exactly what happened: Brain cell fibers had grown across the gap in the cord and made useful connections below the break. The experiment was exciting because it was the first clear-cut evidence of spinal cord regeneration in a vertebrate.

Clues from the sea lamprey experiment, from work with drugs to block the spinal cord's self-destructive behavior, and from other research suggest that the key to regeneration lies within the spinal cord itself. There, the focus has turned to the individual nerve cell.

While neurons differ in size and shape, they generally possess numerous short fine branches and one slightly thicker long branch, the axon. In a brain nerve cell destined to control a toe muscle, the axon may be 3 feet long, extending from the brain to a center in the spinal cord in the lower back. The axon plays a key role in nervous system regeneration because it is through axons that nerve cells link up to one another. The linkage places are called synapses.

Nerve cells and fibers in the spinal cord are arranged in a complex, but orderly, pattern. The cord is round in cross section, with patches of white matter surrounding a gray, butterfly-shaped central region. The white patches are cross sections of axons — millions of them — streaming to and from the brain. The gray matter is nerve cells, each with its own gossamer network of branches and fibers. To mend a spinal cord injury — which usually involves crossing a gap in the cord — not only must numbers of nerve cells and fibers regenerate, but they must also make useful synaptic connections in the cord.

While the problems are monumental, neuroscientists now know that the human nervous system has the potential for regeneration. Among the exciting discoveries in the past decade is that the cell bodies of neurons continually manufacture proteins and other substances. These chemicals flow down the axon in a steady stream to maintain the health of the axon and its synaptic contacts. Similarly, materials from the far end of the axon are returned to the cell body for recycling. This two-way "axon transport" provides a means for repair. But not for long. For unknown reasons, an injured nerve cell starts to regrow, but then stops.

Some neuroscientists think that metabolism in the injured neuron is so altered that the cell can survive for only a short time. Another theory is that the injured cell may regenerate just long enough to make a connection with another cell (no matter whether the connection is useful or not!) and then the growing cell stops working.

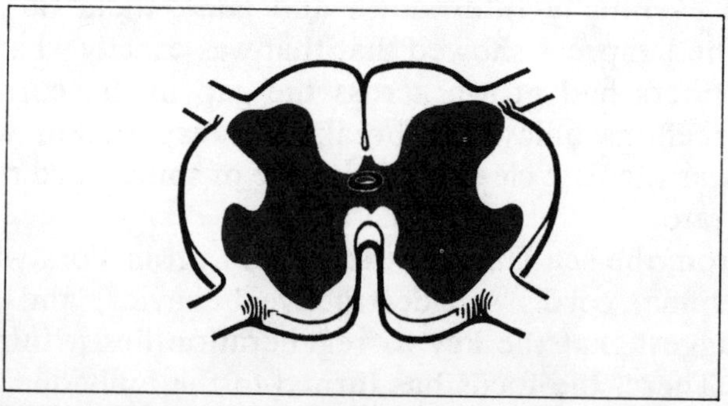

Dark butterfly pattern seen in a typical cross section of the human spinal cord marks the cell bodies of neurons. The surrounding white matter is composed of the long axons of cells traveling to and from the brain.

To aid regenerating cells, some research scientists have tried closing a gap in the cord with a graft of nerve tissue. It acts like a thin tube to guide and support growing axons.

Other investigators are exploring the role of "trophic influences" — chemicals in the nervous system that appear to promote cell growth and lead growing fibers to their appropriate destinations. Scientists are also experimenting with enzymes to attack and destroy scar tissue that may block regrowth. Some scientists are also exploring the possibility that there are growth-inhibitors, perhaps chemicals or electric currents, which prevent the formation of new synapses. Bit by bit, investigators are taking the problem of spinal cord injury apart and isolating the components. This may mean growing nerve cells in tissue culture. It also means fundamental research on how the nervous system normally develops — how its circuits are correctly wired in the first place.

The ingenuity of the nervous system is a constant source of fascination to neuroscientists. Investigators now know that the nervous system can follow an alternate route to recovery once it is injured. This route also involves new growth, not from the injured nerve cells but from nearby undamaged cells. These healthy neurons put out new branches as though to compensate for the severed connections. The process, called "collateral sprouting," may be sufficient to permit recovery from some cases of injury — assuming enough sprouts can bridge the injured area and establish proper connections.

No responsible scientist promises that regeneration of the human spinal cord will become a reality tomorrow. Most are wary, lest enthusiasm lead to premature announcements of success. Recently, for example, scientists in Russia reported using enzymes to treat severed spinal cords in rats. They stated that the cords had regenerated and the rats could move again. The universally accepted rule of science is that, to be valid, an experiment must be repeatable. An NINCDS-supported investigator at the University of Maryland School of Medicine, as well as other American scientists, repeated the Soviet experiment but did not obtain the reported results. It is thought that the Soviet investigators had inadvertently failed to sever the rats' cords completely. Still, the fact that spinal cord injury is a worldwide problem that commands the attention of an international group of scientists is encouraging. The chances of major discoveries being made in science are greater, the more good minds with good ideas and good tools turn their attention to the problem.

Better survivals, richer lives

It is now obvious that much of the damage caused by spinal cord injury can be prevented. Patients need not arrive at hospitals completely paralyzed when, at the outset, there was only partial loss of feeling or mobility. The federal government, through the National Highway Safety Act and the Emergency Medical Services Act, has taken an active role in developing regional systems for handling medical emergencies. The Department of Transportation, in cooperation with the National Institutes of Health and other federal, state, and local agencies, has coordinated efforts to provide ambulance and emergency medical services and to train paramedical personnel at the community level. The agencies have also worked to improve communications from the moment an accident is reported until the victim's arrival at a care facility.

More work needs to be done. Some communities lack adequate emergency services. All communities need ongoing programs to educate the public, as well as paramedical personnel in coping with medical crises.

Communities can do even more: They can work to prevent spinal cord injuries from happening in the first place. They can test the effectiveness of safety devices in cars and motorcycles, and ensure adequate safeguards in operating other vehicles or machinery. They can sponsor driver education and training programs. They can explore the adequacy of current driving laws and enforce traffic and safety rules. We already know that the number of spinal cord injuries goes down when a 55-mile-an-hour speed limit is enforced.

Furthermore, studies of rehabilitation are pointing out how to make the best use of talent and creativity. Spinal cord injury patients can lead productive and satisfying lives. They can have stable marriages and families. Most can and do enjoy sex. The Casa Colina Hospital for Rehabilitation Medicine in Pomona, California, reports, "There is almost always some potential for function."

Where to go for help

There are a growing number of public and private agencies that can advise patients and families in many areas of concern, such as finances, ongoing medical problems, employment, education, and rehabilitation services. Disabled workers who have contributed payments through the Social Security system may qualify for supplemental security income and reimbursements under Medicare. The local Social Security Office can advise individuals and provide handbooks explaining the system.

The Assistant Secretary for Special Education and Rehabilitative Services under the Department of Education is responsible for programs "specifically designed to reduce human dependency, to increase self-reliance, and to fully utilize the productive capabilities of all handicapped persons." Programs include funds to states to expand rehabilitation services. Again, individuals should apply to state or local rehabilitation departments to see what programs are available.

Disabled veterans qualify for compensation and education benefits through the Department of Veterans benefits of the Veterans Administration. Disabled veterans are also legally entitled to priority and preferential service in placement, counseling, and referral to training activities conducted through the United States Employment Service.

The Rehabilitation Act of 1973 was passed to protect the rights of all handicapped persons in areas of employment and access to programs and activities: Section 503 prohibits discrimination against handicapped persons in hiring practices by any employer who receives even minimal amounts of federal funds. Section 504 states "No otherwise handicapped individual in the United States . . . shall by reason of his handicap, be excluded from participation in, be denied the benefits of, or be subject to discrimination under any program or activity receiving federal financial assistance." Implementing the law has meant, among other things, that buildings financed in part by federal funds must be made accessible to persons in wheelchairs.

In addition to government programs and legislation, a number of voluntary health organizations are valuable resources of information and advice for the spinal injured. The principal national organizations are: the National Spinal Cord Injury Foundation; Paralysis Cure Research Foundation; the Paralyzed Veterans of America; the National Easter Seal Society, Inc.; and Rehabilitation International USA (see p. 441).

There are also many local organizations that have sprung up in the past few years in response to the growing demand of disabled persons for independent living, and for opportunities to travel and participate in sports and other recreation (see pp. 441, 442 and 441, 442).

The new emphasis on independent living and participation in activities in part reflects improvements and innovations in technology. Spinal cord injury patients are becoming more mobile. There are stand-up wheelchairs. And stair-climbing wheelchairs. Some wheelchairs can be voice-operated. Others can be maneuvered by breath control. There is a steady stream of ingenious new technical aids to make independent living and movement from place to place more manageable.

But the world is tough. Society, unknowingly, constricts the freedom and offends the feelings of the disabled through indifference or rejection. While laws prohibit discrimination against the disabled, the laws are not always enforced. Some new buildings are being designed so that they are accessible to paraplegics, but others are not so designed. Many older buildings fail to comply with new government standards. Sensitivity to needs of the handicapped is needed, along with respect and understanding.

The world can hardly get tougher than it is for some paraplegics. Some face the complications of repeated bladder infections, spinal cord cysts, or painful skin ulcers. Some suffer agonizing muscle spasms that lead to the continued — and hazardous — use of the muscle-relaxant tranquilizing drugs. Not a few paraplegics have contemplated ending their lives rather than face the unrelenting discomfort that prohibits useful work or rewarding activity.

Yet the vast majority of spinal cord injury patients are survivors: men and women who have had to make radical readjustments in their lives and have emerged with enviable courage, strength, and humor. As a nursing supervisor at the New York University center has said, in order for the patient — or someone close — to come through the experience, "the person has to become almost something he wasn't before."

Dr. Howard A. Rusk, one of the world's best-known rehabilitation specialists, puts it another way:

"Great ceramics are not made by putting clay in the sun; they come only from the white heat of the kiln. In the firing process, some pieces are broken, but those that survive the heat are transformed from clay into porcelain and are objects of art, and so it is with people. Those who, through medical skill, opportunity, work and courage, survive their illness or overcome their handicap and take their places back in the world have a depth of spirit that you and I can hardly measure. They haven't wasted their pain."

Voluntary organizations

The following national organizations are concerned with research, care, and treatment of spinal cord injury and other paralyzing or disabling conditions, and are sources of information, publications, and advice:

National Spinal Cord Injury Foundation
369 Elliot Street
Newton Upper Falls, Mass. 02164
(617) 964-0521

Paralysis Cure Research Foundation
100 Maryland Avenue, N.E.
Washington, D.C. 20002
(202) 547-4777

Paralyzed Veterans of America
Suite 900
4350 East West Highway
Washington, D.C. 20014
(301) 652-2135

Rehabilitation International USA, Inc.
20 West 40th Street
New York, N.Y. 10018
(212) 869-9907

The National Easter Seal Society, Inc.
2023 West Ogden Avenue
Chicago, Ill. 60612
(312) 243-8400

A number of special interest or local groups have formed in response to an increasing demand for access to recreational activities, travel, and other aspects of daily living that concern disabled individuals:

Travel

The Society for the Advancement of Travel for the Handicapped
(SATH)
26 Court Street
New York, N.Y. 11242

(SATH issues a bimonthly newsletter, holds seminars, and offers a free list of travel agencies offering tours geared to the handicapped.)

Athletics

National Wheelchair Athletic Association
4024 62nd Avenue
Woodside, N.Y. 11377

Berkeley Outreach Recreation Program, Inc.
605 Eshleman Hall
University of California
Berkeley, Calif. 94720

Bibliography

Books, reference guides, and periodicals provide valuable information for spinal cord injury patients interested in the latest developments in research and treatment, as well as aids to independent living. (Costs of pamphlets are not listed since they are subject to change.) The following is a sample of publications available:

Spinal Cord Injury: A Guide for Care
by Glenn Goldfinger and Marcia Hanak
New York University Medical Center
Institute for Rehabilitation Medicine
400 East 34th Street
New York, N.Y. 10016

Living with Spinal Cord Injury: Questions and Answers for Patients,
Family and Friends
by Majorie Garfunkel and Glenn Goldfinger
New York University Medical Center
Institute for Rehabilitation Medicine
400 East 34th Street
New York, N.Y. 10016

Directory of National Information Sources on Handicapping Conditions and Related Services (1980)
Office for Handicapped Individuals
Department of Education
Room 3106, 400 Maryland Avenue, S.W.
Switzer Building
Washington, D.C. 20202
(A general guide to organizations and services of interest to handicapped individuals; free upon request.)

Paraplegia News
Suite 108
5201 North 19th Avenue
Phoneix, Ariz. 85015

Rehabilitation Gazette
4502 Maryland Avenue
St. Louis, MO. 63108

Disabled U.S.A.
President's Committee on Employment of the Handicapped
1111 20th Street, N.W.
Washington, D.C. 20036
(free upon request)

Report
National Center for a Barrier-Free Environment
Suite 1006
1140 Connecticut Avenue, N.W.
Washington, D.C. 20036

New World
P.O. Box 1567
South Gate, Calif. 9-280

Rehabilitation Literature
The National Easter Seal Society, Inc.
2023 West Ogden Avenue
Chicago, Ill. 60612

Career Education for Physically Disabled Students: A Bibliography
Products Manager
Human Resources Center
I.U. Willets and Searington Roads
Albertson, N.Y. 11507
(free upon request)

New Life Options, Independent Living and You
Institute for Information Studies
Suite 202
400 North Washington Street
Falls Church, Va. 22046
(free upon request)

Access Travel: Airports
Architectural and Transportation Barriers
Compliance Board
330 C Street, S.W.
Washington, D.C. 20202
(A free list of facilities for the handicapped available at 220 airport terminals worldwide.)

Clothing for Handicapped People: Annotated Bibliography and Resource List
President's Committee on Employment of the Handicapped
1111 20th Street, N.W.
Washington, D.C. 20036
(free upon request)

The Wheelchair Traveler
by Douglas R. Annand
Ball Hill Road
Milford, N.H. 03055
(A guidebook to 6,000 hotels, motels, and restaurants in the U.S., Mexico, Canada, and Puerto Rico, rating their suitability for the handicapped.)

International Directory of Access Guides
Rehabilitation International USA, Inc.
20 West 40th Street
New York, N.Y. 10018
(A listing of access guides for the handicapped available for U.S. and foreign cities, tourist attractions, transportation facilities, etc.)

Chapter 26

Head and Spinal Cord Injury Survey

The National Head and Spinal Cord Injury Survey

What the Survey Found

About Numbers of Head and Spinal Cord Injuries

• In 1 year, an estimated 430,000 Americans were admitted to hospitals with new cases of injury.* Estimates for each category:

Head injury	422,000
Spinal cord injury	10,000

• In 1 year, an estimated 204 out of every 100,000 Americans were hospitalized as a result of traumatic injuries.* Estimated rates for each category:

Head injury	200 per 100,000 population
Spinal cord injury	5 per 100,000 population

• The rate of hospitalized cases of injury which had occurred between 1970 and 1974 — and which still required medical service in 1974 — was 450 per 100,000 population.** Estimated rates for each category:

Head injury	439 per 100,000 population
Spinal cord injury	13 per 100,000 population

About Costs of Head and Spinal Cord Injuries

• In 1974, the estimated economic costs of head and spinal cord injuries sustained through automobile accidents, falls or other trauma in the nation's 48 contiguous states totaled approximately $2.6 billion.

---

* Estimates are for persons first treated for their injuries in hospitals during the years 1970 through 1974 and who still required medical treatmen during 1974. If a person sustained a head and a spinal cord injury, both injuries were counted as one cost.

** Estimates were based on first hospitalization following injury. Persons who suffered injuries to both head and spinal cord were counted only once.

That is $4.8 billion in 1990 dollars.* Approximate overall costs for each category:

Head injury	$2.4 billion ($4.5 billion in 1990 dollars)
Spinal cord injury	$234 million ($437 million in 1990 dollars)

• In 1974, the estimated average health care cost for each American who continued to suffer from a traumatic head or spinal cord injury was $2,715 — or $4,408 in 1980 dollars.** Figured into the average are both direct costs — goods, services, medical care and equipment related to health care — and such indirect costs as the money society loses when the productivity of an injured person is interrupted. Approximate average cost per injured person for each category:

Head injury	$2,534 ($4,731 in 1990 dollars)
Spinal cord injury	$8,863 ($16,548 in 1990 dollars)

• In 1974, the number of new head injuries for males was about twice the number for females.
• In a single year, 15-to-24-year-old males incurred more new head injuries from all causes than any other age group. When only motor vehicle accidents were considered, the number of new head injuries was greatest for this same age group.
• In 1 year, motor vehicle accidents caused nearly half — 49 percent — of all hospitalized cases of head injury. The more severe the head injury, the greater the likelihood that a motor vehicle accident was the cause.
• 1970 through 1974: Head and spinal cord injuries occurred most often on weekends — Fridays, Saturdays and Sundays.

---

* Estimates are for persons first treated for their injuries in hospitals during the years 1970 through 1974 and who still required medical treatmen during 1974. If a person sustained a head and a spinal cord injury, both injuries were counted as one cost.

** Estimates are for persons first treated for their injuries in hospitals during the years 1970 through 1974 and who still required medical treatmen during 1974. If a person sustained a head and a spinal cord injury, both injuries were counted as one cost.

About the Survey

What It Is: This survey is the first reliable statistical picture of head and spinal cord injury problems in the United States. Undertaken in 1974 by the National Institute of Neurological and Communicative Disorders and Stroke (NINCDS), the survey concentrated on head and spinal cord injuries which occurred between 1970 and 1974 through some trauma, and which resulted in admissions to hospitals in the nation's 48 contiguous states. (Alaska and Hawaii were omitted from the survey because of survey cost considerations.) A complete census of all cases was not attempted. Instead, a sophisticated sampling method was applied to hospital records. The survey — the largest of its kind — produced important new information about injuries that are among the nation's most devastating health problems.

Why the Survey Was Undertaken: NINCDS sponsors research on a number of neurological diseases and disorders. Research funds are limited. To determine the best allocation of funds, timely, accurate statistics that describe the national dimensions of health problems are invaluable. Before 1974, such nationwide statistics were scarce. In 1974, to get reliable data for the nation, NINCDS undertook a series of large-scale surveys. One in the series was this first National Head and Spinal Cord Injury Survey.

The Survey's Aims: The overall aim was to determine the magnitude of the problem of head and spinal cord injury in the United States. Specifically, the survey sought to:

- Find out how many new cases of head and spinal cord injury due to trauma were admitted to hospitals in America in a single year.
- Ascertain the number of both old and new cases for 1 year. Old cases of injury are those which had been sustained from 1970 through 1973 and which still required some medical care in 1974.
- Get statistical information about the effects of head and spinal cord injuries on American subpopulations — different age groups, sexes, races and regions.
- Get accurate estimates of economic costs.
- Collect statistical information that might help prevent catastrophic injuries.

Who Many Profit From This Survey:

- Those responsible for planning community medical services. Survey information is likely to be useful in assessing emergency facilities, health care resources, and rehabilitation services needed for head and spinal cord injury victims.

- Those concerned with hiring and allocating medical and paramedical personnel. The survey, for instance, suggests that if a hospital has only one neurosurgeon, he should be on call on weekends.
- Physicians. Survey information may be useful for anticipating health care needs of patients, as well as for research. The survey may also serve as a prototype for studies of other disorders.
- Parents.
- 15-to-24-year-old American males.

How the Survey Was Conducted

Important Note
The "population" in The National Head and Spinal Cord Injury Survey consisted of persons who received inpatient care from hospitals in the contiguous United States from 1970 through 1974. Anyone who was dead on arrival at the hospital or who needed medical treatment just in the emergency room was not included in the survey.

Probability Sampling
Severe head injuries are devastating. Many spinal cord injuries are catastrophic. A practical survey, covering both head injuries and spinal cord injuries, was designed. It was built around a scientific selection of hospitals. The statistical tool selected for the survey was probability sampling. Among its features: it permits one to generalize on the sound basis of statistical theory; it gives all persons in a given population some chance to be included; and it is the only sampling method which allows measures of precision to be computed along with the estimates.

Multistage Sampling Plan
This survey used a "multistage sampling plan" with three stages:

STAGE 1. The contiguous United States was divided into 1,675 groups of counties, called primary sampling units (PSUs). These were stratified by region and by population density. From each stratum, PSUs were selected randomly. Cost dictated the final total: 58 PSUs.

STAGE 2. From the 58 PSUs, 305 hospitals were scientifically selected. Of these, 197 hospitals agreed to participate fully, and 50 more participated in some aspects of the survey. Total studied: 247.

STAGE 3. Discharge records numbering 9,745 were randomly selected from the 247 hospitals for study. Of these, 3,516 were medically eligible for the survey. After a follow-up review, 913 cases were found suitable for inclusion in estimates operations, and 609 interviews on economic costs had been completed.

A Word About Interpretation of Findings

Estimates from The National Head and Spinal Cord Injury Survey, or any other survey, are subject to uncertainties. Some of these uncertainties result from the way the survey was designed; others result from the way the survey was conducted. Estimates will be useful for administrative or scientific purposes only when interpreted in the light of the methods that produced them.

It is beyond the scope of this chapter to detail the uncertainties in estimates from this survey. For more information, refer to the complete report of this survey. The report was printed as a supplement to the Journal of Neurosurgery in November 1980. Copies may be obtained by writing to:

Office of Scientific and Health Reports
National Institute of Neurological and
Communicative Disorders and Stroke
National Institutes of Health
Building 31, room 8A-06
Bethesda, MD 20205
(301) 496-5751

Final Highlights

In 1 year, 1974:

- The estimated rate of new cases of head injury in males was more than twice the rate for females.
- There was no important difference in the number of new cases of head or spinal cord injury between white and nonwhite populations, when the estimates were adjusted for total population figures.
- There was no important difference in the estimated rate of new cases of head injury between various regions of the nation.

Chapter 27

Stroke

Stroke

Each year, 400,000 Americans suffer a stroke. Nearly two-thirds of the survivors may be handicapped: there are right now 2 million people in the United States disabled by stroke.

For these millions, medical research offers hope.

Because of research advances, more stroke victims than ever are surviving. Over the past 20 years, stroke deaths have dropped 40 percent.

And many survivors — even those with severe handicaps — are learning to walk again, to talk again, getting ready to lead independent lives.

Medical research has also done much to prevent strokes from occurring. Scientists now know major risk factors that can lead to a stroke, and have developed ways to treat many of them. Public health campaigns have taught the public that good health habits can help prevent stroke. So can knowing the warning signs of stroke and getting prompt medical care.

Still, stroke remains a major health hazard in the United States, one that increases with age but is by no means restricted to the elderly. Stroke in newborn infants is a major cause of cerebral palsy. A recent survey shows that close to a third of all stroke victims are under age 65 — as were Franklin Delano Roosevelt, actress Patricia Neal, and jazz musician Thelonius Monk when they suffered strokes. Research also shows that the majority of stroke victims are men.

A $14 billion affliction

Stroke is the leading serious neurological disorder in the United States. It ranks third among all causes of death and is a major cause of long-term disability in Americans.

No one can calculate the cost to patients and families in terms of suffering, lost careers, and shortened lives. But the harsh economic realities can be reckoned: When direct medical expenses are combined with lost income and productivity, the total cost of stroke in the United States is estimated to be $14 billion a year.

What causes stroke?

The occurrence of a major stroke is dramatic. A seemingly healthy person is felled by an invisible foe. Describing her near-fatal stroke, a noted dancer and choreographer recalled later that she had suddenly discovered while talking to her dancers that half her body was dead.

In reality, a stroke is not a bolt from the blue. It is, instead, often the symptom of an already existing condition that affects the flow of blood to the brain.

Unlike other organs of the body, the brain cannot store energy. It depends on a continuous supply of fresh blood pumped to it by the heart. A hefty 25 percent of the blood that the heart pumps goes to the brain.

If blood flow to a section of the brain stops for any reason, brain cells in the area lose their source of energy and begin to die. The result is a stroke.

Blood is carried from the pumping heart to the brain and other parts of the body through a network of blood vessels called arteries. In the most common form of stroke, the flow of blood is disturbed as an artery serving the brain gradually becomes clogged. Eventually, the artery may become closed entirely by the formation of a clot.

The mass that forms within the artery is called a *thrombus*, the Greek word for *clot* or *lump*. A stroke produced when blood supply to the brain is blocked because of such a clot is called a *thrombotic stroke*.

A brain artery can also be blocked or plugged by a clot that has formed elsewhere in the body, usually in the heart or the arteries of the neck, and is carried in the body's blood stream to the brain. This kind of traveling clot is called an *embolus* (a Greek word for *plug*). Another word physicians use when discussing different types of stroke is *infarct*. When a clot blocks a blood vessel, the nerve cells served by that vessel are starved of blood-borne fuel and oxygen and, within minutes, begin to sicken and die. The dead cells, other debris, and the clot itself accumulate into a mass of tissue called an *infarct*. Infarct strokes account for two-thirds of all cases.

Another 12 percent of all strokes occur when a blood vessel ruptures and blood pours into the brain. Uncontrolled bleeding of this sort is called *hemorrhage*.

Hemorrhagic strokes are usually more severe than infarct strokes. Not only is the blood supply to the brain cells lost, but the brain tissue itself is damaged by the escaped blood. The stroke experienced by the choreographer mentioned above resulted from a hemorrhage deep in the center of the left side of her brain — an often fatal event.

Certain rare blood diseases, inherited disorders, and birth defects can also cause stroke. Some people, for example, are born with a weak section in the wall of an artery in the brain. The constant pressure of blood being pumped through the artery may cause the weak section to bulge out and form an aneurysm.

The word *aneurysm* is based on the Greek word for a *widening*. An aneurysm is indeed an abnormal stretching or widening of a blood vessel wall. The stretched area is weaker than the other parts

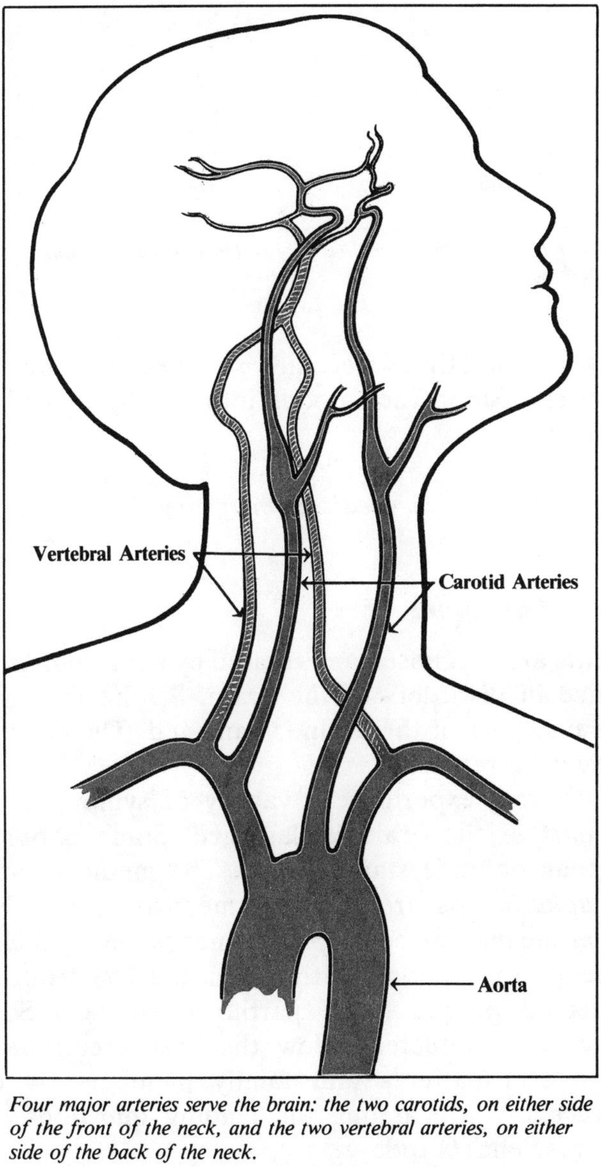

Four major arteries serve the brain: the two carotids, on either side of the front of the neck, and the two vertebral arteries, on either side of the back of the neck.

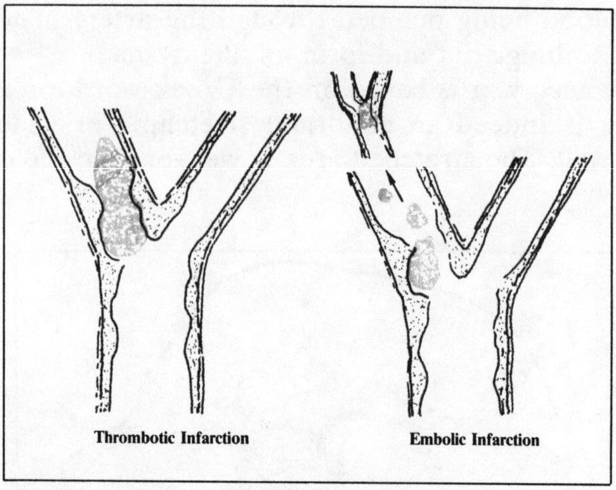

Thrombotic and embolic infarcts in brain blood vessels are major causes of stroke.

of the wall and sometimes becomes so filled with blood that the aneurysm bursts. Blood then floods into the brain and the victim suffers a stroke.

A stroke of any type is a medical emergency. It demands immediate expert care.

A neurological problem

Stroke patients are diagnosed and treated by neurologists, physicians who specialize in disorders of the brain. Stroke is a neurological problem because part of the brain is damaged. The destroyed nerve cells may never be replaced.

Stroke survivors experience a variety of symptoms, depending upon what part of the brain is damaged. Some patients may be unable to speak or understand speech. The medical name for this problem is *aphasia*. As are so many medical terms, this word is Greek: *phasia* means "speech" *aphasia* means "no speech."

Other people are permanently paralyzed by stroke. But even severely affected people make partial recoveries. Some stroke survivors recover completely. How the brain recovers and what physicians — and patients and family members — can do to encourage recovery are among the leading questions challenging research neuroscientists today.

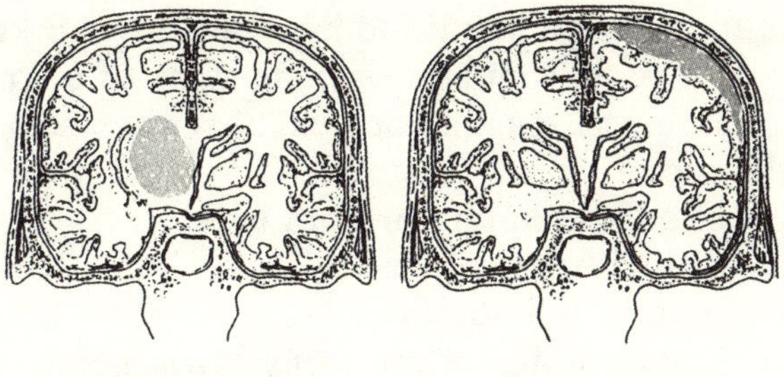

Hemorrhage, either within the brain itself (intracerebral) or in the space surrounding the brain (subarachnoid), is responsible for 12 percent of stroke cases.

Our knowledge of how the brain works has grown enormously in recent years. Many research scientists are now convinced that the brain has the ability to repair itself and to regrow damaged nerve tissue. Scientists are optimistic that they may find ways to restore the stroke-damaged brain.

National brain research institute

The leading federal agency responsible for stroke research is the National Institute of Neurological and Communicative Disorders and Stroke (NINCDS).

The NINCDS is the nation's foremost brain research institute. Through its stroke research program, NINCDS supports studies to find better ways to diagnose and treat stroke and to rehabilitate stroke patients. But the institute has an even more urgent research goal, and that is to find ways to prevent strokes from occurring.

As a unit of the National Institutes of Health in Bethesda, Md., the NINCDS works closely with other institutes concerned with stroke research. Since stroke involves both the brain and the blood vessels (and so is sometimes called "cerebrovascular disease"), NINCDS scientists collaborate with investigators from the National Heart, Lung, and Blood Institute. And since most stroke victims are older, the NINCDS also collaborates with the National Institute on Aging.

Warning signs of stroke

The No. 1 goal of stroke research is to prevent stroke. Fortunately, nature has given science some help. Strokes are often preceded by warning signs that can be identified by a person who knows what to look for. The four most common warning signs of a stroke are:

- Transient numbness, tingling or weakness in an arm or leg, or on one side of the face.
- Temporary blindness in one or both eyes.
- Temporary difficulty with speech.
- Loss of strength in a limb.

These are the symptoms of the transient ischemic attack — the so-called "TIA" — which, left untreated, can lead to a major stroke.

Other danger signals are unusual or unexplainable headache, dizziness, drowsiness, nausea, or vomiting. Abrupt personality changes and impaired judgment or forgetfulness will also warn the alert observer of possible impending stroke.

Such warning signs may be brief. The symptoms of light-headedness, feeling ill, numbness, or memory loss may last only a few seconds, but it is wise not to ignore them even if they go away. The fact that the symptoms have disappeared does not mean that there is no medical problem.

Neither does the fact that TIA symptoms may occur infrequently. "One TIA is as menacing as many," one stroke specialist has warned.

It is best to see a physician immediately and be sure.

Confirming the diagnosis

The physician's job is to determine whether the symptoms you describe mean that you have had a stroke or may have one soon. Often this evaluation can be done in the physician's office. But in an emergency you might go directly to a hospital, where you would report your symptoms and medical history to emergency room physicians. That information, plus routine tests and a neurological examination, might be enough for them to make a tentative diagnosis of a stroke.

But sometimes the patient is unconscious. Sometimes, too, people have symptoms that look like stroke as a result of reactions to drugs, or following an epileptic seizure. A delayed reaction to a head injury and certain kinds of brain tumor can also cause stroke-like symptoms.

Emergency room physicians will discuss these possibilities with neurologists. They will conduct further tests to rule out conditions other than stroke that might be causing the symptoms. The tests will also help them distinguish between a thrombotic and a hemorrhagic stroke (a "plug" or a "leak," as some doctors call them), an important step since treatment for each type of stroke differs.

Stroke Diagnosis

Tests commonly used to establish the diagnosis of stroke include:

- *CT scan.* Many neurologists believe that computerized tomography (CT) scanning has revolutionized the diagnosis of stroke. This painless technique uses a computer to construct black-and-white pictures of the brain obtained from multiple X rays beamed through the head. An area of dead brain tissue as small as half an inch across can be seen and readily distinguished from an area that is bleeding. CT scans can be performed within minutes after a person arrives at a hospital. Physicians can order more scans later to gauge the effectiveness of treatment and to evaluate the course of healing. The CT scan is harmless for patients and gives the physician important information to use in providing the best possible care.
- *Arteriography.* Arteriography produces extremely clear and detailed pictures of the main trunks and fine interconnected branches of the brain's tree-like arteries. These pictures are called *arteriograms.*

The technique requires opening an artery and threading a flexible tube through the artery toward the neck. Then a liquid is injected into the artery. This liquid will show up on X-ray films made as blood circulates in the brain.

If you are to have an arteriogram, you will be advised that there is a small risk of injury, infection, or allergic reaction to the injected material. You should also be told that thousands of arteriograms are performed safely every year. Physicians generally believe that, for most patients, the benefits from arteriography are greater than the risk.

- *DIVA.* A safe new technique of x-raying brain arteries is called digitized intravenous arteriography (DIVA). In this technique, the physician injects contrast liquid directly into a vein.

Veins are the blood vessels that carry blood back to the heart from different parts of the body. So, after the liquid is injected, it is carried along with the blood in the vein back to the heart and through the lungs. By the time the mixture of blood and contrast liquid reaches the brain, the liquid is so diluted that normal X rays will not produce pictures of the brain's arteries. To get around that problem, technicians use the same kind of photo enhancement techniques that enable detailed pictures of Earth to be made from space.

A computer codes the X-ray images in numbers, each number reflecting a different intensity of lightness or darkness. The computer then sharpens or enhances the difference between images taken before and after the contrast liquid is injected.

The pictures that result are not as detailed as arteriograms, but the technique is convenient, fast, and safe. It is especially useful for patients too ill to undergo standard arteriography. It can also be used to screen stroke patients to determine who needs an arteriogram.

- *Ultrasonography*. Many physicians use ultrasound equipment to look for defects in arteries of the neck, for these arteries are major suppliers of blood to the brain.

In this painless technique, a device placed on the patient's neck beams sound waves through the skin. A computer records and analyzes the echoes that bounce back as the sound waves are absorbed and reflected by the tissue.

Investigators at NINCDS-supported cerebrovascular clinical research centers at Cornell University Medical College in New York City and at the Bowman Gray School of Medicine in Winston-Salem, N.C., are using sonograms to study patients with high blood pressure. Groups of these patients are being compared with groups who do not have high blood pressure to see in which group cerebrovascular disease tends to develop, or whether other signs of carotid artery abnormalities appear.

Stroke treatment today

As soon as the physician knows that a patient has had a stroke and can determine what kind, treatment can begin. The physician's main concern is that the brain should suffer no further loss in circulation. Blood flow to the brain must be maintained and steps taken to prevent further damage.

In the case of an infarct stroke, strong drugs like heparin and warfarin may be prescribed for short-term use to prevent blood clots from becoming larger. These drugs are called *anticoagulants*.

Aspirin may also be used by certain stroke patients. But patients who have a history of ulcers should ask their physician whether using aspirin is wise. Usually, aspirin is a help to stroke-prone patients; but, in people with stomach trouble, aspirin can sometimes cause bleeding.

A stroke caused by a ruptured aneurysm — the "hemorrhagic" stroke — may require treatment with drugs that preserve the blood clots that form at the rupture site. These clots are needed to plug the injury. Drugs that reduce brain swelling or control high blood pressure also may be prescribed.

A major part of the National Institute of Neurological and Communicative Disorders and Stroke's research effort on stroke consists of groups of scientists working at a dozen research centers in large hospitals throughout the nation. These scientists evaluate different methods of treating stroke while examining, diagnosing, and caring for patients.

NINCDS-supported investigators at the University of Pennsylvania's center in Philadelphia, for example, are using oxygen chambers to treat stroke patients with high blood pressure. Drugs that increase blood pressure are also being tested to see if they can improve brain blood flow in some stroke patients whose blood pressure is normal.

Stroke's acute stage

The period immediately following a stroke is known as the *acute stage* because of the rapid onset of symptoms and generally unstable condition of the patient. Two or three days after a severe stroke, the brain starts to swell. This may cause further cell damage. Investigators are puzzled about the reasons for this delayed reaction and are exploring the use of steroids and other types of drugs to relieve pressure and swelling.

Some patients rally and steadily improve. Others seem to get worse or show fluctuating symptoms. Some may sink into unconsciousness or be only dimly aware of their surroundings. Speech may come and go; similarly, weakness or paralysis may improve and then worsen.

NINCDS-supported research has shown that many stroke patients become depressed — some only mildly, others to the point of despair. "Everything is so slow," said one stroke patient. "I've never been in a place that I couldn't get out of. What scares me the most is the fear of being a cripple."

This "poststroke depression" is most likely to occur between 6 months and 2 years after the stroke. About half of the severely depressed patients experience such symptoms as anxiety, loss of energy, weight, and appetite, and sleep disturbances. This depression is partially due to the brain's reaction to the stroke, and is partially a psychological reaction. Scientists are now testing a variety of drugs for this problem.

Stroke survivors and their friends and family understandably want to know what to expect. There are no easy answers. But several NINCDS-supported cerebrovascular research centers are compiling data about stroke patients from the moment they enter the hospital, searching for clues to help predict a patient's recovery.

Watching, waiting and prompt intervention are the rule during the acute stage. Patients may be placed in an intensive care unit so that brain function, blood pressure, heart rate, respiration and other vital signs can be monitored around the clock. Neurologists will make frequent checks on reflexes and ask patients what they can feel or what movements they can make. Other questions may sound foolish: Do you know where you are? Why are you here? Who is the president of the United States? But these questions test the patient's orientation as well as the ability to understand and to speak.

Rehabilitation: it takes a team

Once the stroke patient is out of danger and vital signs are stable, rehabilitation should begin. Sometimes stroke survivors lose the benefits of rehabilitative treatment because they don't realize they should have it, they don't know where to find it, or they don't continue treatment long enough to see lasting improvement.

Rehabilitation is a team effort. It involves the coordinated activities of physicians, physical and occupational therapists, social workers, speech and language specialists, and other experts and counselors who work with the family as well as the patient.

After only a week in bed, muscles start to deteriorate. Physical therapy helps the patient strengthen muscles, improve balance and coordination, and relearn the movements necessary for sitting, standing, and walking. When needed, a variety of mechanical aids — walkers, crutches, canes, and lightweight splints or braces — provide additional support.

Some patients experience the bizarre symptoms of "hemispheric neglect." As a result of one side (or *hemisphere*) of their brain being damaged, they ignore half of their body and the corresponding half of their visual world. Sometimes they deny that the neglected half even exists. Asked to put on a robe, the patient may insert an arm in only one sleeve. Asked to draw a human figure or the face of a clock, the patient may draw only half a body, or a clock with the numbers crowded in on one side.

Hemispheric neglect can usually be overcome with training, but it may take the concerted effort of all members of the rehabilitation team and the family.

Speech and language therapists work with stroke patients who have sustained damage in the speech centers of the brain. Occupational therapists concentrate on improving eye-hand coordination and strengthening skills needed in writing, using tools, and preparing food. Occupational therapy rooms are usually equipped with model kitchens and a variety of tools and gadgets designed for use by disabled people. Excellent publications are available to show how apartments and homes can be adapted to give handicapped stroke survivors reasonably independent lives (see page 475).

Rehabilitation has its mysteries. Some patients make remarkable progress, reaching the height of their potential within weeks of the stroke. In other cases, recovery may stretch out over months or years. Patients begin rehabilitation while in the hospital and most continue therapy as outpatients once they go home. Others find it more convenient to attend special rehabilitation institutes located throughout the country.

Rapport and support

"It took six men to move me from the bed to the chair," the woman said. "My back was arched and I was a dead weight." She smiled. "Then the therapist said, 'Why don't *you* try?' and I knew she wasn't going to force me. So I leaned on her arm and stood up for the first time." The speaker was a woman in her sixties who had suffered a severe stroke affecting the right half of her brain.

Her story illustrates an important aspect of rehabilitation: the need for rapport between patient and therapist.

Stroke patients, especially those who are older, may have multiple handicaps as well as other long-lasting conditions. Rehabilitation is likely to be complicated. The process requires patience and the kind of intuitive understanding that tells a sensitive therapist — or relative — how far a stroke patient can be pushed or persuaded.

Rehabilitation experts are finding more and more evidence that a key element in patient rehabilitation is family support and encouragement. Research scientists in comprehensive stroke centers established by the National Institute of Neurological and Communicative Disorders and Stroke have found that training local community members to make home visits to stroke patients, and counseling family members in rehabilitation methods seem to have paid off in better survival rates. Also, stroke patients in the research programs scored higher than expected in such areas as "activities of daily living."

Surgery for stroke

People frequently ask if there are any operations that can help stroke patients. Two operations are becoming increasingly common. Both aim to prevent stroke caused by partial blocking of blood vessels.

• ***Endarterectomy***. In this procedure, surgeons open the carotid artery in the neck and remove clots or other material that is clogging the artery and obstructing the flow of blood to the brain. (The word *endarterectomy* means "excision within the artery.") There is a small risk that not all the material will be removed or that some fragments might be dislodged and travel as clots to the brain. Research studies are still needed to show which patients might best benefit from endarterectomy, and to what extent the procedure actually improves the long-term outlook for stroke patients or those at risk.

• ***Extracranial/intracranial bypass***. When a clogged artery is located within the brain, the surgeon usually cannot operate to remove the obstruction. But sometimes the surgeon may try to reroute blood past the obstruction or clogged area.

One such operation is the extracranial/intracranial or EC/IC bypass.

In this bypass operation, a healthy scalp artery at the top of the head (*extracranial* means "outside the skull") is passed through a hole in the skull to the brain inside (*intracranial*). There it is joined to the clogged brain artery just beyond the obstruction. Blood then flows from the heart through the scalp artery and into the brain artery,

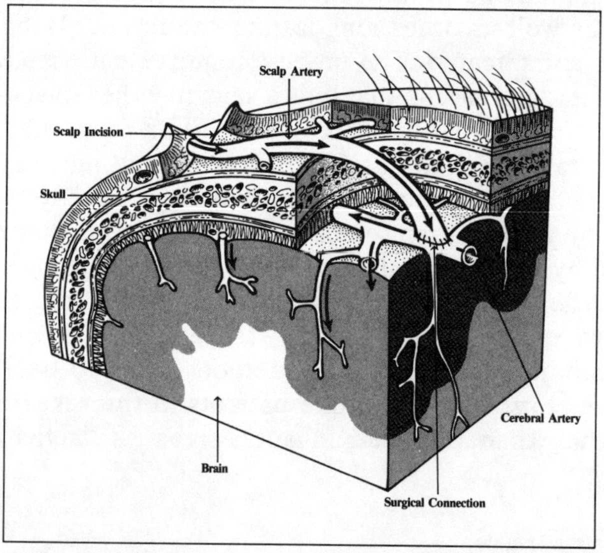

This drawing shows, in simplified form, how a scalp artery is passed through a hole in the skull and joined to one of the arteries serving the brain.

bypassing the clogged area in much the same way that motorists use a detour to bypass a traffic jam.

EC/IC bypass surgery is now the subject of a major NINCDS-supported cooperative research study involving 1,500 patients in the United States, Canada, Europe, and Japan. Scientists do not suggest that the EC/IC bypass is the answer for every stroke patient. But, so far, evidence shows that the operation is safe and well tolerated, and that the newly formed connection between the arteries stays open. The question that remains is whether the operation will significantly reduce the incidence of further stroke or certain warning signs of stroke.

Preventing a first — or second — stroke

In stroke, there is nothing so important as prevention. Survivors of a first stroke do not want to be among the 20 to 25 percent who suffer second or third strokes. Family members may wonder if they, too, will have a stroke, and want to know what to do to prevent it. Fortunately, research scientists have identified several risk factors that can alert you before a stroke occurs.

- *Transient ischemic attack.* The one risk factor that most clearly predicts who will suffer a stroke is a transient ischemic attack or TIA.

Ischemic means lack of sufficient blood. A TIA, therefore, is an assault on the brain resulting from a temporary lack of blood supply.

In a TIA, a person briefly experiences vague symptoms of a stroke — numbness, loss of muscle strength, speech difficulty, even temporary deafness or blindness. The crucial difference between a TIA and a stroke is that TIA symptoms quickly fade. The person returns to normal within moments, or more rarely, within a day.

Unfortunately, too many people ignore TIA symptoms. After all, the symptoms go away. Or else people assume that the episode is due to overwork, lack of sleep, a skipped meal, or some other minor cause. That assumption could be fatal.

A transient ischemic attack is an ominous warning that a serious stroke may be about to occur. Neurologists estimate that about a third of TIA patients go on to have strokes.

Anyone who has symptoms of a TIA should seek medical attention at once.

To discover how frequently TIA's occur and how TIA patients fare in the following months and years, a number of cerebrovascular research centers supported by the National Institute of Neurological and Communicative Disorders and Stroke are establishing TIA registries. At Bowman Gray School of Medicine, for example, patients admitted to the hospital with TIA symptoms are entered into the registry, undergo a battery of tests, and provide detailed medical histories.

• ***High blood pressure (hypertension)***. A common and important risk factor for stroke is high blood pressure, which strains the heart and walls of arteries. High blood pressure is found in 70 percent of hemorrhagic stroke cases. Fortunately, early detection of hypertension and a growing number of medications are helping bring this risk factor under control.

However, many stroke victims do not have high blood pressure. The absence of hypertension is no assurance that one is immune to stroke.

• ***Atherosclerosis***. The disorder that used to be known as arteriosclerosis or "hardening of the arteries" is more accurately called *atherosclerosis*.

The Greek words give a good description of the condition: an *atheroma* is a lumpy tumor; *sclerosis* means "hardness." If a physician says you have atherosclerosis, that means lumps of fatty substances have built up on the inside of your arteries making them thick, rough, and less flexible.

Atherosclerosis may begin in childhood. Examinations of soldiers in their twenties and thirties who were killed in Korea and Vietnam confirmed that, in many, fatty deposits called plaques had already developed around the heart and in the large artery arising from the heart. In time, plaques occur in more distant arteries, bunching up especially at points where the arteries branch. Such a major junction occurs in the carotid arteries in the neck. That is why so much attention focuses on these arteries as sources of clots that can plug brain arteries.

Many neurological scientists are studying how atherosclerosis affects blood circulation within the brain. They have learned, for example, that when stroke is due to hypertensive atherosclerosis, about one-fifth of the survivors are left with varying degrees of dementia. Dementia is the neurological disorder associated with a loss of mental skills.

• ***Heart disease***. Common heart ailments, such as coronary artery disease and valve defects, often result in clots that may break loose and be carried by the blood into the brain.

• ***Diabetes***. Diabetes is commonly considered a disease affecting only the body's ability to use sugar. But it is also associated with destructive changes in blood vessels throughout the body. Diabetic patients are therefore at risk for developing a stroke. Equally serious, if their blood sugar is high at the time of the stroke, brain damage is usually more severe and extensive than when blood sugar is normal or low.

• *Obesity*. Excess weight burdens the heart and blood vessels and increases the risk of heart disease, high blood pressure, and diabetes. If the overweight person's diet is rich in salty foods, fats, and cholesterol, so much the worse, for these ingredients can contribute to high blood pressure and atherosclerosis.

• *Lack of exercise*. A sedentary life may not in itself cause a stroke, but often is a companion to obesity. Even moderate amounts of exercise may strengthen the heart and improve circulation. Exercise may even help dissolve atherosclerotic plaques.

• *Other risks*. Other factors that have been implicated in stroke are:

- Continued high levels of stress
- Hereditary disorders that lead to the accumulation of fat or cholesterol in blood
- Sickle cell anemia
- Other blood disorders.

Use of birth control pills, particularly for a long time and in those who smoke, has also been associated with an increased tendency to form blood clots.

New research gives new hope

An important driving force in stroke research today is the realization that stroke need never happen. "Neurologists are tuned in to the fact that you can identify, intervene, and prevent," says one leading stroke investigator.

At the same time, the new discovery that the brain has unexpected powers of repair and regeneration has inspired scientists to find ways to treat stroke during the acute stage. Major research studies include:

• *PET*. Positron emission tomography is a new technique for producing pictures of the brain. But these brain images are different from the pictures obtained through X rays. X rays show how the brain looks — its anatomy. PET, on the other hand, shows how the brain works — its chemical activity, or metabolism.

PET scanning relies on the need of active brain cells to burn glucose as fuel. Scientists can attach a harmless radioactive tag to glucose. This tagged glucose is injected into a vein and the PET scanner shows where the glucose goes once it reaches the brain.

The most active brain cells use the most fuel. So, they will absorb the greatest amounts of glucose. Without causing the patient any pain, detectors outside the patient's head can identify sites where large amounts of glucose are being used. The detector does this by recording the amount of radioactivity that the cells at these sites give off.

A computer then translates these measurements into a color-coded image of the brain: the most active cells appear as light or bright areas, and less active or diseased tissue appears darker.

Because the NINCDS believes so strongly in the research potential of this new technique, it established a national PET Research Program: major research centers around the country, including a center at its own research facility in Bethesda, Md. All are working to perfect the PET technique, and to use it to conquer brain disease.

Neuroscientists hope that PET studies may shed light on why some stroke patients experience severe mental or emotional changes that seem out of proportion to the size of their stroke lesion. One possibility: large areas of the brain remote from the stroke may have been damaged as a result of broken nerve connections in the brain. A PET scan might show this damaged area as a dark region, indicating low activity.

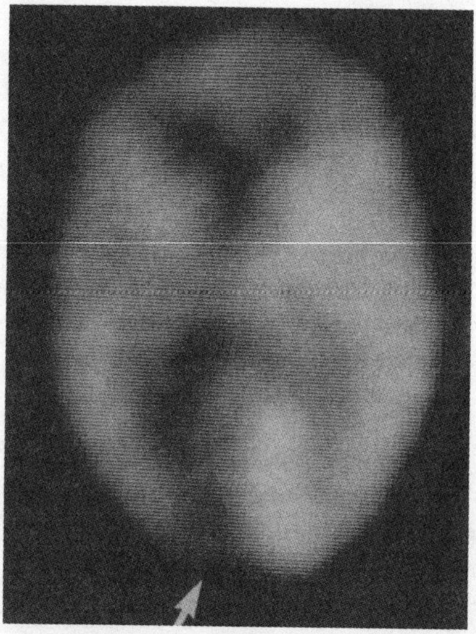

The darker, lower left side of this PET scan of a stroke patient's brain indicates low blood flow and low activity of nerve cells on the injured side. Arrow marks the site of an infarct.

• *New ultrasonic techniques.* The NINCDS-supported cerebrovascular research center at Bowman Gray School of Medicine is considered a world leader in the new science of *neurosonology* — the use of sound waves to study the nervous system.

Devices under development there are expected to provide dynamic images of brain arteries deep within the brain.

At the same time, engineers are refining and perfecting portable ultrasonic equipment that can be used at a patient's bedside to monitor changes in blood flow in the course of stroke.

With other devices under study, scientists can measure the thickness of the several layers that make up the walls of arteries. They can compare the appearance of healthy arteries which have highly flexible walls with arteries that have become stretched and stiff as the result of disease or aging. Studies of normal volunteers already suggest that a two-pack-a-day cigarette habit in a teenager may prematurely stiffen and thicken the arteries in the neck, making the blood vessels of a 16-year-old look like those of a middle-aged person.

• *Aspirin studies.* Several research studies have suggested that small daily doses of aspirin can protect against stroke by lessening the severity or number of transient ischemic attacks.

Normally, a tear or other injury in a blood vessel wall serves as a signal that attracts certain small particles, called blood platelets, to the injury site. The platelets stick to the vessel wall, sealing the leak or covering the injury. They then manufacture chemical messengers that summon still more platelets to the scene, where they clump together.

Aspirin interferes with an enzyme the platelets use to manufacture these messengers. Platelets are then less likely to clump, and a clot less likely to form and obstruct blood flow to the brain.

Atherosclerotic stroke patients appear to have especially "sticky" platelets, ready to clump together at the slightest provocation. That provocation is provided by the fatty plaques that line arterial walls: the plaques dig into the wall, causing injuries that call the platelets into action.

Aspirin has been shown to be effective in preventing thrombotic stroke. But experts have yet to decide what amount of aspirin would be most effective, or even if aspirin is the ideal drug to prevent stroke. In stroke patients with ulcers, for example, aspirin may create bleeding problems.

Aspirin studies have reawakened interest in a chemical called *prostacyclin*. This chemical is manufactured in muscle cells in the artery wall. Like aspirin, prostacyclin inhibits the clumping of platelets. The substance is being studied as a possible treatment for stroke at the NINCDS-supported University of Oregon stroke research center.

• *Fish oil diets*. The cod liver oil you may have had to swallow as a child may turn out to have unexpected benefits in stroke prevention for adults. Observers have long noted that people whose diet is rich in fish, like the Eskimos, seldom suffer heart attacks or strokes. Investigators have turned their attention to a particular ingredient in fish, eicosapentaenic acid. They think this acid may somehow protect against atherosclerosis.

There are many questions: no one knows what a radical change in diet might do to adults. Investigators at Bowman Gray School of Medicine plan to study the effects of adding fish oil to the diet of laboratory monkeys over a 3-year period, and will compare results with monkeys maintained on normal diets.

• *Endorphin studies*. The brain may react to injury by releasing certain natural substances called *endorphins*. The endorphins are chemicals important in the control of pain. Some experiments suggest that they may also lower blood pressure. If so, brain tissue damaged by a stroke — an injury that promotes the production of endorphins — might get less blood and suffer even greater damage. Following that lead, some investigators are experimenting with agents that block the action of endorphins. In this way, they hope to improve blood circulation in the stroke patient's brain.

• *Animal models*. Animal studies are essential to advancing our understanding of what happens to the brain in a stroke. In recent years, investigators have been able to induce stroke in gerbils and rats. One series of rat experiments has been particularly intriguing: it shows striking differences in the degree of brain damage sustained by the rats, depending on whether they had eaten or fasted before the stroke. Fasting rats showed limited nerve cell damage, restricted to certain brain areas. In rats that had eaten, the damage was generalized and often the rats died.

Investigators assume these differences relate to how the brain uses glucose. Nerve cells normally break down glucose, using oxygen available from blood. When deprived of oxygen, as in a stroke, the cells resort to an alternative method of breaking down glucose — a method that produces acids. As the acids accumulate, they may actually poison the cell or create such an acid environment that the cell is unable to carry out normal activities. If this theory holds up, it might lead to new treatments using buffering agents to neutralize acids produced during the acute stage of stroke.

These examples are among the many research attempts being made to analyze the moment-by-moment changes in the brain in response to stroke, and to identify the conditions that favor repair of all damage and restoration of normal brain activity.

At the other end of the spectrum are NINCDS-supported stroke data banks which compile data on large populations of stroke patients. These banks record age, type of stroke, the patient's other medical problems, prior TIA's, and dozens of other bits of information in the hope of discovering which variables are most useful in predicting how well the stroke victim fares.

Where to go for help

The new emphasis on stroke research, on finding better treatments and means of prevention, is affecting the health care system in America as a whole. Someone who needs treatment for stroke might seek out one of the NINCDS-supported cerebrovascular clinical research centers. There are also many excellent stroke units in major research and teaching hospitals, and in smaller community hospitals as well.

Good rehabilitation centers, too, can be found in all 50 states. For recommendations, consult major teaching hospitals in your area or local chapters of the National Easter Seal Society. The Will Rogers Institute, listed below with other stroke-related organizations, can also provide help in locating rehabilitation centers.

It is heartening to know that good treatment and proper rehabilitation can make a big difference in how a stroke patient feels and in what he or she can do. But it is still not clear what happens in recovery. Do patients regain skills because blood vessels near the site of injury have expanded to compensate for the lost blood supply and thus saved nerve cells? Were some nerve cells able to survive the stroke and regenerate? Did healthy neurons nearby grow new axons and restore connections across the damaged area? Or did the brain, by some fancy feat of rewiring, find alternate pathways for brain signals and enable healthy cells to take over for damaged ones?

The answer that Agnes de Mille likes best is what her neurologist told her after her spectacular recovery:

"Your brain didn't get better, Agnes; you did."

Voluntary health organizations

Voluntary health organizations, including the sampling listed here, are excellent sources of help for stroke patients and their families.

The *American Heart Association* supports research and education on heart disease, stroke, and other disorders affecting circulation. Association chapters in many cities sponsor stroke clubs where patients and families can meet to exchange ideas and practical advice, or hear speakers discuss the latest research or stroke treatments. The association also publishes a number of excellent pamphlets and guides, including:

Strike Back at Stroke
Up and Around
Do It Yourself Again — Self-Help Devices for the Stroke Patient
Stroke: Why Do They Behave That Way?
Stroke: A Guide for the Family

For further information, contact:

American Heart Association
7320 Greenville Avenue
Dallas, TX 75231
(214) 750-5300

The *National Easter Seal Society* is concerned with research, education, treatment, and rehabilitation for children and adults with physical disabilities, speech and language problems, and other disabling conditions. Consult local chapters for information or write to the main office:

National Easter Seal Society, Inc.
2023 West Ogden Avenue
Chicago, IL 60612
(312) 243-8400

The *Stroke Foundation* provides information and education on stroke and stroke prevention:

The Stroke Foundation, Inc.
898 Park Avenue
New York, NY 10021
(212) 734-3434

The *Dwight D. Eisenhower Institute for Stroke Research* promotes research in stroke, provides funds for training young physicians interested in careers in stroke research, and provides helpful information. Its pamphlets include:

Stroke: What It Is, What Causes It
Living At Home After A Stroke

For further information, contact:

Dwight D. Eisenhower Institute for Stroke Research, Inc.
785 Mamaroneck Avenue
White Plains, NY 10605
(914) 946-3062

The *Will Rogers Institute* provides information on stroke rehabilitation centers throughout the U.S.:

Will Rogers Institute
785 Mamaroneck Avenue
White Plains, NY 10605
(914)761-5550

U.S. Government publications

The National Institute of Neurological and Communicative Disorders and Stroke offers pamphlets and other materials on stroke and stroke-related conditions:

Aphasia: Hope Through Research
The Dementias: Hope Through Research
What You Should Know About Stroke and Stroke Prevention
List of NINCDS-supported cerebrovascular clinical research centers.

Copies are free in limited quantities from:

Office of Scientific and Health Reports
National Institute of Neurological and
Communicative Disorders and Stroke
National Institutes of Health
Building 31, Room 8A06
Bethesda, MD 20205
(301)496-5751

Stroke Glossary

aneurysm: abnormal stretching or widening of a blood vessel wall. A ruptured aneurysm can cause a stroke.

anticoagulant: substance that reduces blood clotting.

aphasia: loss of the ability to speak or to understand language, including printed words.

cerebrovascular: related to blood vessels of the brain.

embolus: traveling blood clot, which can "plug" a brain artery and cause a stroke.

endorphin: a natural brain chemical that controls pain. Endorphins may also lower blood pressure.

hemisphere: half-sphere; refers to the right or left half of the brain.

hemispheric neglect: tendency among some stroke patients to act as though one side of their body and its functions do not exist.

infarct: mass of tissue consisting of a blood clot and other debris which can block a blood vessel and cause a stroke.

ischemia: lack of sufficient blood.

neurotransmitter: chemical messenger used by the nervous system to move nerve signals from one nerve cell to another.

platelet: small particle in the blood which is attracted to a torn or injured blood vessel wall, sealing the leak or covering the injury. Platelets manufacture chemicals which attract more platelets to the scene of the injury.

stroke: one form of cerebrovascular disease, usually due to an embolus, thrombus, or hemorrhage.

thrombus: clot or lump that forms within an artery, blocking blood flow.

transient ischemic attack (TIA): temporary lack of blood supply in the brain causing brief stroke symptoms. A TIA is a major warning sign of possible stroke. It requires immediate medical attention.

Chapter 28

Stuttering

Stuttering

"What dressing will you have on your salad?" the waiter said.
"R r r r r r-ro-ro-roque-roque-I'll have the roque-I think I'd like to try the ro ro ro ----Thousand Island."

Stutterers laugh at that joke, too. For them, however, stuttering has far more serious consequences than not getting their favorite salad dressing. The frustration and struggle to get the words out can embarrass and exhaust both speaker and listener. Some stutterers avoid the struggle by dodging situations where they have to speak. Children may say "Don't know," to the teacher — even when they do know — rather than face laughter and teasing from their classmates. Other stutterers keep their minds a phrase or two ahead of their mouths. That way, they can pick out problem words and find substitutes. In either case, the stutterer suffers the loss of smooth and easy speech, the spontaneous exchange of feelings and ideas so important at school or work, among family and friends.

"It is like a sharp mmmmmomentary twist of pain that I eexxsss---perience again and again throughout eeeeevery dddddday ah ah of my life. I ss-sssssometimes sssssssssee it as a as a nnnnnnnnail in my shoe that iiiiis thththere and p-p-pro-bab-bly always wwww-ww-wi-ll be there..." says a 36-year-old woman.

Yet there is reason to hope that that woman, and others, particularly younger stutterers, will be able to escape the twist of pain. With therapy — and sometimes without it — many stutterers achieve more normal speech. Studies describing the differences in the way normal and stuttered speech is produced are pointing to new directions in therapy. Spearheading this research is the National Institute of Neurological and Communicative Disorders and Stroke (NINCDS), the leading federal agency supporting research on speech disorders. The institute currently supports investigators who are developing new techniques for the study of normal, as well as abnormal, speech.

Early warning signs

Stuttering is a disorder in which the rhythmic flow, or fluency, of speech is disrupted by rapid-fire repetitions of sounds, prolonged vowels, and complete stops — verbal blocks. A stutterer's speech is often uncontrollable — sometimes faster, but usually slower than the average speaking rate. Sometimes, too, the voice changes in pitch, loudness, and inflection.

Observations of young children during the early stages of stuttering have led to a list of warning signs that can help identify a child who is developing a speech problem. Most children use "um's" and "ah's," and will repeat words or syllables as they learn to speak. It is not a serious concern if a child says, "I like to go and and and and play games," unless such repetitions occur often, more than once every 20 words or so.

Repeating whole words is not necessarily a sign of stuttering; however, repeating speech sounds or syllables such as in the song "K-K-K-Katy" is.

Sometimes a stutterer will exhibit tension while prolonging a sound. For example, the 8-year-old who says, "Ahnnnnnnd---and---thththen I I drank it" with lips trembling at the same time. Children who experience such a stuttering tremor usually become frightened, angry, and frustrated at their inability to speak. A further danger sign is a rise in pitch as the child draws out the syllable.

The appearance of a child or adult experiencing the most severe signs of stuttering is dramatic: As they struggle to get a word out, their whole face may contort, the jaw may jerk, the mouth open, tongue protrude, and eyes roll. Tension can spread through the whole body. A moment of overwhelming struggle occurs during the speech block. The feeling of panic and loss of control is so overwhelming that the stutterer will try to avoid any repetition of the experience in the future. Children may begin to substitute simple words for more troublesome ones; they may giggle before speaking to help get them started, or they may adopt a drawl or other speech mannerism that temporarily displaces the stuttering.

NINCDS is sponsoring a study to analyze the speaking characteristics of young children between 4 and 6 years of age — the time that stuttering most commonly develops. By determining which aspects of speech distinguish those who develop a stuttering problem from those who do not, methods of early detection and improved treatment can be developed.

While the symptoms of stuttering are easy to recognize, the underlying cause remains a mystery. Hippocrates thought that stuttering was due to dryness of the tongue, and he prescribed blistering substances to drain away the black bile responsible. A Roman physician recommended gargling and massages to strengthen a weak tongue. Seventeenth-century scientist Francis Bacon suggested hot wine to thaw a "refrigerated" tongue. Too large a tongue was the fault, according to a 19th-century Prussian physician, so he snipped pieces off stutterers' tongues. Alexander Melville Bell, father of the telephone inventor, insisted stuttering was simply a bad habit that could be overcome by reeducation.

Some theories today attribute stuttering to problems in the control of the muscles of speech. As recently as the fifties and sixties, however, stuttering was thought to arise from deep-rooted personality problems, and psychotherapy was recommended.

Who stutters?

Stutterers represent the whole range of personality types, levels of emotional adjustment, and intelligence. Winston Churchill was a stutterer (or stammerer, as the English prefer to say). So were Sir Isaac Newton, King George VI of England, and writer Somerset Maugham.

There are more than 15 million stutterers in the world today and approximately 1 million in the United States alone.

Most stuttering begins after a child has mastered the basics of speech and is starting to talk automatically. One out of 30 children will then undergo a brief period of stuttering, lasting 6 months or so. Boys are four times as likely as girls to be stutterers.

Occasionally, stuttering arises in an older child or even in an adult. It may follow an illness or an emotionally shattering event, such as a death in the family. Stuttering may also occur following brain injury, either due to head injury or after a stroke. No matter how the problem begins, stutterers generally experience their worst moments under conditions of stress or emotional tension: ordering in a crowded restaurant, talking over the telephone, speaking in public, asking the boss for a raise.

Stuttering does not develop in a predictable pattern. In children, speech difficulties can disappear for weeks or months only to return in full force. About 80 percent of children with a stuttering problem are able to speak normally by the time they are adults — whether they've had therapy or not. Adult stutterers have also been known to stop stuttering for no apparent reason.

Indeed, all stutterers can speak fluently some of the time. Most can also whisper smoothly, speak in unison, and sing with no hesitations. Country and western singer Mel Tillis is an example of a stutterer with a successful singing career.

Most stutterers also speak easily when they are prevented from hearing their own voices, when talking to pets and small children, or when addressing themselves in the mirror. All these instances of fluency demonstrate that nothing is basically wrong with the stutterer's speech machinery.

If the problem is not in the mouth or the throat, is it in the brain? Stuttering can arise from specific brain damage, but only rarely. In general, stuttering is not associated with any measurable brain abnormality and is not related to intelligence.

The new research

To find out what is associated with stuttering, investigators are analyzing how speech sounds are normally produced and what goes wrong when a person stutters.

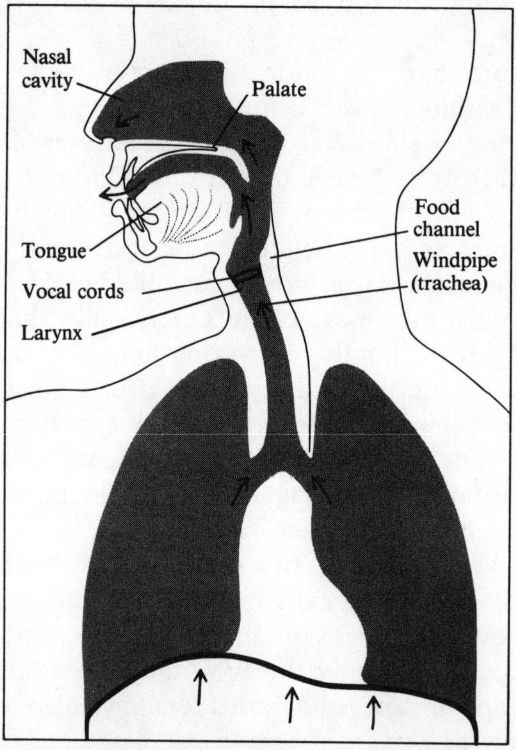

Upward movement of the diaphragm forces air up through the windpipe, setting the vocal cords vibrating. Sounds are shaped into words by movement of other parts of the vocal tract: tongue, lips, teeth, palate.

To produce speech, you must shape the sound that is produced as air moves up from the lungs through the throat and into the mouth. Breathing muscles in the chest provide the pressure that drives air up the windpipe across the voice box, or larynx. At the larynx, the air passes between two folds of tissue known as the vocal cords, and sets them vibrating. Like the reeds of oboes, the vibrating cords convert air flow into audible sound.

The shape and amount of tension of the cords determine the pitch of the voice — how high or low it sounds. The further refining of voice into speech sounds depends on the relative shape and position of other parts of the vocal tract: the lips, tongue, jaws, cheeks, and palate. All told, over 100 muscles are involved in speech production.

Because the larynx is the source of sound, scientists are studying it closely, paying particular attention to the muscles that control the vocal cords. One set of muscles pulls the vocal cords apart, opening the airway. Opening allows you to take a deep breath, for example. An opposing set of muscles closes the vocal cords, allowing you to produce voice. The vocal cords are also in a fully closed position when you swallow. That helps prevent food from getting into the airway and causing choking.

Normally, the laryngeal muscles work in a coordinated and reciprocal manner: one set of muscles relaxes while an opposing set of muscles contracts. When NINCDS-supported investigators at

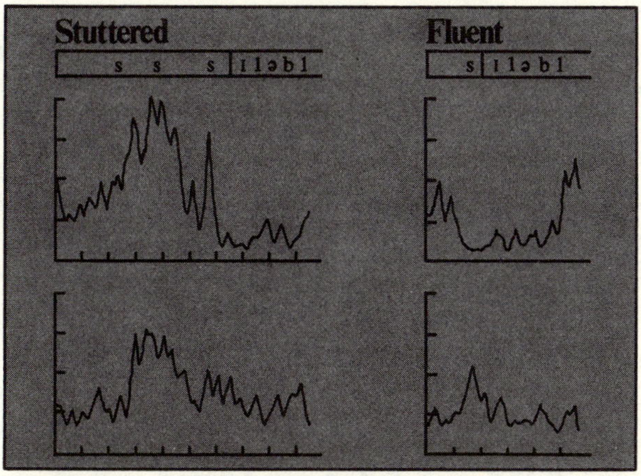

Similar-shaped graphs on left indicate that opposing vocal cord muscles both contract when a person stutters on the word "syllable." Under fluent conditions (right) the graphs are mirror images: when one muscle relaxes, the other contracts.

Haskins Laboratories, New Haven, Conn. studied the behavior of the laryngeal muscles during stuttered speech, however, they were astonished to find that both sets of muscles contracted — setting up a virtual tug of war for control of the cords. This striking difference between normal and abnormal muscle behavior can be observed in the same speaker when speaking fluently and when stuttering.

Scientists have also noted excessive muscle activity during stuttering. Not only do both sets of opposing muscles contract during stuttering, but they also contract as hard as they can.

Ingenious techniques have enabled scientists to record the abnormal muscle movements. Investigators can hook wires directly into throat and neck muscles, for example, and pick up the electrical activity associated with muscle movement. They can also observe the movements of the vocal cords directly by using special fiber-optic equipment, transmitting light through a flexible narrow tube which is inserted into the subject's nose.

In some cases, the inappropriate muscle activity prevents the vocal cords from coming together long enough to make a normal sound. In other cases, the vocal cords are so tightly locked no sound at all can emerge: the speaker is totally blocked. Unusually high levels of muscle activity have also been discovered in stutterers' tongue muscles. Whether the extreme muscle contractions cause the failure of coordination of the muscles of speech, or are a reaction to the failure, is not known. Conditions that reduce muscle activity, however, appear to ease stuttering.

The muscle activity associated with partial or complete verbal blocks is not the only aspect of stutterers' speech scientists have analyzed. Both trained and untrained listeners can distinguish the voices of stutterers, when speaking fluently, from normal speakers. A slower rate of speech and an abnormal rhythm were the cues that identified the stutterers. Such differences may result from the stutterer's habit of planning words ahead to avoid a block and consciously trying to control the speech muscles.

Experiments in several laboratories have shown that stutterers are slower than normal speakers to begin vocalizations (for instance, when they are told to make a sound as soon as a signal goes on). Stutterers are also slower to make transitions from voiced sounds (when the vocal cords vibrate) to unvoiced sounds (when the vocal cords do not vibrate). When a stutterer switches from ordinary speech to some nonstuttering mode, such as choral speaking, the rate of speech also tends to decrease. So, some scientists speculate that stutterers have a lower than normal maximum speaking rate. Their everyday speech frequently exceeds that limit, however, and trips them up.

Improved techniques have led to a more detailed description of stuttering and the conclusion by some scientists that what we call stuttering may be more than one condition. Each condition, in turn, may have a different cause. Another conjecture is that stuttering results from the interaction of several factors. For example, a child may inherit a tendency to stutter, but certain environmental conditions may have to be present for stuttering to develop.

Stuttering does seem to run in families, and it affects boys more than girls. NINCDS-supported scientists at Yale University have studied 555 stutterers and more than 2,000 of their close relatives. The results support the idea that a susceptibility to stuttering is inherited, but just how is not clear. Certainly the inheritance pattern does not follow the simple rules that explain how eye color, hair color, or colorblindness is inherited.

To search for a clue to a cause of stuttering — genetic or otherwise — investigators are adopting newly available techniques to investigate brain activity in stutterers. Since the brain is the master regulator and coordinator of all body activity, it is possible that some slight brain dysfunction might disturb the clockwork coordination of the organs of speech. On those occasions when stutterers do speak fluently, the coordination task is usually simplified. Whispering, for example, does not involve vibration of the vocal cords at all.

A subtle brain dysfunction might also affect our ability to hear what we're saying as we say it. Alterations in that hearing "feedback" system, or in similar systems monitoring other parts of the speech production machinery, may also be involved in stuttering. Scientists are also just beginning to examine the brain areas that are active during normal and stuttered speech. Important, too, are studies of how the two halves of the brain, the cerebral hemispheres, interact in speech activities.

New treatments and old schools

While research has yet to explain why stuttering occurs, some of the new findings have been applied to therapy:

- ***Biofeedback.*** One recent approach uses biofeedback techniques to help stutterers relax their throat muscles. The stutterer hears a tone that becomes louder with increased muscle tension, and he or she is instructed to quiet the tone. Usually when the person succeeds in reducing the tension of the throat muscles, he or she is able to speak without stuttering.

• ***Larynx control.*** Some treatment programs emphasize modifying sound production at the larynx itself. Stutterers are taught to speak with lower levels of laryngeal activity, slower rates of vocal cord opening and closing, and loose, rather than tight, vocal cord closure. The resultant voice is somewhat lower, softer, smoother, and slower than average speech. To evaluate this technique, as well as other approaches to stuttering therapy, long-term studies will be necessary.

• ***Regulating speech rate.*** Some patients are taught to slow their overall speech rate. Devices used in such training include ear receivers that play back the speaker's words with a few seconds' delay (delayed auditory feedback). Sometimes, a slow "pacing" tone is presented to one ear to provide a rhythm for the stutterer to follow in pronouncing syllables. Although both devices reduce stuttering, they often result in monotonous speech. However, for some patients, monotonous but fluent speech may be better than severe stuttering.

In general, therapists employing the new techniques in treating stuttering belong to one of two traditional schools. One school believes that stutterers and non-stutterers fall into two distinct groups and that no adult stutterer can be completely cured. Therapists of that conviction teach their clients to stutter easily. Stutterers learn to reduce the tension and struggle so that they do not become completely blocked in speech. Once a person gains confidence in the skill to stutter easily, the frequency of stuttering often drops dramatically. Because normal speakers do stutter occasionally, recipients of the "stutter easy" therapy can learn to speak without noticeable hesitations.

Charles Van Riper, the leading proponent of that approach and a stutterer himself, says, "Stuttering is not the world's worst of all curses . . . about 99.9 percent of the problem is in the way you respond to the thing!"

The other major school of therapy believes that any stutterer can be taught to be completely fluent. Therapists use methods such as breath control and soft, gentle attacks on words to create fluent speech with no stuttering. Preventing relapses of stuttering once fluency is reached is the most difficult problem with this approach.

A variety of training devices are used by both groups to allow a stutterer to experience fluent speech. A metronome can repress stuttering by setting a slower than normal rate for speech. A relatively new instrument called a masker prevents the stutterer from hearing his or her own voice during a conversation. The portable model consists of earphones and a microphone that rests on the throat near the larynx. Whenever the wearer speaks, the device makes a humming noise in the earphones so the wearer cannot hear his or her words. The device is successful in preventing stuttering even in difficult situations, and some stutterers have found that by using it they eventually learn to speak more fluently unassisted.

The hope for children

Therapists from both schools agree that the development of stuttering in young children is reversible. Treatment often includes the parents as well as the child. Parents are cautioned to listen to the content of the child's speech rather than to how he or she speaks. They are encouraged to be patient, and make speech enjoyable by playing word games and by reading or telling stories. The parents themselves are taught to speak slowly, quietly, and calmly, attacking their words gently. Overall, parents are advised to create pleasant and rewarding situations in which the child can communicate, and to reduce stress in the child's life that can disrupt fluency.

Therapists from both schools also agree that motivation is a key to success. The stutterer who feels frustrated and deprived of normal participation in speech is ripe for therapy. Usually, it is best for the stutterer to specify exactly what he or she wants to change rather than just express a vague desire to stop stuttering. Results are more likely to be satisfactory if individuals decide that they most want to reduce their physiological struggle, for example, or change their speaking pattern, or lower anxiety.

Where to go for treatment

In some places in the world, anyone can hang out a shingle as a speech therapist. But in the United States, more than 20 states have laws governing the credentials of speech therapists, who also are called speech-language pathologists. The American Speech-Language-Hearing Association, through its standards board, certifies or accredits individual practitioners, educational programs, and service agencies. Approximately 24,000 speech pathologists work in U.S. schools, hospitals, clinics, private practices, and health departments. Selection of a licensed or certified speech therapist does not guarantee an expert on stuttering therapy, but the therapist should be able to refer the stutterer to an appropriate practitioner.

Evaluating the treatments available for stuttering is a particularly frustrating problem. For one thing, a fraction of stutterers improve with little or no treatment. For another, investigators must follow their subjects for years to see whether any improvement is long lasting. Over a period of 5 to 10 years, therapy techniques continue to evolve. So, by the time the results of therapy are evaluated, newer methods may have supplanted those being evaluated.

From another standpoint, the very fact that new techniques are developing and older ones are undergoing revision or refinement is encouraging. Stutterers who quit trying to improve their speech years ago should be advised to try again.

To make a decision about treatment or to exchange ideas and opinions, it may be helpful to join one of the self-help groups for persons who stutter. These groups discuss the problems stutterers face in their daily lives, as well as developments in stuttering research and therapy. They also help stutterers to understand how other people react to them. The National Council of Adult Stutterers and the National Stuttering Project may be able to refer a stutterer to a nearby group.

If you have a friend who stutters or if you come into contact with stutterers, there are ways to ease the embarrassment and frustration. First, try to be patient, though you have other demands on your time. Second, try to maintain eye contact, even when the stutterer looks away during a stuttering block. Finally, never fill in words for the person who stutters. That reinforces a feeling of time pressure and takes away the triumph of finally saying the difficult word.

One scientist who works on stuttering calls it the most fascinating and most frustrating communicative disorder. After years of research, the feeling persists that the missing pieces of the stuttering puzzle are close at hand. Rather than having a simple cause — thick tongue or black bile or weak breath control — stuttering may be so complex that scientists will unravel the wonders of normal speech as they search for effective treatment.

For additional information:

American Speech-Language-Hearing Association
10801 Rockville Pike
Rockville, Md. 20852
(301) 897-5700

National Council of Adult Stutterers
c/o Speech and Hearing Clinic
Catholic University of America
Washington, D.C. 20064
(202) 635-5556

National Stuttering Project
4438 Park Boulevard
Oakland, Calif. 94602
(415)530-1678

National Easter Seal Society, Inc.
2023 W. Ogden Avenue
Chicago, Ill. 60612
(312) 243-8400

Division for Children with Communication Disorders
The Council for Exceptional Children
1920 Association Drive
Reston, Va. 22091
(703) 620-3660

National Association for Hearing and Speech Action
Suite 1000
6110 Executive Boulevard
Rockville, Md. 20852
(301) 897-8682

Speech Foundation of America
152 Lombardy Road
Memphis, Tenn. 38111
(901) 452-0995

Three good films on the prevention of stuttering were underwritten by the Speech Foundation of America: Part 1 — *Identifying the Danger Signs*, Part II — *Parent Counseling and the Elimination of the Problem*, and Part III — *Ssstuttering and Your Child. Is it you? Is it me?* The films are available for purchase or rent to self-help groups, schools, and other organizations interested in speech disorders. Write to:

Seven Oaks Productions
9145 Sligo Creek Parkway
Silver Spring, Md. 20901

Specific inquiries concerning programs on stuttering may be directed to:

NINCDS Office of Scientific and Health Reports
Bldg.31, Room 8A-06
National Institutes of Health
Bethesda, Md. 20205

Chapter 29

Torsion Dystonia

Torsion Dystonia

What is torsion dystonia?

Torsion dystonia — also called dystonia musculorum deformans, or DMD — is an incapacitating neurologic disorder which causes patients to twist or writhe in repeated and uninterrupted involuntary movements. The movements may affect a single muscle; a group of muscles such as those in the arms, legs, or neck; or the entire body. Experts have lately been referring to this disorder as "the dystonias," indicating a group of related diseases rather than a single disorder.

What are the symptoms?

Early signs can be very mild and may be noticeable only after prolonged exertion, or with stress or fatigue. Handwriting may deteriorate after the patient writes several lines; there may be foot cramps, and one foot may tend to pull up or drag after the patient has run a distance or walked home from school. The neck may turn or pull involuntarily, especially when the patient is tired. There may be other involuntary movements. Other possible symptoms are tremor and speech difficulties. Over a period of time, the movement disorders may become more noticeable and widespread; sometimes, however, there is little or no progression.

What causes torsion dystonia?

The cause of torsion dystonia is as yet unknown. Some investigators and physicians believe the disorder results from an abnormality in an area of the brain called the basal ganglia. They suspect a defect in the body's ability to process a particular group of chemicals which help transmit nerve impulses.

How many forms of torsion dystonia are there?

Dystonia has been classified into three forms. Two are inherited and one is acquired.

A *recessively inherited* form results when both parents, who appear normal, but carry a defective gene, pass it on to their child. All the children of such parents are at risk of inheriting the defective genes. About one-quarter of them inherit one defective gene from each parent — the so-called "double dose" — and so develop dystonia.

The existence of this recessive form has been confirmed by scientists at the National Institute of Neurological and Communicative Disorders and Stroke (NINCDS) who are studying the genetics and epidemiology (occurrence and distribution) of dystonia. The recessive form is found most often in persons of Ashkenazic Jewish (eastern European) ancestry. One in every 100 Jewish persons of this origin in the United States carries the defective gene.

A *dominantly inherited* form of torsion dystonia can be passed on by one parent. A parent who carries the gene for this form generally has dystonic symptoms, and any child born to such a parent has a 50 percent chance of also developing dystonia.

There is also an *acquired* form of dystonia resulting from environmental causes. Birth injury (particularly due to lack of oxygen), certain infections, reactions to certain drugs, intoxication with heavy metals or carbon monoxide, trauma, or stroke can cause torsion dystonia.

How do these three forms differ?

With the *recessive* form, dystonic symptoms generally appear between the ages of 5 and 16, usually in the patient's foot or, less often, in the hand. The involuntary dystonic movements may progress quickly to involve all limbs and the torso, but the rate of progression slows noticeably after adolescence. People with this type of dystonia may have higher than normal intelligence, suggesting that the gene for recessive torsion dystonia has some relationship to intellectual potential.

The *dominant* form strikes people in a wider age range, but usually symptoms emerge late in adolescence or early in adulthood. The torso is generally involved early, and patients often have involuntary movements of the neck muscles (called torticollis) as well. Symptoms may progress slowly, but their progression continues beyond adolescence.

Studies of dominant dystonia strengthen the suspicion that there is an abnormality in one or more of the chemicals involved in the transmission of impulses from one nerve cell to another. It is still not certain whether these abnormalities are present in people who carry the gene but do not get the disease, or in people who have not yet shown any symptoms but will later on.

In the *acquired* form of dystonia, people often have abnormal movements of just one side of the body, which begin at the time of the brain injury. Symptoms generally do not get worse, and do not spread to other parts of the body.

What are the stages of dystonia?

Dystonia often progresses through various stages. During the first stage, dystonic movements are sporadic and appear only during voluntary movements or stress. Later, patients may show dystonic postures and movements while walking, and ultimately even while they are relaxed. Dystonic motions may lead to permanent physical deformities by causing tendons to shorten and connective tissue to build up in the muscle.

Is there any treatment?

As yet, there is no known treatment for the underlying disorder, but mild dystonic symptoms can sometimes be controlled by drugs such as diazepam (Valium®), which relaxes muscles. Some patients have been helped by drugs such as Artane®, which affect the metabolism of the chemicals that transmit impulses from cell to cell. Another drug, L-dopa, can cause dystonic symptoms in some patients with Parkinson's disease, yet, ironically, can help alleviate symptoms in some patients with dystonia. Fortunately, more and more scientists are joining the search for effective drugs.

In a few cases, advanced dystonia has been helped, at least temporarily, by surgery on the thalamus, a structure that lies deep within the brain.

What research is being done?

The ultimate goals of research are discovering the cause of dystonia so the disorder can be prevented, and finding a cure or improved treatment for people now afflicted. Several organizations, including NINCDS and voluntary health agencies established to help dystonia patients and their families, are supporting basic and clinical studies, both by scientists at the National Institutes of Health and at medical centers throughout the country.

These studies are providing physicians and other health workers with clues for identifying people who are at risk for developing dystonia. These clues should lead to better genetic counseling. Meanwhile, scientists are continuing the search for drugs that may help treat dystonic symptoms. Investigators are also seeking better surgical techniques to treat symptoms, including implantation of electrical stimulating devices, which aid in normal nerve impulse transmission.

Is more information available?

Patients can keep informed of current research advances by maintaining close contact with their private physicians.

Three privately supported voluntary health agencies are working in the field of dystonia:

The Dystonia Foundation, Inc.
425 Broad Hollow Road
Melville, New York 11747
(516) 249-7799

Dystonia Medical Research Foundation
Suite 416
9615 Brighton Way
Beverly Hills, California 90210
(213) 272-0353

National Foundation for Jewish Genetic Diseases
Suite 1200
609 Fifth Avenue
New York, New York 10017
(212) 753-5155

All of these organizations will supply literature about their activities and services.

Chapter 30

Tourette Syndrome

Tourette Syndrome (Multiple Tic Disorder)

What is Tourette syndrome?

Tourette syndrome is a neurological disorder characterized by involuntary muscular movements, uncontrollable vocal sounds, and inappropriate words. These multiple tics usually begin when the patient is between the ages of 2 and 16. Males are afflicted about three times more often than females.

What are the symptoms?

The first symptoms of Tourette syndrome are usually facial tics: the patient blinks his eyes excessively, twitches his nose, or grimaces. As the condition progresses, he may repeatedly stretch his neck, stamp his feet, or twist and bend his body.

The Tourette patient eventually produces strange uncontrollable and unacceptable sounds. He may continuously clear his throat, cough, sniff, grunt, bark, or shout. Some patients involuntarily shout obscenities (coprolalia), or constantly repeat the words of other people (echolalia). Victims may touch other people excessively, or repeat actions obsessively and unnecessarily. A few patients bite their lips and cheeks, bang their heads against hard objects, and develop other self-destructive behavior.

Can patients control their tics?

Tourette syndrome patients can sometimes control tics for a short time but, eventually, tension mounts and the tics once again appear. Tics become worse during periods of stress. They improve when the patient is not anxious, or is absorbed in an activity. In most instances, tics disappear during sleep.

What causes Tourette syndrome?

The basic cause of Tourette syndrome is unknown. Current research has focused on the possibility that a chemical abnormality is involved which affects neurotransmitter systems used by the brain to regulate movement and behavior. Neurotransmitters are chemicals that carry signals from one nerve cell to another in the brain and spinal cord and along the nerves.

How is Tourette syndrome treated?

Physicians have had some success treating Tourette syndrome patients with haloperidol. This drug, also known as Haldol, suppresses symptoms for many patients, but does not cure the condition. The long-term side effects of Haldol are not yet known. Some short-term side effects, such as muscular rigidity, drooling, and restlessness, can be reduced by drugs commonly used to treat Parkinson's disease — Artane or Cogentin, for example. Other side effects such as fatigue, depression, anxiety, weight gain, and difficulties in thinking clearly may be more troublesome. Patients with mild Tourette syndrome symptoms may be able to do without any medication.

Haldol should be administered by a physician familiar with the drug and with Tourette syndrome. Haldol is given in very small doses that are increased slowly, usually every fifth day, until the best possible balance between symptoms and side effects is achieved.

Do Tourette patients need psychotherapy?

Psychological problems do not cause Tourette syndrome, and psychotherapy does not help suppress the patient's tics. However, psychotherapy may help the patient cope with his disorder, and deal with the social and emotional problems that sometimes accompany it.

What research is being done?

Research on Tourette syndrome is being supported at major medical institutions throughout the country by the National Institute of Neurological and Communicative Disorders and Stroke, and is under way at its laboratories at the National Institutes of Health. The National Institute of Child Health and Human Development and the National Institute of Mental Health are also supporting research of relevance to Tourette syndrome.

- Pharmacologic studies. New drugs are being tested that might help patients who do not respond to Haldol or who cannot tolerate the drug's side effects.
- Genetic studies. Families of Tourette syndrome patients have a higher than normal incidence of tics, and some families have more than one member suffering from the disorder. Scientists believe that there is a familial form of Tourette syndrome.
- Neurotransmitter studies. Abnormally low levels of brain

chemicals called neurotransmitters have been found in patients with Parkinson's disease, and effective drug therapy to counter the deficiency has been developed. Scientists hope this avenue of research will prove equally fruitful in solving some of the mysteries of Tourette syndrome.

Research also focuses on the synapse — the essential junction where neurotransmitter chemicals carry impulses from one nerve to another. Together, neurotransmission and synaptogenesis account for about half of the research dollars currently being devoted directly and indirectly to Tourette syndrome.

Scientists seeking grant support for research in Tourette syndrome are urged to contact the National Institute of Neurological and Communicative Disorders and Stroke at the National Institutes of Health. Inquiries may be addressed to:

Joseph Drage, M.D.
Chief, Developmental Neurology Branch
Convulsive, Developmental, and
Neuromuscular Disorders Program
NINCDS
Federal Building, Room 816
Bethesda, Maryland 20205
Telephone: (301) 496-6701

What is the prognosis?

Patients with Tourette syndrome can expect to live a normal life span. Although the condition is generally lifelong and chronic, Tourette syndrome is not a degenerative disorder. Intelligence is normal. In a handful of cases, complete remission occurs after adolescence.

What is the best educational setting?

Students with Tourette syndrome should be placed in educational settings according to their individual needs. Many patients function well in the regular classroom. Others, whose symptoms greatly interfere with their academic or social adjustment, may need smaller classes, special classes, or special schools.

All Tourette students require a tolerant and compassionate setting that encourages them to work to their full potential and that is flexible enough to accommodate their special needs. This setting may need to include a private study area, exams outside the regular classroom, or even oral exams, if the child's symptoms interfere with his ability to write. Time limits are a major source of stress for Tourette students.

Psychological problems and, frequently, minimal brain dysfunction may compound educational problems for Tourette patients. Investigators believe that more than half of Tourette patients suffer from some degree of minimal brain dysfunction. Children with minimal brain dysfunction have a normal range of intelligence, but their short attention span, low frustration tolerance, hyperactivity, poor coordination, and specific areas of learning disability make it probable that they will need special attention in school. Psychological problems that may arise as a consequence of Tourette syndrome, and symptoms of minimal brain dysfunction must be treated on an individual basis.

Is there a voluntary agency to help Tourette patients and families?

Yes. The Tourette Syndrome Association, Inc., is a voluntary, nonprofit organization of patients, their families and friends, and health care professionals. The goals of the association are:

- To education physicians and the general public about Tourette syndrome, with a view toward promoting more accurate diagnosis and better treatment.
- To stimulate and support research on Tourette syndrome.
- To be of service to patients and their families.

For further information write:

Tourette Syndrome Association, Inc.
41-02 Bell Boulevard
Bayside, New York 11361
Telephone: (212) 224-2999

Chapter 31

Tuberous Sclerosis

Tuberous Sclerosis

What is tuberous sclerosis?

Tuberous sclerosis (TS) is a genetic disorder that causes a variety of neurological and physical symptoms, including seizures, mental retardation, and tumors of the brain, kidneys, eyes, or other organs.

Other signs of the disorder include

- White spots on the skin of the trunk and limbs
- Characteristic bumpy skin rash over the cheeks below the eyes
- Delayed development of speech and language skills
- Physical handicaps such as motor difficulties (rare)

Patients may have one or more of these conditions in varying degrees of severity. In its most devastating form, TS renders the patient completely helpless and dependent.

Tuberous sclerosis was first identified in the late 1800s by Dr. Désiré-Magloire Bourneville, a French neurologist. Despite being one of the more common genetic disorders, TS remains poorly understood. The disorder is present at birth, but the clinical signs may be subtle and full symptoms may take considerable time to develop. As a result, TS frequently goes unrecognized or misdiagnosed for many years.

How common is tuberous sclerosis?

The true incidence of TS is unknown. Estimates of new cases of TS each year (the incidence rate) range from 1 in 10,000 to 1 in 30,000 births. However, the incidence could be greater, since many cases probably go unrecognized. The disorder affects both sexes and all races.

What causes tuberous sclerosis?

Tuberous sclerosis is caused by a defective gene that is usually inherited from a parent who has the disorder. In some cases, however, the parent does not have TS, but passes on a defective gene that has resulted from a spontaneous change or mutation. The cause of such a gene mutation is unknown.

The disease is inherited as an autosomal dominant disorder. This means that each child of an affected parent, or of a parent who is unaffected but carries the defective gene, has a 50 percent chance of developing symptoms.

What are the signs?

The signs of the disorder may vary according to the extent to which a particular body system is involved. Seizures, motor difficulties, developmental delay, mental retardation, hyperactivity, and behavioral abnormalities reflect brain involvement. Small benign tumors called angiofibroma some times form on the face. More commonly, white spots appear on the skin. These spots are of great importance in early diagnosis since they are present at birth in up to 90 percent of affected infants. The white spots are less pigmented than the adjacent skin, and can occur anywhere on the body.

What research is being done?

The National Institute of Neurological and Communicative Disorders and Stroke, a part of the National Institutes of Health, supports basic laboratory studies that may lead to a greater understanding of the causes of TS. Several scientists are searching for improved methods of treating the symptoms. Other investigators are trying to identify the location of the defective gene responsible for the disorder. Such a discovery would aid in diagnosis and treatment.

Clues about tuberous sclerosis may come from research on another genetic disease, neurofibromatosis. The two diseases — both of which cause tumors and skin spots — are believed to result from similar disruptions in the development of the central nervous system. Some scientists are studying a naturally occurring fish model of neurofibromatosis in the hope of finding the cause of the disease. Other investigators are evaluating the effect of certain drugs on tumor growth. Advances achieved through such studies might benefit TS patients as well as those who have neurofibromatosis.

Is there any treatment?

Although there is no cure for TS, there are various forms of treatment for its symptoms. Recent studies have led to treatment advances in several areas. New anticonvulsant drugs are controlling seizures more effectively. Children with learning disabilities and speech and language difficulties are being helped through more sophisticated educational techniques. Teams of neurologists, orthopedists, physical therapists, occupational therapists, and other professionals are helping handicapped patients learn daily living skills and ways to improve mobility. With these and other advances, the outlook for tuberous sclerosis patients continues to improve.

Prognosis

The effect of tuberous sclerosis on a person's life varies according to the symptoms shown. Patients with the mild form of this disorder may live a normal and productive life. In the more severe forms of TS, the disabilities may be serious, and premature death may occur as a result of infections, seizures, or tumors in vital organs.

How can I help research?

The National Institute of Neurological and Communicative Disorders and Stroke and the National Institute of Mental Health support a national human specimen bank at the Wadsworth Veterans Administration Hospital in Los Angeles. This bank supplies investigators around the world with tissue from patients with neurological and psychiatric diseases. The bank needs tissue from tuberous sclerosis patients to enable scientists to study this disorder more intensely. Prospective donors should write to:

Dr. Wallace W. Tourtellotte, Director
Human Neurospecimen Bank
VA Wadsworth Medical Center
Building 212, Room 31
Los Angeles, CA 90073
Telephone: (213) 824-4307 (Call collect.)

Sources of information

Parents and patients who have TS can be kept informed of current research and medical advances by their physicians.

In addition, there are two nonprofit, tax-exempt organizations which provide information and support to families affected by the disorder;

American Tuberous Sclerosis Association
P.O. Box 44
Rockland, MA 02370
(617) 878-5528 or (toll free) 1-800-446-1211

National Tuberous Sclerosis Association
P.O. Box 612
Winfield, IL 60190
(312) 668-0787

For additional information concerning research supported by the National Institute of Neurological and Communicative Disorders and Stroke, contact:

Office of Scientific and Health Reports
National Institute of Neurological and
Communicative Disorders and Stroke
Building 31, Room 8A-06
National Institutes of Health
Bethesda, Maryland 20892
(301)496-5751

PART TWO

UNDERSTANDING THE BRAIN AND THE NEUROLOGICAL SYSTEM

Chapter 32

The Brain — A Mysterious Jewel

The Brain — A Mysterious Jewel

For centuries, scientists have been fascinated by the mystery of the brain. Protected by a bony skull and cushioned by cerebrospinal fluid, this three-pound organ is the crown jewel of the human body. Yet, its appearance is far from lustrous, and its value cannot he measured in carats.

The brain orchestrates behavior, movement, feeling, sensing. It controls automatic functions like breathing and heartbeat. Without it, you cannot fall in love, lift a pencil, or enjoy a concert.

Brain health and disease

When the brain is healthy, it functions quickly, automatically, precisely. But when problems occur, the results can be devastating. Some 50 million people in this country lead lives diminished by a damaged nervous system. They suffer losses that only the most determined research efforts can restore or prevent.

Fortunately, advances in neuroscience research have ushered in a new era of discovery about the nervous system. At the forefront of this new age is the National Institute of Neurological and Communicative Disorders and Stroke (NINCDS). Through its support of brain research, new ways are being found to compensate for neurological loss, restore function, and prevent future nervous system disease.

Features of the brain

The brain's most obvious features are its two hemispheres (1). Some brain functions, such as hearing and vision, are served by both hemispheres, but certain activities originate in one side or the other. The left hemisphere, for example, controls movement and receives sensations from the right side of the body. The right hemisphere controls those same functions on the left side. Generally, the left hemisphere controls language.

Each hemisphere is divided into four lobes. The frontal lobe (2) and the temporal lobe (3) help you regulate your behavior and learn new things. Without the frontal lobe, you could not plan a picnic or decide to move indoors when a rainstorm threatens. The temporal lobe is the seat of memory and strong emotions: your first kiss is stored there, but that's also where the pangs of jealousy originate. The parietal lobe (4) receives information from the eyes, ears, nose, and tongue, and sends messages to move muscles. This is also the part of the brain that helps you mimic and orients you in space: you use the parietal lobe to play "Simon says" or read a map. At the back of your head, the occipital lobe (5) coordinates vision.

Descending from the brain, inside the backbone, is the spinal cord (6). Nerves connect the brain and spinal cord with the sensory organs, muscles and skin, and all the organs of your body.

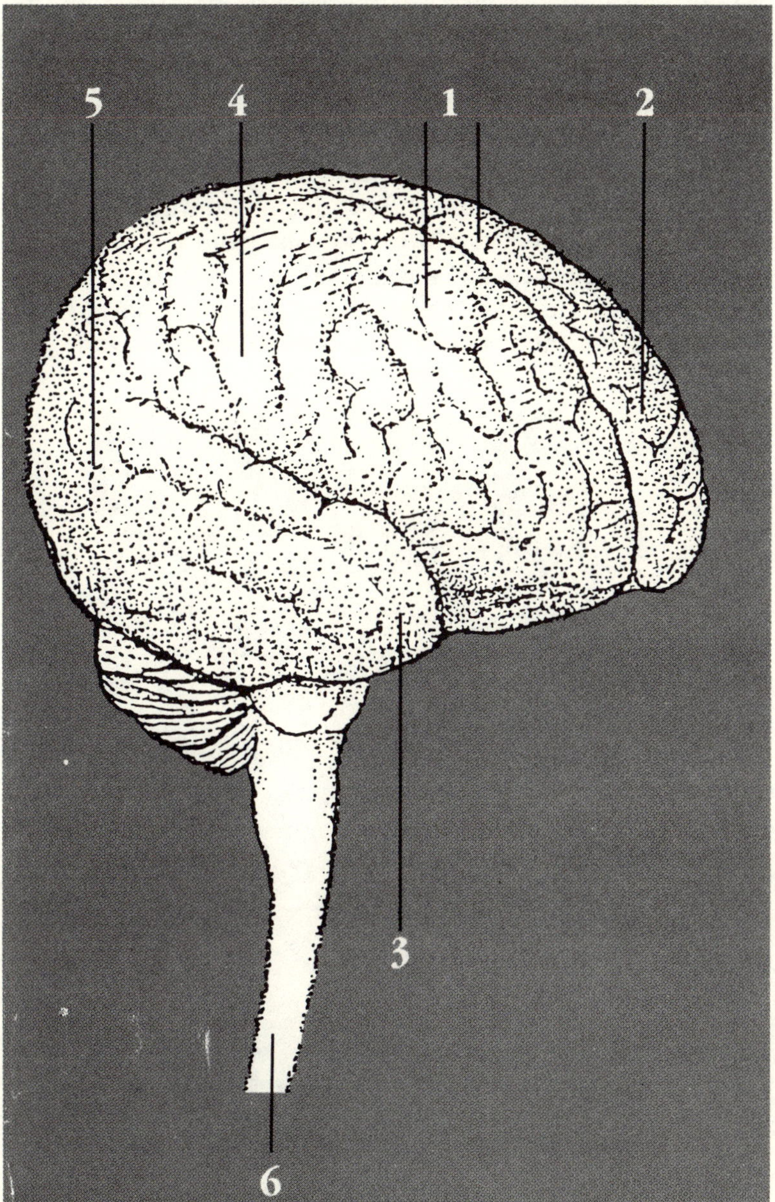
5
4
1
2
3
6

The Vital Link

A nerve is a group of nerve cell fibers bound together like an electrical cable. Individual nerve cells, called neurons, are the basic units of communication in the body.

Nerve cells consist of three parts: the cell body (**1**) which contains the nucleus (the nucleus of each of the body's cells is where the units of heredity known as genes are located) as well as the the machinery for making proteins and producing energy to power nerve cell activity; many dendrites (**2**) extend out from the cell body, like branches from a tree, to receive messages from other nerve cells; messages then pass through the nerve cell body and down the single long axon (**3**) to another nerve cell, a muscle, or an organ.

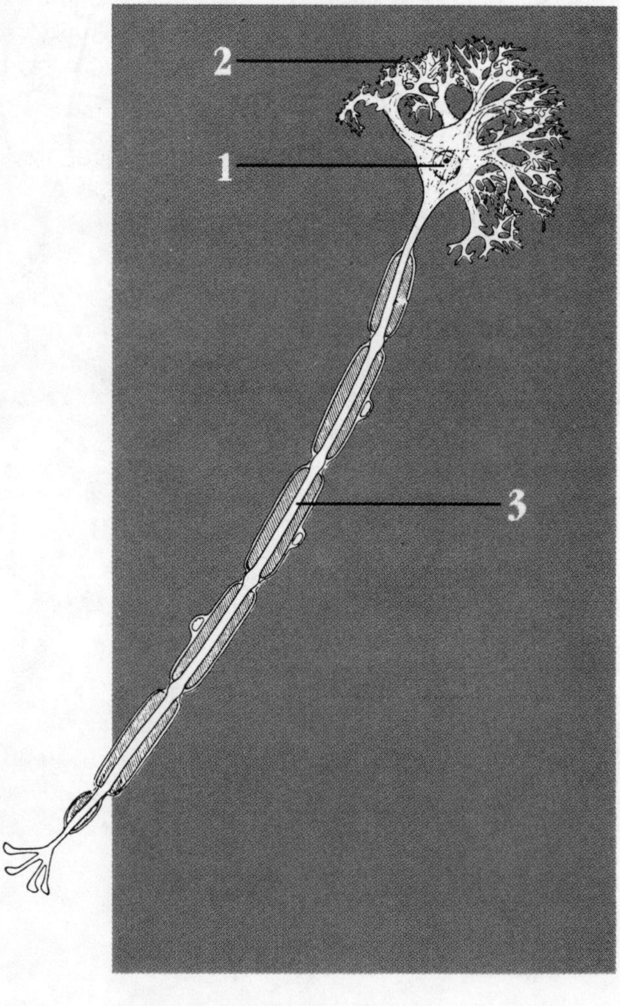

The Forebrain. By far the largest area of the brain, the forebrain contains the two hemispheres that control complex mental activities. Forebrain structures help regulate vital body functions like temperature and blood pressure. The forebrain also governs drives like the "fight or flight" reaction and sexual desire.

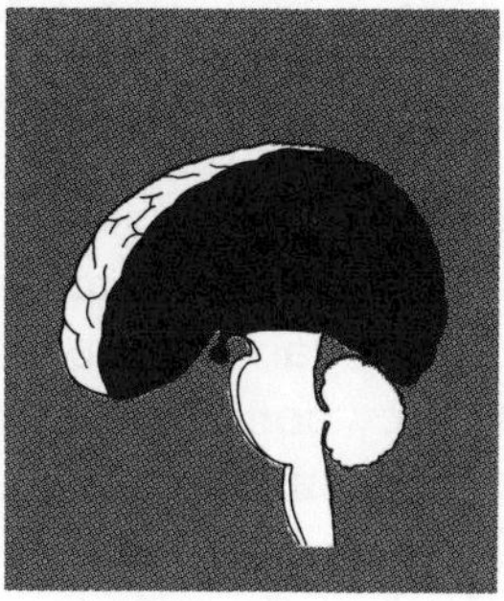

The Midbrain. The small area of the midbrain acts as a relay station for information about sound and sight, and for almost all other messages coming into or out of the forebrain. The midbrain also contains nerve fibers that play a major role in regulating movement.

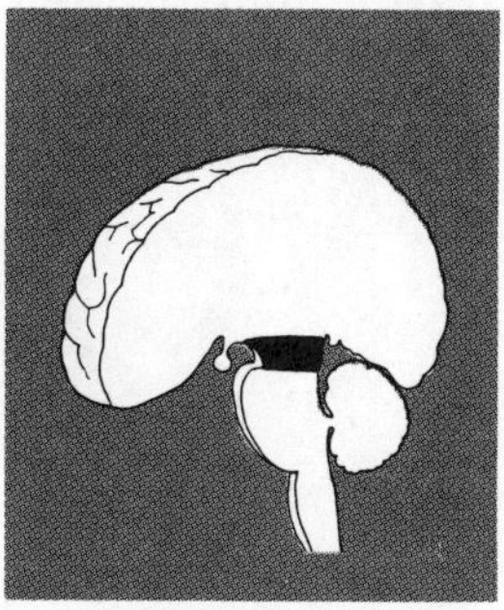

The Hindbrain. The hindbrain controls breathing and heartbeat, and helps you with the fine muscle control needed to put together a model airplane. From the hindbrain come messages to sneeze and swallow.

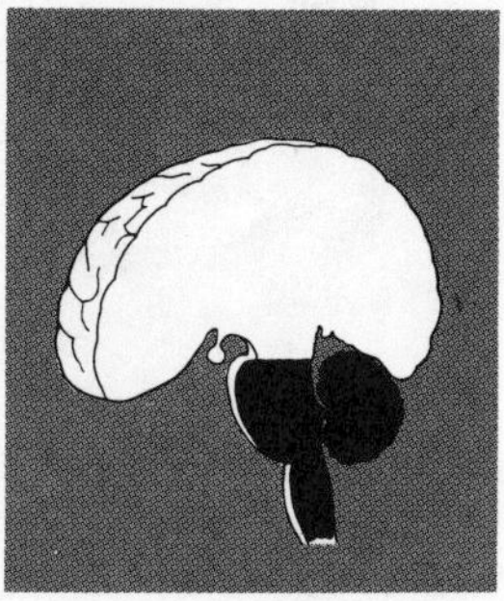

The Cerebral Cortex. This major part of the forebrain is the brain's command center. It contains more nerve cells than any other brain structure. There are so many cells that the cortex is bunched up in folds to fit within the skull. The folds make the surface of the brain look something like a walnut.

Certain areas of the cortex have been named after the body functions they control. The motor cortex **(1)** is responsible for every movement you make voluntarily, from a handshake to the winking of an eye. Lying behind the motor cortex is the sensory cortex **(2)**. This area of the brain receives a flood of different sensations. It lets you know when you are being tickled. It identifies heat and pain, the feel of velvet, the scratchiness of steel wool.

The auditory cortex **(3)** allows you to pick out the sound of a saxophone from a jazz recording. To transform your thoughts into words, you need the help of the Brocas area **(4)**, which coordinates the many complex movements required for speech. At the back of the brain lies the visual cortex (not shown), whose nerve cells recognize a green traffic light turning red.

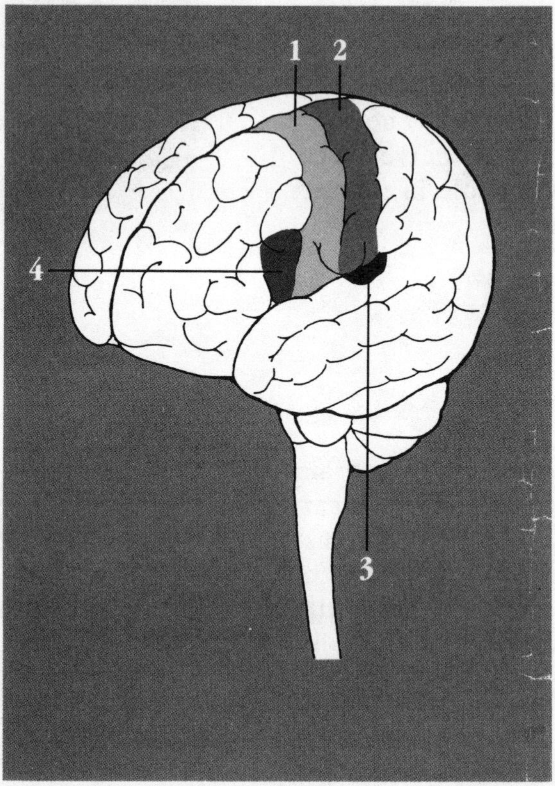

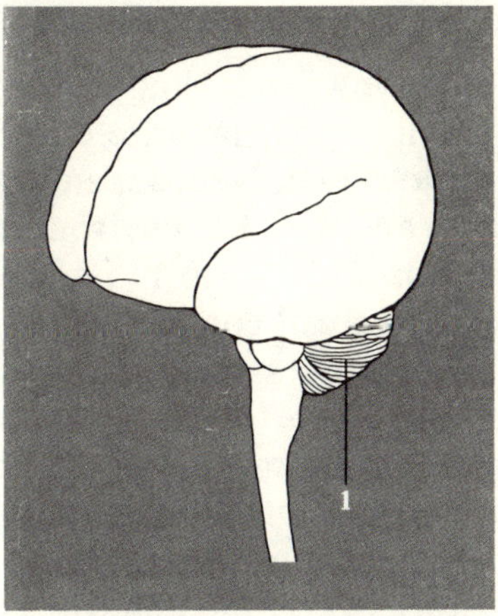

The Cerebellum. The cerebellum (1) is perhaps the most easily recognized part of the hindbrain. It helps coordinate movement. Without your cerebellum, you would not be able to run, walk, or even step off a curb without falling over. It lets you perform intricate movements like threading needles and buttoning your shirt.

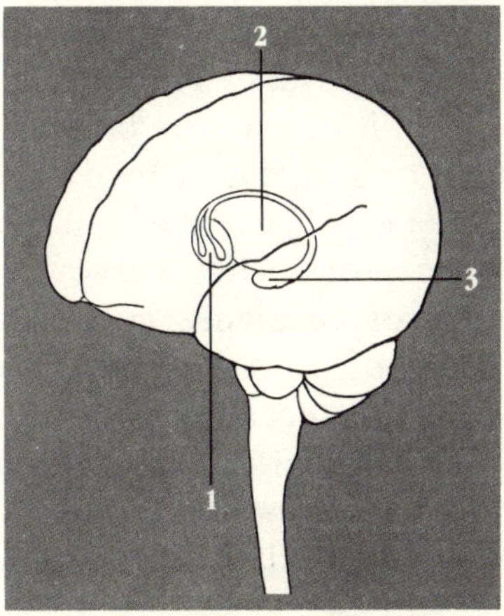

The Inner Brain. Deep within the brain lie the structures that define your highly developed mental, emotional, and motor capacities. The hypothalamus (**1**), about the size of a pearl, directs a multitude of important functions. It wakes you up in the morning, reminds you how hungry you are, and gets your adrenalin flowing for that job interview you've been worried about. The hypothalamus is also the brain's emotional center, controlling the hormones that make you feel exhilarated, angry, depressed. Above it lies the thalamus (**2**), a major relay station for messages arriving from the muscles and sense organs.

When you recall the nursery rhymes taught to you as a child, you probably are relying on your brain's hippocampus (**3**). Essential to learning, this structure also helps you commit a new phone number to your long-term memory bank. The basal ganglia (not shown) lie deep in the forebrain, and help with voluntary movement. If your basal ganglia malfunction, you may have tremors in the arms and legs, find yourself moving rigidly or ungracefully, or be unable to speak normally.

Neurotransmission: Getting the Message Across

Whether you are raising a glass, counting pocket change, or enjoying the smell of your favorite dinner dish, you have nerve cell communication to thank. Neurons interact with each other, with muscles and organs, and with the environnient through touch and other senses to help your body perform its many functions.

A nerve cell communicates with another cell through an electrochemical process called neurotransmission. An electrical message from the brain travels down the length of the nerve cell axon and stimulates tiny sacs (1) at the axon's tip. These sacs release chemicals known as neurotransmitters (2) into the gap or synapse (3) between nerve cells. The neurotransmitters cross the synapse and lock onto receptors (4) on the dendrites or other parts of a neighboring nerve cell.

This meeting of neurotransmitters and receptors sparks a second electrical message. The new message then travels along other nerve cells until it reaches its target and carries out the brain's orders: you stretch, or scratch, or turn off the television.

But not all receiving nerve cells "fire" after neurotransmitters find receptors. One nerve cell may have thousands of receptors capable of receiving conflicting neurotransmitter messages from hundreds of other nerve cells. Some neurotransmitters (excitatory) may tell the receiving nerve to fire; others (inhibitory) may modify the fire command. The particular mix of excitatory and inhibitory neurotransmitters determines whether firing takes place and whether messages are relayed or stopped.

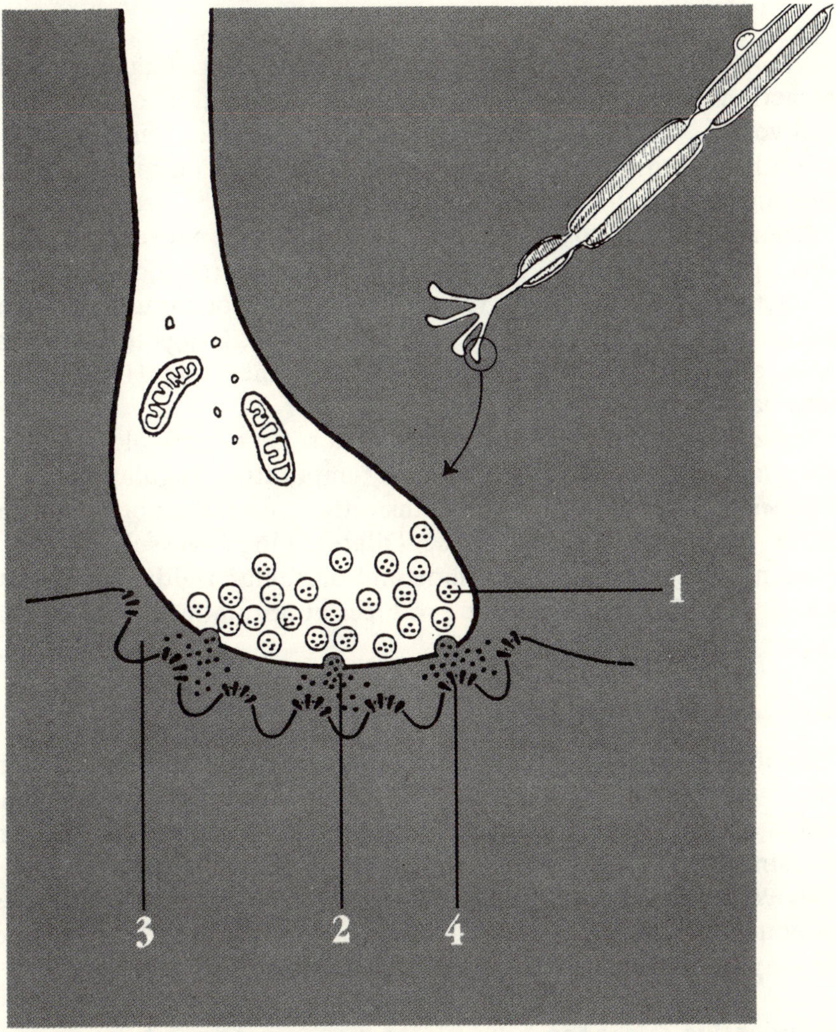
1
3
2
4

Some Neurotransmitters at Work — How They Affect You

Acetylcholine — An excitatory neurotransmitter. Causes muscle contraction and regulates smooth muscle contraction of the heart, blood vessels, and gut. Stimulates glands to secrete. Lack of acetylcholine has been linked to the muscle weakness seen in myasthenia gravis and memory loss in Alzheimer's disease.

GABA (Gamma-aminobutyric acid) — Inhibitory neurotransmitter. Helps maintain muscle control and visual perception. Loss or malfunction of GABA could result in seizures, poor muscle control, anorexia, or unusual sensitivity to heat or touch. Drugs that increase GABA are used to treat uncontrolled movements in Huntington's disease and seizures in epilepsy

Serotonin — Inhibitory neurotransmitter. Constricts blood vessels and brings on sleep. Also involved in temperature regulation.

Dopamine — Inhibitory neurotransmitter. Influences behavior and control of complex movements. Dilates blood vessels. Loss of dopamine gives rise to the tremor and muscular rigidity of Parkinson's disease. Excess dopamine produces abnormally increased body movement.

Neurogenetic Diseases

Huntington's disease — A fatal, progressive brain disorder of uncontrolled movement and intellectual and emotional impairment. Scientists have identified a genetic marker for the disease. They are now using the marker to develop a test for people at risk.

Muscular dystrophy — A family of inherited neuromuscular diseases. The gene for Duchenne muscular dystrophy was recently located. This may lead to prenatal diagnosis and therapeutic interventions.

Degenerative Diseases

Alzheimer's disease — A progressively dementing disorder whose hallmarks are loss of memory and mental skills. Scientists have isolated the gene responisible for an abnormal substance characteristically found in the brains of Alzheimer's patients.

Parkinson's disease — A chronic condition characterized by tremor and rigid muscle movements. Investigators are now experimenting with tissue implants as a way of reversing Parkinson's symptoms.

Metabolic diseases

Gaucher's disease — An inherited and sometimes fatal condition marked by the dangerous buildup of fatty material in body tissues. NINCDS scientists discovered the enzyme responsible for Gaucher's disease, and pioneered an experimental therapy. They recently cloned the gene for the enzyme — a major step toward improved diagnosis.

Communicative Disorders

Otitis media — A common childhood ear infection. Studies of treatment for this condition have shown the ineffectiveness of popular decongestant and antihistamine drugs, and value of the antibiotic amoxicillin.

Hearing loss — A cochlear implant that will allow the profoundly deaf to hear is being refined.

Cerebrovascular Disease

Stroke — Stroke is an interruption in the brain's blood flow that threatens to starve brain cells of food and oxygen. The third leading killer in the U.S., stroke can be caused by a blocked or ruptured brain blood vessel. Many patients have been spared the risk and expense of a brain bypass procedure because research has shown aspirin and blood pressure control to be as effective as such surgery in preventing stroke.

Trauma

Spinal cord injury — Investigators are testing ways to prevent scar tissue from forming at the site of spinal injury and blocking nerve cell regrowth. Prosthetic devices are being refined to help disabled people regain the use of their hands and to restore bladder function.

Convulsive Disorders

Epilepsy — Doctors are better able to help patients control their seizures with new drugs, and techniques of intensive monitoring and brain imaging developed with NINCDS support.

Infectious Diseases

AIDS (Acquired Immune Deficiency Syndrome) — This is a deadly infection that destroys the immune system and sometimes causes dementia. Recent research has shown that the brain can harbor the AIDS virus. This discovery points to the importance of developing drugs that can penetrate the blood-brain barrier.

Chapter 33

The Brain in Aging and Dementia

The Brain in Aging and Dementia

Editor's note: The Clinical Center of the National Institute of Health sponsors a series of lectures by distinguished physicians intended to aid the lay public's health awareness. The text which follows was delivered, as a part of that series, by Dr. Stanley Rappaport, Chief of the Laboratory of Neurosciences of the National Institute on Aging. The original lecture was illustrated with a series of slides, some enhancing the supporting statistics, some providing graphic metaphors to clarify processes, etc. Since colored, continuous tone slides are not reproducible in this book's format, some — the ones deemed crucial to the text — have been convertered to black and white line format for use here. The others have been omitted, while the slide numbers were rearranged to reflect it. The Clinical Center has reprinted the lecture with all colored slides intact as NIH publication 83-2625 for those wishing to access the totality.

The problems of brain aging and of the dementias of old age are relatively new concerns to medical science. As recently as 1850, the average life expectancy in the western world was only 40 years. People rapidly wearied and died because of hard work, disease, malnutrition, and — for women — childbirth. But aging, with its associated diseases, was rare.

Montaigne, the 16th-century French philosopher and writer, who lived to the then uncommon age of 61, made early observations on aging, particularly of the intellectual faculties:

> Since I was 20 years of age, I am certain that my mind and body have deteriorated more than they have developed. It is likely that knowledge and experience increase with aging, but activity, alertness, strength and other important qualities nevertheless decline. Sometimes the body capitulates first to age, sometimes the mind. I have seen many men in whom the brain becomes diseased before either the stomach or the limbs.
>
> — *Michel Eyquem de Montaigne, 1581, "Essay On Aging"*

In the early 20th century, when life expectancy rose to the seventh decade, scientists first clearly recognized mental impairment in the elderly. Their observations supported Montaigne's early insight that intellectual faculties dependent on accumulated information and experience increase with age, whereas faculties related to immediate memory and speed of information processing decline.

In order to examine the brain during aging and in diseases of old age, we first should understand something about the normal anatomy, physiology, and function of the brain in youth, and about the qualities of intelligence and behavior.

Brain anatomy and physiology

Brain regions. The cerebrum is the largest part of the brain, and has a mantle, or cortex, of gray matter and a core of white matter containing gray matter regions (nuclei). It is separated into almost identical halves (the right and left cerebral hemispheres), which are each further subdivided into four cortical lobes that control specific mental and body functions. They are the frontal, parietal, temporal and occipital lobes (figures 1A and 1B).

The frontal lobe controls voluntary motor movements — both fine motor functions such as those involved in speaking and writing, and gross movements required for walking, for example. This lobe also contains associated regions critical for planning, establishing the identity of the personality, and regulating the complex emotions and intellectual tasks that define human behavior.

The parietal lobe receives information from the various sense organs in the body, and regulates coordinated motor movements, whereas the occipital lobe is the screen on which visual images are displayed. The temporal lobe contains an auditory cortical area, and a specific region called the hippocampus, which is critical for memory. When the hippocampus is damaged, the ability to recall facts — even if presented just a moment before — is lost. The cerebellum, at the back of the brain, controls posture and coordination. The brain stem influences autonomic functions such as respiration, heart rate, and blood pressure, and the spinal cord is the site of communication between the central nervous system and the muscles and sense organs.

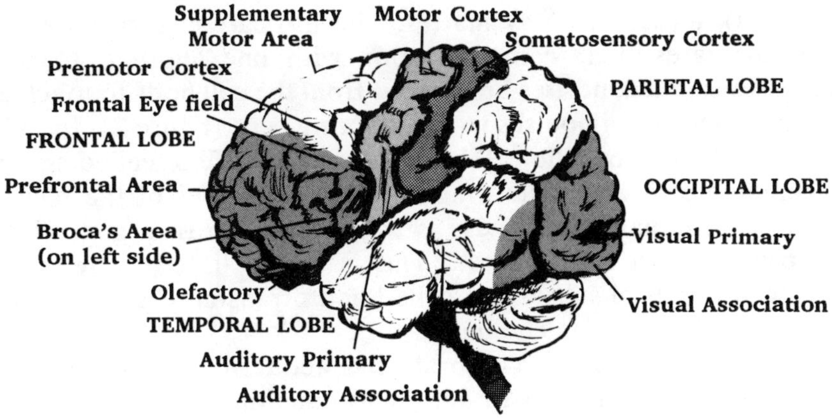
Supplementary
Motor Area
Motor Cortex
Somatosensory Cortex
Premotor Cortex
PARIETAL LOBE
Frontal Eye field
FRONTAL LOBE
Prefrontal Area
OCCIPITAL LOBE
Broca's Area
(on left side)
Visual Primary
Olefactory
Visual Association
TEMPORAL LOBE
Auditory Primary
Auditory Association

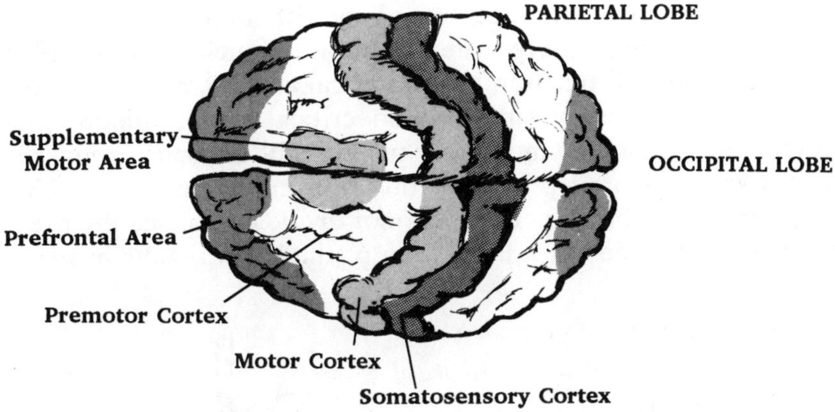
PARIETAL LOBE
Supplementary
Motor Area
OCCIPITAL LOBE
Prefrontal Area
Premotor Cortex
Motor Cortex
Somatosensory Cortex

Brain cells. All the complex functions of the brain — emotions, memory, sensation, motor movements — are controlled by nerve cells (neurons), located in gray matter. The intricate structure of these cells facilitates their communication with one another. Complex processes called dendrites branch out from the cell body to touch and transmit electrical impulses to neighboring cells (figure 2). Impulses may also travel from the cell body down a long fiber called an axon to communicate with distant nerve cells or muscles of the face. At the axon terminal, the impulse is transmitted across a gap called a synapse to affect the next cell. This is accomplished by release of packaged chemical substances called neurotransmitters (figure 3), a typical one being acetylcholine.

Energy for the brain. The brain has about 10 billion nerve cells that require vast amounts of energy to function. Although the adult brain comprises only two percent of total body weight, it uses 20 percent of the body's energy resources and oxygen. Energy for the brain must be in the form of a simple sugar called glucose. Blood carries glucose and oxygen to the brain, where glucose is metabolized (burned with oxygen) in the nerve cells to produce carbon dioxide, water, and heat. A fraction of the energy within the glucose molecule is converted to high-energy chemical bonds which then are used to maintain nerve cell function and electrical activity, and for synthetic processes. This energy supply is so critical that if blood flow is interrupted for only 1 minute, a person will become unconscious. After 4 minutes of deprivation, the neurons begin to die. Unlike other cells in the body, neurons cannot divide or replace themselves. Deprivation of blood in a large area of the brain results in *stroke.*

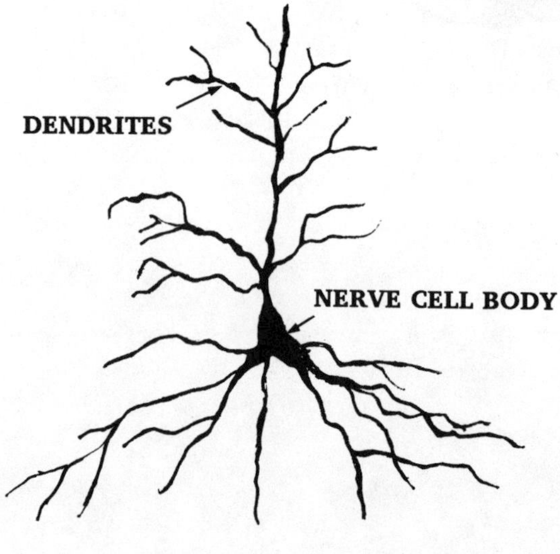

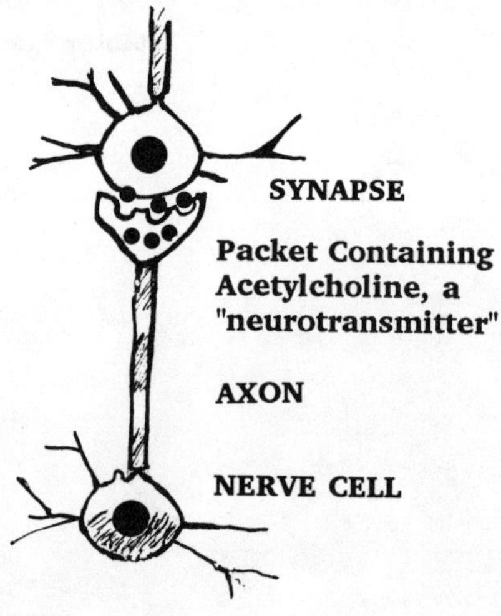

Brain blood flow. The heart pumps blood to the brain via the carotid and vertebral arteries, which branch out in a network of smaller arteries that feed various regions of the brain. The regional rate of flow is coupled to local nerve cell activity, based on concentrations of oxygen and carbon dioxide within the brain. Flow increases with increased brain activity and decreases with decreased activity. This coupling can be demonstrated by radionuclide studies. A radioactive gas, ^{133}xenon, is injected into the carotid artery and is rapidly taken up by the brain. Sensitive detectors on the skull measure the concentration of xenon in the form of small amounts of gamma radiation on the brain's surface. With this information, it is possible to calculate the rate of flow in specific brain regions.

When the data are converted to an image on a display screen, the varying concentrations in parts of the brain are represented by different colors, with red indicating the greatest flow, and diminishing to yellow, blue, and green. For example, in a resting individual with eyes closed and ears plugged, blood flow is greatest in the frontal lobe, indicating greatest activity in the centers concerned with emotions and association processes. When the same individual is asked to speak, the pattern changes. Flow is redirected to brain regions involved in speech — the motor area in the frontal cortex that activates throat and mouth muscles, an area between the frontal and parietal lobes used in formulating speech, and the auditory area in the temporal lobe, which represents the person hearing himself speak. The flow patterns change according to specific tasks.

Glucose consumption. Another way scientists look at brain activity is through the consumption of glucose. If the glucose molecule is altered slightly by removing an oxygen atom from the second carbon position, a new compound — deoxyglucose — is formed, which also is taken up by the brain but is not burned. Its rate of accumulation can be measured and used to calculate how rapidly native glucose is burned, by a procedure called "positron emission tomography*," or PET scanning.

Radioactive fluorine (F^{18}) is attached to the deoxyglucose and injected into a vein. The fluorine emits a positive electron (positron) which combines with a negative electron to produce two gamma rays moving in exactly opposite directions. Detectors on the skull measure this radiation and, as with the blood flow studies, reconstructed images of the brain (this time in transverse "slices" rather than

* See special chapter explaining Positron Emission Tomography (PET scan)

surface areas) are displayed on a screen. The varying color intensities tell scientists the location and extent of glucose utilization, which indicates brain activity.

These precision instruments and sophisticated diagnostic methods enable scientists to examine brain function and scrutinize changes that occur with normal aging and with disease.

The Brain in Aging

The human brain grows tremendously in the first 4 years of life and reaches its maximum weight at age 20. Its cells number 10 billion. Then the aging process begins. Brain weight decreases gradually — by about 10 percent over a normal life span, largely because an average of 50,000 cells are lost each day. Moreover, the dendritic branching of many of the surviving cells becomes sparser and the amounts of neurotransmitter decrease. In view of these changes, neuroscientists at first were not surprised to find that brain blood flow and oxygen consumption — measurements of energy metabolism — also decreased with aging, commensurate with the fall in cell number.

This interpretation of brain aging was not seriously challenged until about 20 years ago, when scientists at the National Institutes of Health doubted the inevitability of a major loss of brain function with aging. They suggested that most of the previous clinical studies showing this loss were defective because the subjects examined were not healthy, but suffered a variety of illnesses that might affect brain function, such as hypertension, atherosclerosis, diabetes, psychosis, or other organic disease. Thus, they designed a carefully controlled study to discover the true functional significance of the brain changes that occur with aging.

The investigators examined two groups of healthy male volunteers — one group around age 20 and the other around 70 years old. After carefully screening the participants to rule out the possibility of brain disease or factors that might contribute to disease, they measured blood flow and oxygen consumption in all the men. As a whole, blood flow and oxygen consumption, which is tied to glucose utilization, differed little in the two groups, and the scientists concluded that overall brain functional activity in normal healthy men does not change over a 50-year period. PET studies by the National Institute on Aging's Laboratory of Neurosciences clearly show, furthermore, that glucose utilization in specific brain regions of healthy men under resting conditions does not fall with age.

Psychological testing. Brain function also can be studied with a battery of psychological tests of memory, vocabulary, and other parameters designed to examine how clearly elderly people think as compared with younger individuals. These psychological tests have shown that some functions of intelligence decline with age while others increase. Fluid intelligence, represented by memory span and the ability to process information rapidly, decreases with age. On the other hand, crystallized intelligence, measured by extent of vocabulary, general information, and accumulated aspects of intelligence that depend on knowledge and experience, increases with the years and can frequently compensate for the loss of rapid information processing in healthy elderly people.

Thus, scientists have found that the physiological parameters of brain competence and function — glucose utilization, blood flow, and oxygen consumption — do not decline with aging, and, moreover, that certain aspects of intelligence increase with age. Faced with the knowledge that the adult brain loses thousands of nerve cells each day, and that the complexity of the remaining cells decreases as well, scientists are seeking to understand why brain blood flow and metabolism and aspects of the human intellect do not decline correspondingly.

Redundancy and plasticity. The first suggestion in solving this paradox is that the brain at 20 years may contain an overabundance of cells needed for the intellectual processes critical to the personality. This concept, is known as a *redundancy*. If we diagrammed this concept and portrayed the young brain as having six cells in a particular area, our diagram could indicated that only three of six cells must be active to carry out a specific task. A similar diagram of the elderly brain suggests that if three cells are lost, a sufficient number remain to function normally — perhaps with a smaller margin for error or for responding to stress.

Second, scientists recently learned that even though brain cells cannot divide and replicate, many of the active undamaged cells in the elderly brain can grow more dendrites and axons, enhancing intercommunication. This phenomenon is called plasticity. The combined compensatory mechanisms of redundancy and plasticity probably account for maintenance of much normal intellectual functioning and brain metabolism with aging.

The Brain in Dementia

Characteristics of dementia. Plasticity and redundancy work wonderfully, but their capabilities are limited. In some disease processes, cell death is accelerated, and plasticity is inhibited. The result is a serious disturbance of brain function and a consequent appearance of signs and symptoms of dementia, or alteration of the normal mental state.

The behavioral characteristics of dementia may include general deterioration of mental function, marked memory loss, disorientation, impairment of learned skill movements, disturbance of language, and loss of ability to recognize objects. These characteristics can be progressive and irreversible. They are associated with disorganization of the personality and progressive loss of the person's identity, and are distinct from changes of normal aging.

The affected population. The dementias of aging frequently affect people around 65 years or older, although younger individuals are affected as well. As the average life expectancy increases, so does the incidence of dementia and the problems it brings. In the United States, dementias affect 10 percent of people over 65. Intellectual and bodily functions are impaired so severely in 5 percent as to require institutional care. Only about 5 percent of the elderly between 65 and 69 are affected, but of those over 80 years of age, 20 percent are seriously demented.

In numbers of people, about 1 million elderly in this country require hospitalization due to dementia. Another 1 to 1.5 million who are not hospitalized present enormous physical, financial, and emotional burdens to their families and communities. The cost of treatment for this population — which will more than double by the year 2030 — is currently $6 billion a year. It is critical, therefore, to try to identify the causes of dementias and design appropriate treatments.

Types of dementia

Efforts to identify and study the dementias began in earnest at the turn of the 19th century. Alois Alzheimer, professor of psychiatry at the University of Breslau in Germany, identified the two major types of dementia in the elderly: vascular dementia, which develops secondary to interruption of blood flow to the brain and subsequent cell death; and a primary disease characterized by loss of brain mass, which is now called Alzheimer's disease.*

Vascular dementia (also called multiple infarct dementia) constitutes 30 percent of the dementias of old age. Small arteries in the brain (arterioles) become blocked by plaque buildup from atherosclerotic disease or by emboli (pieces of clot from the heart or elsewhere) which lodge in these arteries and prevent blood flow to the brain region they normally supply (see figure below). Without

---

* A full discussion of Alzheimer's disease appears elsewhere in this book. See CONTENTS for location.

oxygen and glucose, the brain cells die and the area of cell death — the infarcted area — softens and stops functioning. Progressive deterioration leads to the behavioral characteristics of dementia.

The second type of dementia, which accounts for 50 percent or more of cases, does not involve interference with blood flow. For reasons yet unknown, the disease process simply leads to accelerated cell death, for which plasticity and redundancy can in no way compensate. If we look at the atrophied brain of an individual who has died of Alzheimer's disease and compare it with that of an age-matched control, we see significant loss at the cellular level. Cells from the Alzheimer brain are much sparser than those of the normal aged brain, and frequently are abnormal. Some normal cells can be seen, but many are filled with a black fibrillary material that accumulates and accelerates their death. In specific regions, axon endings from cells become abnormal, leaving "senile" plaques of degenerated networks of axon terminals. These plaques form in the hippocampus and temporal lobe of the Alzheimer patient, and progressively involve the frontal and parietal lobes. An enzyme used to synthesize the neurotransmitter, acetylcholine, is also severely reduced in Alzheimer's disease, especially in the hippocampus and frontal lobe.

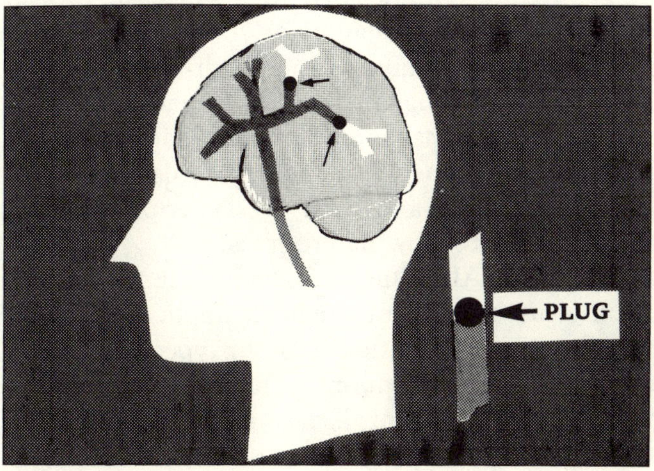

Functional deterioration of the Alzheimer brain is dramatically demonstrated by studies of blood flow and glucose consumption. A typical image generated by a PET scan of the brain would show a bright, active pattern of blood flow in a normal individual. Comparing that with a similar scan of an Alzheimer's affected brain, the Alzheimer's brain would show far less blood flow. It would appear as a desolate landscape by contrast with the activity visible in the scan of the normal brain. Similarly, a comparison of glucose utilization in the brain of an Alzheimer patient would be very different quantitatively. In a typical study, active glucose utilization will be seen in both the front and back of the normal brain, whereas, in the Alzheimer brain, the frontal aspects are quiet and non responsive. Only the occipital lobe, which receives visual images, lights up on the Alzheimer brain. Even so, the patient cannot interpret or identify the images.

Causes of dementia

Although a great deal of information is being gathered on Alzheimer's disease, its cause and treatment are not known. Researchers are investigating several factors that appear related to development of the disease. The first is genetic. Alzheimer's disease, especially when it afflicts individuals younger than 65 or 70, frequently occurs within families. By studying families with a high incidence of disease, scientists hope to find biological "markers" that identify the disease and the pathological process, and which may lead to identification of high-risk individuals. Then, when therapy is developed, physicians may be able to recognize and treat these people early enough to prevent the disease or to slow its progress.

A second theory in Alzheimer's disease centers on a "slow virus." Although such viruses have not yet been implicated in Alzheimer's disease, they have been identified in other types of dementias. Slow viruses can live in brains of apparently healthy people for 20 years or more before leading to signs of disease and dementia.

Tied in with the virus theory is a possible immunological factor. As people get older their immune defenses weaken and they are less able to resist viral and other infections. This may explain why the disease is seen more frequently in the elderly.

Finally, it has been suggested that substances in the environment, like aluminum, may contribute to development of the disease.

Other dementias

Alzheimer's disease and multiple infarct dementia, neither of which is currently curable, constitute about 80 percent of the dementias in the elderly. About 20 percent of the dementias, however, are curable. For this reason, physicians must be scrupulous when diagnosing symptomatic patients to rule out diseases that can be reversed. For example, a common cause of dementia-like symptoms in the elderly is drug intoxication. Older people often are prescribed several medicines for various ailments. These drugs, either singly or in combination, can cause untoward effects similar to the symptoms of dementia. Cessation or substitution of the drugs may quickly reverse the symptoms. Depression also is common with advancing age, and may carry with it forgetfulness and confusion that could be treatable. Hyper- and hypothyroidism and vitamin B12 deficiency also can cause reversible dementias. Bleeding at the brain surface, resulting from even a minor blow to the head, can contribute as well.

Directions in research

Basic research on laboratory animals is crucial in the search for the causes of dementia and, ultimately, a treatment. The clinical methods described above to study glucose metabolism and blood flow in the human brain may provide ways to diagnose Alzheimer's disease, to examine its natural history, and to distinguish it from other diseases which may or may not be treatable. These methods also will permit physicians to evaluate responses to new therapies and perhaps, by identifying individuals at risk for the disease, to initiate prophylactic treatment.

Studies to develop effective drug therapies continue. Scientists are trying to find substances that can speed the synthesis of neurotransmitters — especially acetylcholine — or slow their breakdown within the brain to compensate for their decline.

Finally, environmental therapy is critical for the care of the demented elderly. It would be tragic to remand to long-term nursing care people afflicted early on with a disease without first altering their environment to compensate somewhat for the loss of memory, disorientation, and other changes associated with the early aspects of disease, and reduce their suffering.

William Wadsworth Longfellow wrote, "For age is opportunity no less/than youth itself, though in another dress/ And as the evening twilight fades away/ the sky is filled with stars, invisible by day." For a substantial fraction of the elderly, however — about 5 to 10 percent — age is not filled with stars nor even the memory of daylight. These are demented individuals and the infirm who may be our parents and our friends. And it is to them that we must commit our efforts as physicians and as civilized men and women.

Questions and Answers on the Brain in Aging

Q. Dr. Rappaport, what is your view on the use of physostigmine in Alzheimer's disease?

A. As far as I know, physostigmine, which slows the breakdown of the neurotransmitter acetylcholine, and other drug therapies have not been proven effective in treating Alzheimer's disease.

Q. Could you explain what prophylactic therapy is?

A. Prophylactic therapy, or therapy initiated prior to signs of disease in subjects at risk, has not yet been successful. It is designed, however, to compensate for early loss of acetylcholine. Lecithin and other precursors of acetylcholine have been used in animal experiments to increase the brain concentrations of acetylcholine, sometimes alone or together with physostigmine, which interferes with the enzyme that breaks down acetylcholine. Perhaps a combination of both approaches will prove useful. Some changes have been reported, but at this time there is no accepted treatment for the disease.

Q. What is the role of chelation in treatment?

A. Environmental factors might contribute to Alzheimer's disease. Dr. Donald Crapper McLachlan and his colleagues have suggested that aluminum may be involved. High concentrations of the element have been found in the pathologic nerve cells within the brains of Alzheimer's subjects. Whether they are the cause or the result of damage and fibrillary changes, however, is not clear. A therapeutic approach based on the aluminum hypothesis is to give a chelating drug, such as EDTA or EGTA, which binds or sequesters the aluminum in the blood and accelerates its loss through the kidneys, and may perhaps deplete the brain of aluminum. As far as I know, chelation therapy has not shown any positive results.

Q. Should aluminum cooking pots be avoided?

A. With all the proposals relating to nutrition and environmental toxicity, one might wish to avoid virtually every harmful influence in life. The aluminum hypothesis has not been validated, and I personally would not avoid aluminum cooking pots. Bauxite miners — who come into contact with aluminim containing ores — don't get a significantly higher incidence of Alzheimer's disease. There is an atypical dementia associated with renal dialysis, which is probably caused by extremely high plasma aluminum concentrations, but a blood-brain barrier normally prevents access of aluminum to the brain.

Q. How does one go about finding a qualified physician to diagnose and treat dementia?

A. The first step would be to ask your physician to recommend a board-certified neurologist, who will establish a probable diagnosis with the skills available to him. If Alzheimer's disease is diagnosed, the neurologist should refer you to an association of families of Alzheimer's patients, where you can obtain information on treatment, diagnosis, and new research lines. The Alzheimer's Disease and Related Disorders Association (ADRDA) is becoming progressively more active and effective in gathering families and informing them of new research and of facilities available in the community. Information can be obtained from the ADRDA at 360 N. Michigan Avenue, Suite 1102, Chicago, Illinois 60601.

Q. Would a geriatrician, who specializes in care of the elderly, identify and diagnose Alzheimer's disease more readily than other doctors?

A. Geriatricians are aware of the diseases that increase in frequency with aging and should be helpful in making a tentative diagnosis by excluding the possibility of drug toxicity, vitamin B12 deficiency, depression, hyperthyroidism, or bleeding due to head trauma. Outpatients eventually would have to be referred to a neurologist in a hospital setting, because the diagnosis requires specific technologies, such as computer assisted tomography (CT scan) and other methods available only in medical centers.

Q. Could the changes in the elderly brain cause physical problems such as weakness in the legs and unsteady gait?

A. Yes. Areas of the brain, such as the motor cortex, contain specific motor cells called Betz cells. These cells send long axons along the spinal cord to spinal motor neurons, which then communicate through peripheral nerves to the muscle. In some normal elderly brains, as many as 80 percent of Betz cells are lost. Furthermore, sensory function is reduced as well. So motor coordination and function (the brain works by balancing extensor and flexor muscles) may be dramatically changed in aging, causing weakness, pain, muscle contractions, and tremor. Also, peripheral nerves lose many of their axons with aging. The very large axons, which communicate rapidly to muscles for contraction, are lost preferentially. Finally, muscles themselves become atrophic. They lose their ability — in many cases, perhaps, through disuse — to contract as adequately as they do in the young. For muscles, at least, much of the atrophy might be reversed through activity and training.

Q. Can that be reversed if it's due to a change in the brain cells?

A. The combined changes in brain and spinal cord cells, the axons within large peripheral nerves, the neuromuscular junction, and the muscles themselves can be additive, leading to tremor, weakness, and many of the neuromuscular disorders that occur with aging. The peripheral nervous system, like the central nervous system and muscles, is plastic and may respond to greater demands by increasing its growth and capability of action.

Q. How was it determined that 50,000 brain cells die each day beginning age 20?

A. Experimentally, with cell counters applied to human brain specimens. Scientists look at cross sections of brain regions in individuals between 20 and 70 and count the number of cells in a given volume. Brain cells are not lost at equal rates throughout the brain. Some specific regions may lose very few cells, whereas others, such as the motor cortex, may lose proportionally more.

Q. Do you know what the rate of loss is in the cerebral cortex and the thinking areas of the brain?

A. On an average, it's 50,000. I don't know the exact numbers in different areas.

Q. How does the pattern of glucose utilization and oxygen utilization in the sleeping brain compare with that of the resting brain?

A. Brain glucose utilization in the monkey during sleep, in the absence of rapid eye movements, has been shown by C. Kennedy and colleagues to be generally reduced throughout the brain, without any specific structure selectively affected. As far as I know, no one has used PET scanning for sleep studies with humans.

Q. Does the sleeping brain look more like the demented brain or the elderly brain?

A. Glucose utilization in the elderly brain, in the absence of sensory stimulation, is not reduced as compared to use in the young brain. Sleep in the young monkey reduces glucose utilization but to a much lesser extent than seen in dementia in man. A large amount of energy is consumed during sleep. Sleep is not a quiescent state.

Q. Does diabetes in an elderly person contribute to dementia? If a diabetic maintains a low sugar intake, will the dementia process speed up?

A. Diabetes would not affect Alzheimer's dementia, but could increase the likelihood of multiple infarct dementia because it is associated with blood vessel disease. However, if well-treated, the condition may have no effect whatever. Close correlations have not been worked out yet, but we do know that diabetes can affect blood vessels throughout the body.

Q. You explained that deterioration of the brain can lead to physical malfunction in the body. Can we assume that, conversely, "a healthy body houses a healthy brain"? I was taught that if a healthy human is exposed to starvation, the bodily functions deteriorate before the brain does. Is it true that the brain still functions when the body is practically dead?

A. First, I'd like to address the issue of a healthy body housing a healthy brain. In Alzheimer's disease, the brain is affected despite the health of the body, and the tragedy is that the body may remain very healthy.

On the other hand, the issue of interaction between the body and the brain is a subject for current research. For example, Drs. Marion

Diamond and Arnold Scheibel studied the effects of environmental stimulation and deprivation on brain anatomy of young and old rats. They found that brain cells in the cortex of rats, which were caged with other rats or with toys, or in an "enriched" and active environment, seemed to have more extensive dendritic arborizations than did brain cells of older rats which were caged singly in a quiet environment with little to do. The brain also was enlarged. This suggests that environmental and physical stimulation can lead to brain growth and maintenance of brain structure and probably of function, even in old rats. The issue then arises as to whether activity can alter cell structure to some extent in elderly humans as well.

Q. Do you mean that general health and physical activity will keep the brain healthy as well? Is the brain somehow protected in disease?

A. The brain is a critical organ, which must be preserved. In liver or kidney disease, toxins within the blood might get into the brain and damage it. Elevated temperature will accelerate brain demands and may kill certain nerve cells. It's important, as much as possible, to avoid disease states that can contribute to brain damage.

In starvation, brain function is preserved at the expense of the muscle tissue, the fat mass, the liver, or blood protein. In severe protein deficiency, which we call "kwashiorkor," the legs may swell, blood protein may decline, the liver mass may be reduced, the muscles may be atrophic, but brain function continues until the very end. Under these conditions, the body is making very little glucose. This is an exception to the rule that glucose is the major food for the brain. As fats are broken down when carbohydrates are depleted, the body makes "ketone bodies," beta hydroxybutyric acid and acetoacetate, which partially substitute for glucose in the starved state. The other body organs contribute to the maintenance of brain function. Without an intact brain, the rest of the body's existence is not very important.

Q. Does regular physical or mental exercise have any effect on reducing the rate of brain cell loss or on promoting plasticity?

A. I pointed out that in rats, environmental stimulation, through plasticity of the brain, can lead to increased complexity of nerve cells and dendrites. These are exciting experimental issues that can be studied in rats and then interpreted in human conditions.

Q. Are women more prone to dementia, and is it a "sex-linked" genetic disease?

A. Women are not more prone to Alzheimer-type dementia and the disease is not sex-linked. Even if a genetic predisposition is present, the disease may not appear. This critical factor is apparent in identical twins, in which one will get Alzheimer's disease and the other — with the identical genetic makeup — will not.

Q. Is genetic counseling advisable for families with a history of Alzheimer's disease?

A. Genetic counseling should be considered in families with a high incidence of disease. Most often, the disease is thought to be sporadic. If Alzheimer's disease occurs in a parent before the age of 70, as well as in siblings within a family, then genetic counseling should be considered.

Q. How do you determine the etiology? Can it be determined at autopsy?

A. We don't know the etiology. At autopsy we make the diagnosis by looking at brain plaques, neurofibrillary tangles, cell number and brain size. Taking into account the clinical history, we then decide whether these factors characterize Alzheimer's disease. Because other dementias may have similar symptoms, the final diagnosis can be made only at autopsy. Diagnosis in the living patient is now only 70 percent accurate, largely because we don't have sensitive measures of brain function or peripheral markers of the disease. PET* scanning may enable us to increase the accuracy of diagnosis in life, to initiate early treatment if available, and to identify other dementias that might be treatable.

Q. Is it possible to differentiate drug intoxication from another cause of dementia?

A. Yes. You examine the time course of the dementia, and the incidence of toxicity of all drugs which may be administered. For example, if a patient started a drug on October 3 and became

---

* PET scanning is discussed in detail elsewhere in this book. See CONTENTS for location.

disoriented October 5, but normal when the drug was stopped, he probably was intoxicated.

Q. Does Alzheimer's disease appear suddenly or build up gradually so that it can be recognized in its early stages?

A. It builds gradually and might be recognized early if we could develop techniques to identify it in the early stages. Disease processes, leading to accelerated cell death, do not simply appear one day. They are slow and progressive. There could be memory loss, emotional disturbance, or motor dysfunction years before the disease becomes full-blown. With PET scanning and other sensitive biological and neuropsychological techniques, we may be able to identify the disease at an early stage.

Q. It seems to me that there is probably a strong correlation between emotional problems and Alzheimer's disease. Is that true?

A. The correlation is because the disease causes emotional problems; emotional problems don't cause the disease.

Chapter 34

The PET Scanner (Positron Emission Tomography)

The PET Scanner (Positron Emission Tomography)

Editor's note: In many of the foregoing chapters, the authors have referred to the PET scan (PET is an acronym for Positron Emission Tomography) as one of the key diagnostic and treatment aids in neurology. The lay person may be a bit mystified by the term, when it is used without clarification — as it usually must be because of PET's technical nature. Many readers will not be satisfied with that. Wishing to understand modern medicine's approach to their own or a loved-one's neurologically focused illness, they will seek to learn at least the general idea of PET scanning — where it came from — and its use in neurological medicine. To serve that need, this book takes the space to provide a definitive report, in lay language, on the PET concept. This text was prepared by researchers and writers at the National Institute of Neurological and Communicative Disorders, and is quite readable by any educated lay person. A currentness note: While there may be some refinements on the PET scan, which have occurred since this material was gathered, the text, nevertheless, portrays well the overall technology of positron emission tomography, and how it is being used to improve neurological treatment.

What inspired PET scanning technology?

In centuries past, the human brain — the body's control center — has been an enigma to those who wished to probe its workings. Enclosed in a bony skull and surrounded by a barrier that repels chemical intruders, it has resisted most attempts at visualization or intervention. Today, however, new ways of studying the brain are uncovering the intricate pathways through which its messages flow.

Modern brain imaging was born in the early 1900s with the advent of skull X-rays. Scientists were quick to realize that more powerful techniques for studying brain function were possible. In 1927, neurologist Egas Moniz developed *cerebral angiography*, which relied on an injected contrast agent to capture on film the distribution of the brain's tissue, blood, and fluid. The next decade saw this exciting technology produce thousands of successful diagnoses.

Brain research leapt forward in the 1940s and 1950s when neurosurgeon Wilder Penfield recorded a remarkable series of observations about the brains of patients who were candidates for neurosurgery. By stimulating various areas of the brain while the patient was conscious, Dr. Penfield identified regions of the cortex that activated specific movement — the raising of an arm, for instance. But Dr. Penfield's "maps," as remarkable as they were, were limited to the *surface* of the brain. They could not illuminate subtle brain activities such as maintenance of consciousness, nor could they be used to study deficits in most patients with neurological diseases.

At about the same time, Nobel Laureate Roger Sperry, studying persons whose brain hemispheres had been separated by trauma, identified dominant control centers for particular brain functions on different sides of the "split" organ. While today electroencephalography (EEG) — a technique that measures electrical brain waves — can better identify a malfunctioning area of the brain, EEG is of limited usefulness in explaining why the brain fails.

Then came *computerized tomography* (CT), a remarkable technology for producing images of the brain's anatomy. CT scans can detect malignant tumors of a certain size. A scan can identify dead and necrotic areas of the brain deprived of oxygen by a stroke or injury. But this information may be gained too late to help physicians treat the disorder or identify the cause of the defect.

Scientists still needed a way to study the function of the living brain itself, even in the absence of gross structural damage. A potential answer was positron emission tomography.

Viewing the brain as it works

Positron emission tomography (PET) is the first imaging technique that shows, in the living, awake human being, ongoing metabolic activity in various regions of the brain. PET's advantages spring from the knowledge that active nerve cells consume oxygen and glucose. In fact, the brain is one of the most metabolically active organs, consuming 80 percent of the glucose that the body uses. PET measures this activity in specific areas of the brain, detecting subtle increases or decreases in glucose use during tasks such as listening or remembering, or in persons who have brain diseases.

It is the unique ability to observe brain function that allows PET to reveal fundamental information about the healthy and diseased brain. This new research tool is helping scientists understand how the normal brain works and what alterations lead to brain diseases, both neurological and psychiatric.

The National Institute of Neurological and Communicative Disorders and Stroke (NINCDS), the focal point for brain research in the federal government, was an early champion of PET technology. Because the NINCDS believed so strongly in the research potential of this new technique, it established a national PET Research Program: major research centers around the country, including a center at its own research facility in Bethesda, Maryland, all working to perfect the technique and using it to understand neurological disease. Today, these centers are uncovering new information about the nervous system that, without PET, might nave remained unknown.

Putting together the pieces

At the center of PET's unique abilities is a small family of radioisotopes* — O^{15}, C^{11}, N^{13}, F^{18} — that decay by emitting a subatomic particle called a positron. These positron-emitting isotopes, joined to harmless chemicals that are then dispatched to the brain, have three properties that endow PET with its impressive imaging capabilities.

The isotopes all have very short half-lives, emitting half of their radioactivity between 2 minutes (O^{15}) and 110 minutes (F^{18}). Such rapid decay allows research patients to be studied after receiving a very low dose of a radioactively tagged chemical. Because the radioactivity dose to the subject is so low, PET can be used for repeated studies in the same patient to follow the course of a disease. It can also be used safely to study healthy persons. This latter capability enables scientists to gather information on how the healthy brain works:

Positron-emitting isotopes produce a unique radioactivity event: an emitted positron shortly collides with its antimatter particle, an electron, producing mutual annihilation. The energy released in the annihilation takes the form of two photons which fly apart at approximately 180@ Thus, each positron decay sends a two-directional signal. *These photons register virtually simultaneously on the opposite sides of a ring of detectors*, each detector being geographically positioned to record the time and location of a positron annihilation. A specially programmed computer then picks up, stores, and correlates the information from many different annihilations and reconstructs from that data *an image* of a narrow sector of the brain.

But these favorable physical properties would mean nothing were it not for these isotopes' biochemical advantage: since each is a variant of an element that is intrinsically associated with the life process,

---

* Oxygen^{15}, Carbon^{11}, Nitrogen^{13}, and Flourine^{2}

the isotopes can be attached to compounds involved in the brain's metabolism. Oxygen, carbon, and nitrogen are found in most important biochemical compounds, while fluorine can be attached to many biochemical substances without substantially altering function.

Scientists used these isotopes for decades before PET scanning evolved. What made possible the exciting, powerful technique known as positron emission tomography was the development of scanning computer programs by Nobel Laureate Geoffrey Hounsfield in England. Hounsfield's programs permitted the tomographic reconstruction of three dimensional structures from a series of two dimensional measurements — a most remarkable development.

Not the same as the CT scan

PET scanning, however, differs from CT scanning in a major way. Where CT detects transmitted X rays, PET detects emission of photons from a previously administered compound — an isotope-labeled biochemical compound (as noted above). In the PET scanning equipment itself, detectors are arranged in a ring, much like a flat doughnut, and produce images in a series of up to 14 brain "slices," individual two-dimensional views at various levels of the brain. (The root *tomos* in *tomography* is greek for *slice*.) This information is integrated by the computer into a composite picture of the brain at work.

The computer reconstruction into a detailed image actually *shows the distribution in various regions of the brain of the organic compound containing the positron-emitting atom*. Each compound administered to the subject yields a different kind of information about brain activity. With labeled carbon dioxide, the picture represents the flow of blood throughout the brain. If the subject breathes labeled oxygen, the distribution will indicate the brain's metabolic utilization of oxygen. Following injection of deoxyglucose, an analogue of glucose, the scan reveals the brain's use of glucose. The aspect of metabolism measured is limited only by the ingenuity of physiologists in figuring out which compounds will trace the function they want to study, and the ingenuity of nuclear chemists in synthesizing these compounds.

One beneficial property of isotopes — their short half-life — may paradoxically limit the growth of PET scanning. Because these isotopes release their positrons so very quickly, they must be swiftly transported to the center where the study is to be done and rapidly incorporated into the carrier compound. This means only institutions having close access to a cyclotron can perform PET scanning.

With the advent of smaller, less expensive medical cyclotrons, this barrier may eventually be somewhat overcome, but PET experts generally doubt that the technology will ever become common in clinical settings. Where PET excels is in research. Already PET images are revealing urgently needed information about both normal and abnormal brain function; from this research will come the improved diagnosis and treatment that will benefit the patient.

Observing the healthy brain

Although clinical investigators are using PET to study pathology in many disease states, they are also asking the intriguing and fundamental question PET must first answer: How does the normal brain perform its awesome range of everyday activities? This question underlines the importance of being able to study healthy persons, to see the brain unaltered by disease.

Research on normal brain function also emphasizes the value of studying the brain in living human beings. Examining animal models and animal or human brains from autopsy gives little information about the hierarchical organization that underlies such complex human abilities as speaking and understanding speech. Several research groups have now begun to combine PET with complex experimental paradigms to dissect human communication.

For example, NINCDS grantees at the University of Pennsylvania are focusing on how we understand spoken language. Normal healthy subjects listened to a story in either English or Hungarian, played into either the right or left ear. What was common in all situations was that the temporal lobe on the right side of the brain responded with an increase in glucose metabolism. The increased burning of glucose indicates greater brain activity in that region, and suggests that the right temporal lobe is involved in extracting meaning from spoken information.

At UCLA, subjects listening to a story also showed increased physiological activity in a specific brain area. But when instructed to remember certain details from the story, they showed increased metabolism in another brain area as well. Such manipulation of simple tasks shows promise of identifying brain regions responsible for the separate, but related, functions of hearing, understanding, remembering, and speaking.

The University of Pennsylvania team pursued the processing of information by having subjects perform two types of tasks: one requiring spatial analysis, the other verbal analysis. The two classes of activity affected many brain regions similarly. But in 3 of 35 areas examined, there were consistent differences in glucose metabolism while the subjects performed the two disparate tasks. This finding supports the theory that different tasks are assigned to individual brain regions, and suggests that PET analysis can localize these functional areas.

At UCLA, one of the most enigmatic acts of the human mind — thinking — is also being examined. While subjects wrote their names, metabolic brain patterns reflected activity in the motor control regions, as expected. But when people were told simply to think about writing their names, the pattern of glucose consumption was quite different. Similar research may help determine which brain cells are responsible for organizing and planning our actions.

Research at UCLA has also shown that PET is very sensitive to the changes in brain metabolism that occur with slight changes in external stimuli. Subjects resting in a quiet environment had metabolic patterns different from subjects with their eyes covered or ears blocked. In addition, metabolic activity in the visual cortex quantitatively increased with an increasingly complex series of visual cues, ranging from the simple darkness of closed eyes to the complexity of a picture of an outdoor scene.

Locating the epileptogenic lesion

Beyond the realm of the normal brain, PET technology is being used in research on neurological diseases. PET scans, for example, are already guiding treatment for a special class of research patients with epilepsy. These are persons who have partial complex seizures that do not respond to medicines but can sometimes be treated satisfactorily by surgery.

NINCDS scientists and institute-sponsored investigators at the University of California, Los Angeles, have been using PET with EEG and CT scanning to study these patients before surgery. Initial observations were that, in many of these patients, PET could identify an area of abnormal brain metabolism. Between seizures, the focus displayed decreased glucose metabolism. In the patients who had seizures while being examined, this same area showed activity above normal levels during the seizure.

In a group of 25 patients at UCLA studied by PET and CT, and who subsequently had surgical removal of a suspected epileptogenic focus in the temporal lobe, PET's predictive value was evident. In the study, scientists first located the source of seizures with depth EEC. Later CT scans detected lesions in the correct hemisphere in only two patients. PET, however, showed a metabolic abnormality in 22 patients, 19 of whom were found at surgery to have a corresponding pathological lesion.

At NINCDS, PET is also being used to study how antiepileptic drugs affect the brain. Preliminary results suggest that some drugs, such as phenobarbitol, may reduce brain glucose metabolism.

Taking the measure of brain tumors

The first PET studies of central nervous system malignancies in the late 1970s showed that the technique could be used to study these tumors. This result was to be expected, since a tumor is not only a mass, but a mass with radically altered metabolism.

More specifically, theory predicts that malignant tissue has an increased metabolic rate, and that the degree of increase in metabolism can be used to determine the degree of malignancy. NINCDS investigators have verified this prediction, and are using this information to improve studies evaluating new therapies for brain tumors.

PET can also provide a complete "profile" of the tumor's characteristics. When the metabolic rates of glucose and of oxygen are compared, these values yield an estimate of the amount of anaerobic and aerobic glucose breakdown occurring in the tumor tissue. Combining this information with measurement of blood flow in and around the tumor gives a more complete characterization of the malignancy. Eventually, these data may help determine the most appropriate therapy for different categories of tumors.

Pet in the study of stroke — from ischemia to infarct

A problem ready-made for investigation by PET is stroke, a disease condition that involves a decrease in blood flow with impairment or death of brain tissue. PET's forte is that it allows scientists to identify changes both in blood flow and metabolism, and to examine the effects of stroke at an early stage. Metabolic changes have been found within a few hours of a stroke, as early as patients could be studied. In addition, metabolic alterations following a stroke can be correlated with functional losses, bringing a better understanding of how strokes cause their tragic consequences.

Because PET scans entail minimal radiation exposure, a series of studies can be done to correlate metabolic changes with waxing and waning of neurological deficits. Another application, one with far-reaching consequences, will be to evaluate blood flow and metabolism in patients receiving cerebral bypass surgery to determine which patients benefit most from this procedure.

Since 1975, NINCDS grantees at the Massachusetts General Hospital in Boston have been studying blood flow and oxygen metabolism in stroke patients. These studies were some of the first to suggest that our knowledge of stroke damage was incomplete. Emphasis had always been on blood flow as the primary cause of stroke damage. Thus, a stroke had been termed an "ischemic insult" and long-term neurological deficits resulting from stroke had been considered signs of "chronic ischemia." In addition, potentially effective treatment for stroke is a surgical cerebral bypass, which is intended to restore blood flow to the nutrient-starved area.

Observations with the PET scanner at Massachusetts General Hospital and elsewhere have demonstrated that the true clinical picture is more complicated. Although a sudden drop in blood supply is no doubt the initiating event in stroke, decreased blood flow may not be the most important factor over the long term. Once the ischemic insult has occurred, the Boston scientists found, values of cerebral blood flow alone are not as important as the rate of oxygen metabolism or of oxygen metabolism and blood flow combined. In fact, the most important unfavorable factor in the first few days after a stroke appeared to be the slowed rate of oxygen metabolism in the presence of normal blood flow. Although early CT scans of patients with this combination of factors appear normal, almost invariably a CT scan taken a few months later shows death of the affected brain region. This finding verifies the assumption that underlies many scientists' enthusiasm for PET: *metabolic changes often precede structural changes, so a technique that detects altered physiology can allow study of the very early stages of brain lesions.*

The new information about stroke will help in determining prognostic categories. More important, it can also point to rational new therapies and provide accurate evaluation in tests of these therapies.

PET scans are already enabling scientists to determine the true effectiveness of extracranial-intracranial cerebral artery bypass surgery as a technique to prevent stroke. In the procedure, an external scalp artery is connected to a blocked internal cranial artery beyond the point of blockage. The objective: to furnish a blood supply to parts of the brain that have been cut off by the blockage. According to previously held concepts of stroke damage, this new blood supply should relieve the chronic ischemia and allow the brain tissue to function again.

But, as we have seen, PET studies have thrown the simple interpretation of stroke damage into question. Now, with NINCDS support, PET scans are being applied in a serial manner at Washington

University in St. Louis to see whether cerebral bypass achieves its objective in all patients, or whether patients can be selected who are more likely to benefit from this procedure.

The Washington University scientists have found that only one group of patients has benefitted from the surgery. These are patients who have had transient ischemic attacks — so-called small strokes — with no lasting neurological losses. These patients, and others now being entered into the study, will be observed to see if postsurgical changes in oxygen metabolism and blood flow predict clinical outcome.

PET scanning in studying Alzheimer's and other dementing diseases

Many scientists are predicting that Alzheimer's disease could become the nation's premier public health problem. Alzheimer's disease is a major cause of mental incapacity in people over age 65 — a segment of the U.S. population that will continue to increase.

Because mental dysfunction is the primary symptom of Alzheimer's, PET is now being used in metabolic studies to determine the characteristics of the disease. Scientists also feel that PET technology will prove helpful in exploring any associated changes in neuroreceptor distribution and blood flow.

PET studies of some patients with Alzheimer's disease have revealed a distinctive pattern: a reduction of metabolic activity in particular parts of the cortex. These parts include the area responsible for mental association, as one would predict from the difficulties with language and visual-spatial cognitive functions that occur so prominently in Alzheimer's patients. Studies at NINCDS and elsewhere have demonstrated that the decrease in metabolism is greatest in an area at the back of the brain, the parietotemporal region. This area has not been emphasized in previous work on Alzheimer's, but dysfunction here might explain many of the major symptoms of the disease.

A well-known theory about disease suggests that metabolic changes in certain parts of the body precede severe symptoms. In the Alzheimer's brain, this theory can be explored with PET. If early metabolic changes are present, PET research may provide the information needed to identify the first stages of Alzheimer's disease. It is at these early stages that testing of drug therapy is most likely to be fruitful, scientists believe.

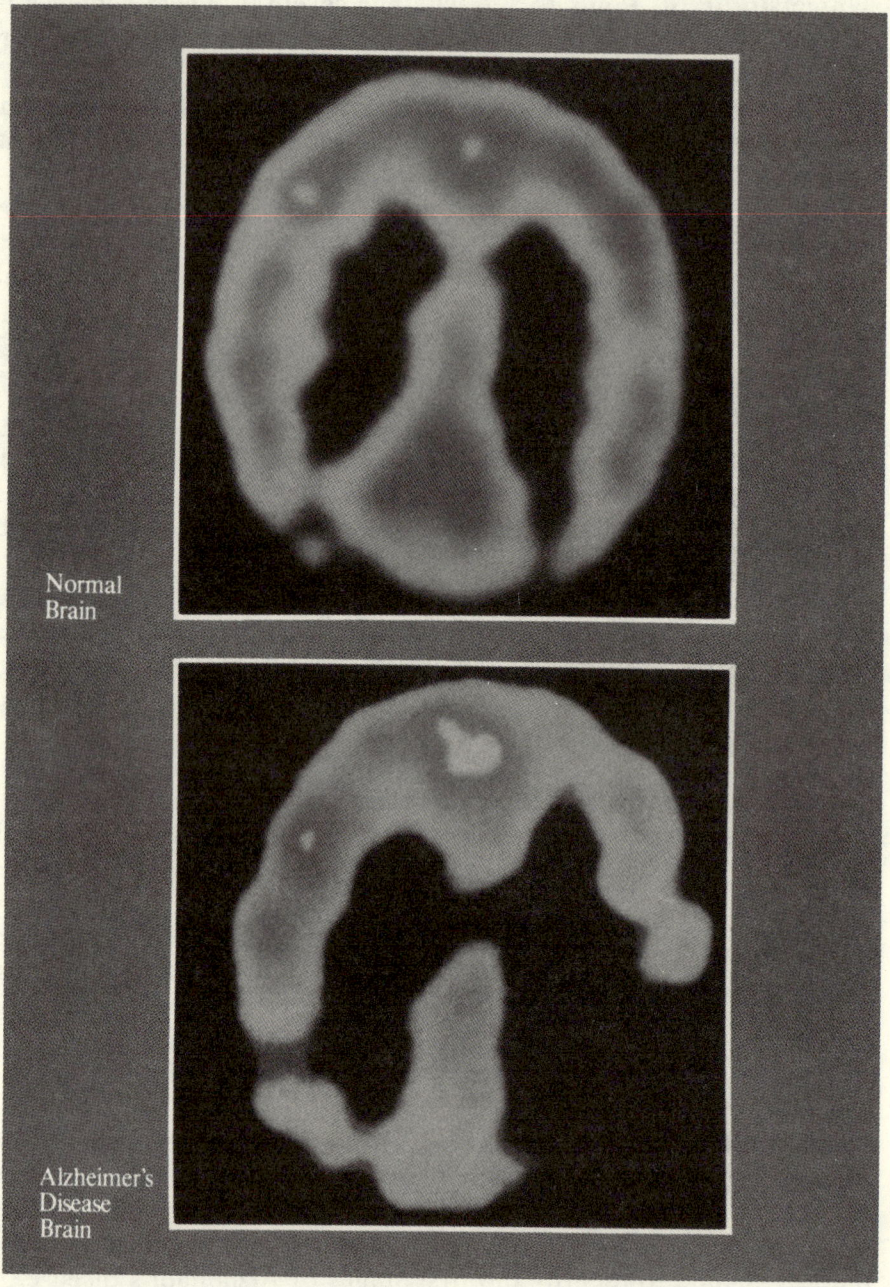

The Brains of Alzheimer's disease patients show distinctive patterns when imaged by PET. The scan of a normal brain is pictured at the top. Below, the scan of a 65-year-old woman with Alzheimer's who could no longer set a table or make a bed, reveals loss of activity in the right hemisphere, where spatial relationships are controlled.

The NINCDS-sponsored PET team at UCLA has also obtained important information about metabolic changes in patients with dementia due to Huntington's disease. In these patients, changes were seen in the striatum, an area deep within the brain. This remarkable finding verifies the ability of PET to yield information about structures beneath the cortex — the first imaging technique that can do so. The ability to view underlying structures is especially important in Huntington's disease, because this illness is characterized by uncontrollable movements and there is good evidence that deep areas of the brain, including the striatum, coordinate motor impulses.

Equally important, PET showed metabolic changes in patients with early Huntington's disease in whom CT scans were normal. Again, these results demonstrate that in this disease metabolic dysfunction precedes structural change, such as cell loss that can be seen with CT. PET clearly is a promising tool for studying the early stages of Huntington's disease and, perhaps, for finding the first sites involved.

Probing psychiatric disorders with PET's help

One of the amazing success stories of the last few decades has been the development of drugs that alleviate the symptoms of acute psychosis. This success implies that at least some psychoses involve abnormal brain chemistry. Current studies with PET scanning are seeking to unravel some of these chemical abnormalities.

One promising area for study is schizophrenia. In a combined project, scientists at the NINCDS-supported New York University-Brookhaven National Laboratory PET Center detected what they call "hypofrontality" in a group of newly diagnosed schizophrenics not yet taking medicine. This term refers to a general decrease in metabolism in the frontal cortex. When medication was given and the patients' psychiatric symptoms improved, metabolism in the frontal cortex increased but remained significantly below normal. This alteration may be a fundamental characteristic of the disease.

The investigators do not believe that hypofrontality can be used as a diagnostic indicator of mental disease. It cannot, for example, help to differentiate schizophrenia from manic-depression. But it may offer valuable clues to the control of mood and help answer questions about the contribution of brain dysfunction to psychiatric symptoms.

Neurotransmitters — PET helps to understand them

While metabolism of glucose and oxygen is necessary for neuronal activity, studies of metabolism do not give direct information about nerve cell activity, in which nerve cells communicate with others through chemical messengers called neurotransmitters. Quantifying that communication activity would increase our understanding of the brain and brain disease.

Neurotransmitters have been successfully studied in laboratory animals by examining brain tissue and measuring the amount of the transmitters in various regions, or by looking at the effects of adding various chemicals to a nerve preparation in a test tube. But these tests were of limited value in investigating the function of the transmitters in the living human being.

In the last few years, scientists supported by NINCDS have learned how to use PET to observe neurotransmitter activity in man. Chemists have synthesized positron-containing analogues of neurotransmitters, such as spiperone, a chemical that competes with the neurotransmitter dopamine. With these analogues, scientists can use PET to explore communication among nerve cells in the living animal, starting first with primates and then proceeding to humans.

A disturbance of neurotransmitter function underlies Parkinson's disease, in which inadequate amounts of dopamine are thought to hinder motor function. NINCD-supported scientists at the Johns Hopkins University used PET to produce the first images of dopamine receptors in the brain. With PET technology, investigators may further be able to determine whether loss of dopamine activity follows or precedes degeneration of the neurons that synthesize this transmitter. They may also be able to differentiate reduction in release of dopamine from inability of receptors to bind the substance.

Moreover, scientists will be able to study a peculiar phenomenon: after 3 to 5 years of dopamine replacement therapy with the dopamine precursor L-dopa, the drug either loses its effectiveness or works erratically. These changes have been explained as an alteration in the sensitivity of the dopamine receptors. With PET, this hypothesis can be tested directly.

Another exciting group of transmitters are "the body's own morphines": enkephalins and endorphins. Scientists have suggested that these chemicals are involved in many useful functions, the most important being analgesia. With newly synthesized positron-bearing enkephalin analogues, such ideas can be tested in normal healthy humans, perhaps providing a basis for improved management of pain.

More advances in PET technology ahead

Future advances in knowledge from PET research will depend on devising new strategies for separating the individual components of normal brain function and extending ongoing studies to more subjects. PET scientists will also be using the technology to get an earlier look into the disease state of patients with neurological or psychiatric diseases, and to test the effects of pharmacologic agents.

Such advances will be hastened by improved instrumentation. NINCDS scientists have developed an advanced scanner known as Neuro-PET with assets such as increased resolution and sensitivity. At Washington University, a new PET scanner with improved speed has been developed. With increasing technological advances such as these, PET scanners will continue to provide a depth of information about brain function that scientists of even 20 years ago could not have imagined.

PART THREE

INDEX